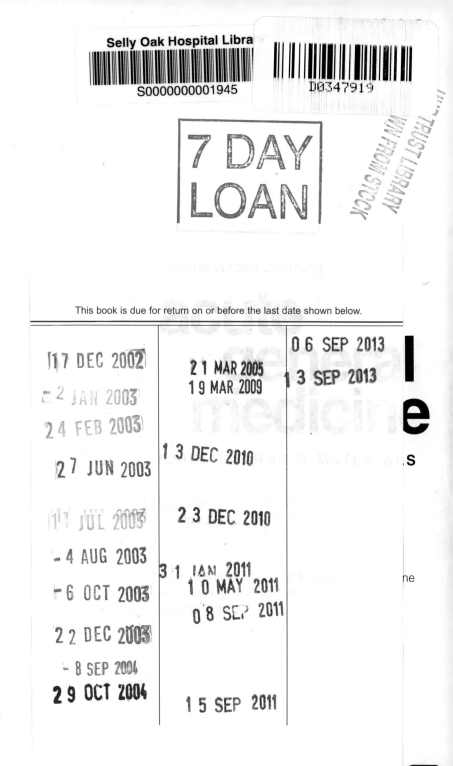
7 DAY
LOAN

This book is due for return on or before the last date shown below.

17 DEC 2002

2 JAN 2003

24 FEB 2003

27 JUN 2003

17 JUL 2003

4 AUG 2003

6 OCT 2003

22 DEC 2003

8 SEP 2004

29 OCT 2004

2 1 MAR 2005
19 MAR 2009

13 DEC 2010

23 DEC 2010

31 JAN 2011
10 MAY 2011

08 SEP 2011

15 SEP 2011

06 SEP 2013
13 SEP 2013

**acute general medicine**
is available from:

Reed Healthcare Publishing
Quadrant House
The Quadrant
Sutton
Surrey SM2 5AS

Telephone 020 8652 8789
Email: Hospital.doctor@rbi.co.uk

ISBN 1 873207 02 6

Published by:
Reed Business Information
Quadrant House
The Quadrant
Sutton
Surrey SM2 5AS

Illustrations by: Andrew Bezear
Laid out and typeset by: Brian Cronk Design
Origination by: JJ Typographics Limited Southend-on-Sea Essex
Printed by: Interprint Limited Malta

# Contents

# Foreword

*'Service Based Learning for Acute General Medicine'*

This volume represents a further approach to improving learning opportunities and methods for physicians in training. Service Based Learning is recommended by the GMC and colleagues felt that this provides an excellent model for young physicians to learn about common conditions found in acute medicine in a practical, relevant way.

Many people have contributed to the final product. This includes more that 40 Fellows and Members who have generated the Service-Based Learning Materials at weekend retreats or from home – most are busy practising clinicians and the notes reflect their day-to-day practice. Funding has also been collaborative – the surplus on postgraduate courses, and a major contribution from Hospital Doctor for which we are extremely grateful.

The pocket book format of the Brief Learning Materials will, we hope, be particularly helpful, so that doctors in training will have the book with them as they work. There are also self-assessment questions (and model answers!) in a companion Workbook. The latter can then be used for further discussion with senior colleagues.

I feel that this is another step forward in improving the learning opportunities for doctors in training especially SHOs, and am confident it will prove useful.

Professor Sir George Alberti

President, Royal College of Physicians

February 2000

# Preface

The first introduction we had to 'Service Based Learning' was when a leaflet from the Open University Centre for Education in Medicine came across our desk in the Postgraduate department at our own hospital. As the study leave budget was always tight it seemed a good idea to invest in a 'learn on the job' programme – but was it possible on such a large subject as General (Internal) Medicine? We therefore undertook a pilot study in some General Medicine and Accident and Emergency Departments and the doctors in training and their consultants received the idea with enthusiasm.

'Serviced Based Learning (SBL) is an essential component in balancing education and service during SHO training'. This quote is taken from 'The Early Years' the GMC booklet for doctors in medical training. We have tried to produce guidance for young doctors and students on how to manage general medical problems in a systematic way which will also help them in discussion with their senior colleagues. The materials consists of two parts – Brief Learning Materials (BLMs) which are short pieces ('bites') to help in the immediate understanding and management of a patient and secondly a companion workbook, short answer question (SAQs) and model answers which will help in the revision of the topic.

The BLMs have all been written by Members and Fellows of the Royal College of Physicians, all of whom undertake acute medical work. Each chapter has been written by a group of specialists. All physicians gave their time unstintingly to bring this project to a conclusion. The Editors have used 'Clinical Medicine' (Eds Kumar, Clark) extensively and we would like to thank Harcourt–Brace Publishers for allowing us to quote the text and to use some illustrations.

**Prof Parveen Kumar,** director of continuing professional development, Royal College of Physicians, and professor of clinical medical education, St Bartholomew's and the Royal London School of Medicine and Dentistry

**Dr Michael Clark,** honorary senior lecturer, St Bartholomew's and the Royal London School of Medicine and Dentistry

# Acknowledgements

Serviced Based Learning in acute general medicine could not have been developed without the hard work of all involved in defining the topics of the Brief Learning Materials (BLMs), writing the BLMs, short answer questions and answers and in piloting the scheme. All are Members and Fellows of the Royal College of Physicians.

We would like to thank the postgraduate department of Barts and the London NHS Trust and the Director of North Thames, Dr Elisabeth Paice, for the initial financing of the project. Hospital Doctor took over the funding and the production of the final materials. The Open University Centre for Education in Medicine, who started the concept of SBL, co-ordinated the project on a daily basis. We would like to particularly thank Claire Waring, Julian Mack and Clare Jennings for their enormous hard work, help and continued enthusiasm. The Royal College of Physicians helped to establish the project by hosting the initial meeting and reviewing each of its stages.

**Project team**

| | |
|---|---|
| Project director | Prof Janet Grant |
| Editors | Prof Parveen Kumar, Dr Michael Clark |
| Project manager | Claire Waring |
| Production co-ordinator | Phil Johnson |

# List of Authors

Dr Simon Alywin

Dr Roger Amos

Dr Janet Anderson

Dr Veronique Bataille

Dr Mark Caulfield

Dr Charles Clarke

Dr Craig Davidson

Dr Christopher Davidson

Dr Keren Davies

Dr David DíCruz

Dr Noemi Eiser

Dr Ian Fawcett

Dr Tim Gluck

Dr Martin Hurst

Dr Gordon Jackson

Dr Ramesh C Joshi

Dr Mark Kinirons

Dr John McAuley

Dr Adam McLean

Dr Karim Meeran

Dr Heather Milburn

Dr David Paige

Dr K John Pasi

Dr Stephen Patchett

Dr Drew Provan

Dr M R Qadiri

Dr G S Raj

Dr Mark Rake

Dr Armine Sefton

Dr David Trash

Dr David Watson

Dr Mark Weaver

Dr Peter White

Dr Peter Wilkinson

# Other contributors

Dr James Ahlquist

Dr John Amess

Dr David Blainey

Dr Bob Bown

Dr T Briggs

Dr Mac Cochrane

Dr Mark Cottee

Dr Lucy Goundry

Dr Des Johnston

Dr Peter Kopelman

Dr David Leaver

Dr Brian Livesley

Dr Fiona Moss

Dr Christina Williams

Dr Jennifer Worrall

# List of Figures

# List of Tables

# Introduction to Service-Based Medicine

Service-Based Learning for Acute General Medicine is based on the Royal College of Physicians' Core Curriculum for Senior House Officers in General (Internal) Medicine, looking specifically at the cases that would be encountered on-take.

Service-Based Learning is a way of organising your training so that:

• You get the most educational benefit from the post

• You review your practical experience systematically

• There are practice-related learning materials available to you

• You have the opportunity for self-assessment of your learning

Service-Based Learning consists of four types of learning which are based on your service experience and relate to the curriculum.

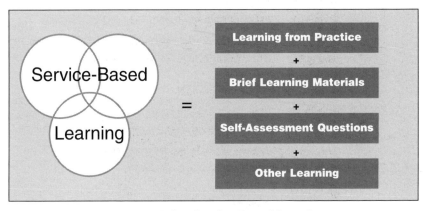

## Using Service-Based Learning

To get the most from Service-Based Learning you will need to use both the Brief Learning Materials and the Workbook. This Workbook (editor/designer - change to The Workbook for front of BLMs) provides a checklist linked to the topics for Acute General Medicine for you to keep a record of your four types of Service-Based Learning which are explained below:

## Learning from Practice

We are aware that doctors in training learn most from the patients they see when they see them, in preparation and with follow-up.

You can use the list of topics at the front of the Workbook to keep a record that you have seen a particular acute case.

## Brief Learning Materials (BLMs)

These materials are organised into groups to cover all acute general medicine topics. Each short piece should take around 10-15 minutes to digest and is designed to help in the immediate understanding and management of a patient. With this in mind their presentation is practice based with examples. They can also be used in preparation and follow-up as well as for learning about a new topic.

You can use the list of topics at the front of the Workbook to keep a record of the BLMs you have used.

## Self-Assessment Questions (SAQs)

The Self-Assessment Questions and Model Answers relate directly to each group of BLMs and are contained in the Workbook. You can use them to check your understanding of the topics covered by the BLMs in a number of ways. They are valuably used in weekly educational meetings where the answers are discussed amongst all members of the team. They are also frequently used for home study and on their own to test gaps in learning.

You can use the list of topics at the front of the Workbook to keep a record of the SAQs you have completed.

## Other Learning

You will also find a column in the list of topics for other learning, You can put a mark here if you'd like to record other types of learning such as observations, educational meetings and events or personal study time.

**GROUP 1:**

**ITEM 1:**

# Infectious diseases
# Pyrexia of unknown origin (PUO)

## CASE HISTORY

A 25-year-old male is seen in the A & E department at the request of the GP, with a history of fever and malaise. He had returned from a month's backpacking trip around India the previous week. He had lost 5kg in weight in the last month. The casualty officer asks you to see this patient with a diagnosis of PUO. The preliminary blood investigations by the GP were normal.

He was found to be febrile with a temperature of 39.5°C. He had no lymphadenopathy or pallor of mucous membranes

BP 110/70. Pulse 90. Heart sounds normal.

Chest – clinically clear

Examination of abdomen – slim, slight generalised tenderness. Liver, kidneys and spleen not palpable

Examination of CNS – unremarkable

### What is meant by the term PUO?

Pyrexia of unknown origin – classically of over three week's duration observed in hospital.

Not all cases of PUO are due to infection. In fairly acute PUO approximately two-thirds of cases are due to infection compared to only about one-third of cases in chronic infection. Other causes include malignancy, connective tissue disorders.

### Where would you manage this patient?

In a side room until an infectious aetiology has been ruled out.

### What questions should you specifically ask when you see a patient with PUO (in addition to routine questions)?

- Full travel history including exactly where patient has been and type of accommodation they have stayed in
- Vaccination/prophylaxis history
- Contact with animals/sick people
- Occupation – exactly what do they do
- Water exposure – occupational/recreational
- Food history – shellfish, drinking dirty water, re-heated/raw foods
- Risk behaviour – drug addiction, unprotected sex
- Factors which may predispose to infection

---

**Investigations**

- FBC
- Urine analysis and microscopy, culture and sensitivity
- CXR
- U&Es
- Liver biochemistry
- ESR and/or CRP
- Blood cultures – repeated
- Stools for ova, cysts and parasites and culture and sensitivity
- Store serum for future serological tests if required
- If any wounds swab these and culture them
- Additional investigations in this man because of travel abroad:
  Thick and thin blood films for malaria.

---

## *i* Information

CAUSES
• Infections
• Neoplasms
• Collagen diseases
• Other including granulomas, drug reactions, factitious

### Infective causes

GENERAL
Abscesses e.g. liver, abdomen, pelvis, ear, sinus or dental infection
Infective endocarditis
Urinary tract infection
SPECIFIC
Bacterial
– *Mycobacterium tuberculosis*
– *Salmonella typhi* or *S. paratyphi*
– *Brucella* spp
– Leptospirosis
Viral
– Epstein-Barr
– Hepatitis
– Cytomegalovirus
– HIV
– Dengue fever
Protozoal diseases
– Malaria
– Amoebiasis
– Leishmaniasis
– Toxoplasmosis
– Trypanosomiasis
Rickettsial diseases
– Typhus
– Q fever
Chlamydial
– Psittacosis

## What initial investigations should you perform in a patient presenting with PUO?

Perform minimally invasive tests prior to highly invasive and expensive ones. It is always worth repeating previously performed tests. (see box on previous page)

### Results

• WCC – slightly raised at 12,000 x 10 $^9$/l
• ALT – 92 iu/l (normal range 5 – 40 iu/l)
• Alkaline phosphatase 190 iu/l (normal range 25 – 115 iu/l)
• All other initial investigations were normal

## What should you do now?

• Recheck his history of travel
• Recheck his risk factors for hepatitis and HIV
• Send blood for viral markers
• Arrange liver ultrasound

The ultrasound shows a liver abscess and in view of his travel an amoebic abscess is a likely possibility. Fortunately you had sent off an amoebic CFT sample and you ring the reference laboratory urgently. The test is positive (always in a liver abscess).

## Action

Treatment is with metronidazole 400 – 800mg x3 daily for five to ten days followed by diloxanide furoate 500 mg x3 daily for ten days.

## Beware

• Take a careful history – ALWAYS REPEAT
• Examine the patient thoroughly – ALWAYS REPEAT

Initial investigations often give a clue to the diagnosis – may need repeating

• Be patient and don't give antibiotics until diagnosis is made unless the patient is very sick
• Only do invasive and/or expensive investigations when appropriate, e.g. ECHO, CT scan/MRI, bone marrow and culture, lymph node/liver biopsy

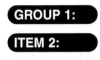

**GROUP 1:**

**ITEM 2:**

# Infectious diseases
# Septicaemia

### CASE HISTORY

A 70-year-old lady was admitted to hospital with fever, confusion and hypotension. She lived on her own and was unable to give a history.

She was clinically dehydrated, confused and had cold clammy peripheries. She was hypotensive with a BP 90/50 and a temperature of 39°C.

### What are the commonest causes of septicaemia in patients presenting from the community?

Commonest organisms isolated are *E coli, Staphylococcus aureus, Streptococcus pneumoniae* and pyogenic streptococci – especially Group A streptococci.

In hospitalised patients, coagulase negative staphylococci may also cause sepsis in immunosuppressed patients with IV lines in-situ.

### What factors predispose to septicaemia?

In both Gram-positive and Gram-negative septicaemia impaired host defences and surgery or instrumentation including intravenous cannulae predispose to septicaemia.

**Table 1.2.1 Additional predisposing factors for septicaemia**

| Gram negative sepsis: | Gram positive sepsis: |
|---|---|
| • Urinary tract infections | • IV catheters |
| • Nosocomial pneumonia – especially ventilator associated | • Skin/wound infections |
| • Pre-existing abdominal sepsis, biliary tract infections | • Bone and joint infections |
| • Severe burns | • Drug addiction |
| | • Respiratory tract infections/pneumonia |
| | • Obstetric or neonatal infections |
| | • Meningitis, Endocarditis |

### What is the differential diagnosis of septic shock?

Non-infective disorders such as acute myocardial infarction, pulmonary embolism or drug reactions must be excluded. Toxic shock may also present in a similar manner.

## What would be your initial management of this lady and what investigations would you do?

The patient would require supportive therapy e.g. fluid replacement as she is dehydrated, oxygen, inotropes and broad spectrum antibiotics after relevant cultures have been taken. The extent of antibiotic therapy will vary according to local hospital policy and if there is thought to be a likely focus of infection. The severely shocked patient will need transfer to ITU (see Group 12, Item 1).

Further investigations may include ultrasound, CT scan and in some instances a lumbar puncture.

If a urinary tract infection is thought to be the likely source a broad spectrum cephalosporin is often appropriate e.g. cefuroxine, cefotaxime, ceftriaxone, ±gentamicin.

If there is no obvious focus of infection, blind therapy must be broad spectrum and cover streptococci, staphylococci, and coliforms.

Suitable choices are:

- A broad spectrum cephalosporin such as IV cefuroxime or IV cefotaxime or IV ceftriaxone ±gentamicin

- Metronidazole should be added if an anaerobic infection is considered likely

- A broad spectrum penicillin with a β lactamase inhibitor ±gentamicin e.g. piperacillin/tazobactam (tazocin) ±gentamicin

- Carbapenem e.g. imipenem (a restricted antibiotic in many trusts)

### Beware

- If you give gentamicin remember that you need to monitor levels. Combining it with a cephalosporin may potentiate its toxicity

- Cefuroxime, ceftriaxone and cefotaxime have fairly good activity against staphylococci and streptococci. Ceftazidime has poor activity against streptococci and staphylococci but excellent activity against *Pseudomonas* spp and other gram negative organisms

- If a patient develops sepsis while they are in hospital it is possible that it may be due to resistant organisms e.g. methicillin resistant S. aureus (MRSA) or resistant gram-negative rods

- If MRSA infection is considered likely and the patient is very sick consider adding IV vancomycin 1g x 2 per day (assuming normal renal function) given over at least 100 minutes while awaiting culture results

A urine sample was obtained from this patient. Microscopy found it to contain 1000 wcc/mm$^3$ and ++ bacteria.

---

### Investigations

- FBC and differential
- U and Es, blood sugar, liver biochemistry
- ESR/CRP
- Blood cultures
- Blood gases
- Urine for microscopy, culture and sensitivity; sputum for microscopy, culture and sensitivity (if any being produced)
- Swabs of any infected-looking lesions (including throat swab if throat appears inflamed)
- Pus – if present for microscopy, culture and sensitivity
- High vaginal swab in women
- CXR
- ECG

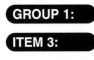

**Remember**
Many hopsitals have specific guidelines for antibiotic usage – ALWAYS CHECK or get microbiological advice

The patient had already been given IV cefuroxime and was continued on this. On admission she was also given a single dose of gentamicin. The following day both her urine and blood cultures grew an *Eschericia coli* which was susceptible to cefuroxime and gentamicin but resistant to amoxicillin. The patient made a good recovery.

**In your hospital do you know the approximate percentage of organisms causing urinary tract infections which are susceptible to commonly used antibiotics?**

In many areas in the UK approximately 50% of *E. coli* causing urinary tract infection are resistant to amoxicillin and about 20 to 30% resistant to trimethoprim. More than 90% are susceptible to cefuroxime, ciprofloxacin and gentamicin. You need to know local resistance patterns.

**GROUP 1:**

**ITEM 3:**

# Infectious diseases
# Meningococcal meningitis and septicaemia

### CASE HISTORY

An 18-year-old girl is brought into A&E collapsed. The previous day she had apparently been well apart from symptoms of a minor upper respiratory tract infection. She woke up feeling very unwell and asked her flatmate to call the emergency doctor. The flatmate noted that her friend had a couple of spots on her chest but by the time the doctor arrived she was developing a more widespread petechial rash. The emergency doctor transferred her immediately to hospital after giving her a single dose of benzyl penicillin.

The patient was febrile with a temperature of 38ºC.

• Petechial rash present

• Hypotensive and shocked

• Minimal neck stiffness present

### What do you think is the most likely diagnosis?

The girl probably has fulminant meningococcaemia which has a worse prognosis than meningococcal meningitis and usually has an extremely rapid downhill course. Other causes of fulminant septicaemia with disseminated intravascular coagulation need excluding as do other causes of meningitis.

## What should the immediate management be?

Take blood and throat cultures and then start antibiotics immediately. Give intravenous benzylpenicillin initially 2.4g four-hourly or IV cefotaxine 2gx 6 hourly *or* IV ceftriaxone 2g/day for presumed meningococcal meningitis/septicaemia.

## General principles

If it is thought that a patient could have bacterial meningitis caused by *S. pneumoniae* you should commence treatment on cefotaxime or ceftriaxone and not on IV benzylpenicillin since 5-10% of *S.pneumoniae* in the UK have decreased susceptibility to penicillin. If *Haemophilus influenzae* is suspected as a possible cause (rare in children over the age of five years and also now uncommon in the UK due to vaccination) cefotaxime or ceftriaxone should also be given. If other causes of septicaemia cannot be excluded broader spectrum antimicrobial therapy may be required. It is currently advised that a doctor who sees a suspected case of meningococcal disease at home should start antibiotics immediately and not wait until the patient gets to hospital. Provide supportive therapy.

## What investigations should be performed?

Relevant investigations are shown left. Other causes of meningitis/septicaemia should be excluded.

## Who should be informed and what further action should be taken?

The consultant (or his/her deputy) in charge of communicable disease control (CCDC) should be informed immediately by phone if a clinical diagnosis of meningococcal disease is made. Formal notification should then be done in writing. Notification books should be kept on all wards. Rifampicin prophylaxis can then be arranged for any close contacts.

## Contacts who should receive prophylactics are:

- People who live in the same household as the case or who have lived there in the previous week
- Sexual partners
- Work fellows sharing a small office i.e. an office for two
- Staff carrying out mouth to mouth resuscitation on the patient or 'specialing' him/her especially in the first 24 hours
- The patient herself at the end of her parenteral therapy
- School contacts if more than one case in a school

Once the CCDC has been informed he/she will usually arrange for chemoprophylaxis and vaccination if appropriate but they may ask the hospital doctor to do it for the patient's relatives.

### Investigations

- FBC and differential
- Urea and electrolytes
- Liver function tests
- ESR/CRP
- Blood cultures – always before starting antibiotics
- Throat swab to look for meningococcal carriage
- Culture of petechial lesions
- Lumbar puncture (not indicated in meningococcal septicaemia)
(Note – Lumbar puncture is contraindicated in meningitis if the patient has raised intracranial pressure. A CT scan should always be performed first)
- Serum to send to reference laboratory for meningococcal PCR if meningococci not grown

### Remember

NOTIFICATION OF INFECTIOUS DISEASES
Do not forget to notify. If in doubt check immunization against infectious disease: (1996) HMSO London or ask microbiology

### Vaccination

There is an effective vaccine which can be given to contacts of meningococcal meningitis/ septicaemia due to Group A and C infections. Unfortunately N meningitidis Group B is the commonest type found in the UK and there is no effective vaccine against this.

**Remember**

The patient should have rifampicin 600mg x2 daily for two days after she has finished her parenteral antibiotics in order to eradicate carriage of N. meningitidis from her nasopharynx.

**Remember**

In pregnancy – seek expert advice. If chemoprophlaxis is thought appropriate, ceftriaxone is usually given

**Table 1.3.1 Recommended chemoprophylaxis of meningococcal meningitis**

| *First choice:* | |
| --- | --- |
| Rifampicin | |
| Adults and children over 12 years | 600 mg x2 daily for two days |
| Children 1-12 years | 10 mg/kg x2 daily for two days (maximum dose 600 mg x2 daily for two days) |
| Infants, 12 months | 5 mg/kg x2 daily for two days |
| | |
| *Other options:* | |
| Ciprofloxacin | |
|     Adults | Adults – 500 mg single dose |
|     Children | not recommended |
|     Pregnancy/breastfeeding mothers | not recommended |
| | |
| Ceftriaxone: | |
|     Adults | 250 mg IM as a single dose |
|     Children, 12 years | 125mg IM as a single dose |

### What should you tell people who are taking rifampicin prophylaxis?

That it may interfere with the effectiveness of the oral contraceptive if they are taking it. Hence they should take additional contraceptive measures for the remainder of the cycle

That their secretions – tears etc. may turn orangey pink – and that their soft contact lenses will also be permanently stained unless they remove them!

The patient was treated with intravenous ceftriaxone 2g IV once per day in the intensive care unit. After a stormy course she made a full recovery. There were no secondary cases.

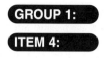

# Infectious diseases
# Pseudomembranous colitis

## CASE HISTORY

A 40-year-old man who has been on the Intensive Care Unit for three weeks with a head injury following a road traffic accident develops severe diarrhoea. He is ventilated and currently finishing a course of a third generation parental cephalosporin for nosocomial pneumonia. According to the nurses, one other patient on the ITU currently has diarrhoea.

### What other questions do you want to ask?

You would want to know what the diarrhoea was like – were the stools liquid, or bloody? How long has the patient been on broad-spectrum antibiotics? Has any other patient/member of the staff got diarrhoea? (One of the ITU nurses informs you that another patient did have loose stools and you need to ascertain if this is really the case and if there were any obvious reasons for this.)

### What is your differential diagnosis?

It would include:

• Antibiotic associated diarrhoea particularly pseudomembranous colitis

• Diarrhoea due to enteral feeding

• Other bacterial causes, e.g. *Salmonella* spp, *Shigella* spp, *Campylobacter* spp; less likely as patient hasn't been eating but could occur due to cross-infection

• Viral gastroenteritis

### What investigations would you perform?

You would need to send a stool from the patient to the microbiology laboratory (and also from any other patient/staff member with diarrhoea) for microscopy, culture and sensitivity.* In addition, you would specifically need to request examination for *Clostridium difficile* (toxin and culture) – the organism responsible for pseudomembranous colitis. Do a sigmoidoscopy to look for the typical pseudomembrane seen in pseudo-membranous colitis and to exclude inflammatory bowel disease by rectal biopsy.

*If several patients/members of staff are affected, stools should also be sent to the virology department to look for a viral aetiology, e.g. small round viruses.

The patient was thought, on clinical grounds, to have pseudomembranous colitis. This was later confirmed by the Microbiology Department, who found the stool to be positive for *C. difficile* toxin.

**Remember**

Culture of C. difficile in a stool is insufficient evidence that a patient has pseudomenbranous colitis: it is only toxin producing strains which cause this.

### How would you manage the patient?

The patient should be isolated in a side room to prevent cross-infection. You need to ensure that the patient is adequately hydrated. In patients with antibiotic-associated diarrhoea, if it is at all possible, any broad spectrum antibiotics that they are taking, should be stopped. Specific first-line therapy is oral metronidazole 400-mg x3 for seven to ten days or oral vancomycin 125-250mg x4 for seven to ten days. Note, you do not need to do vancomycin levels in patients receiving oral vancomycin since it is not systemically absorbed.

Normally metronidazole is tried first because there is a worry that use of oral vancomycin may predispose to development of vancomycin-resistant enterococci in the gastrointestinal tract and in some parts of the world vancomycin resistance in enterococci is becoming a major problem.

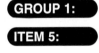

**GROUP 1:**

**ITEM 5:**

# Infectious diseases
# Food poisoning – *E.Coli* 0157

### CASE HISTORY

A 15-year-old girl is admitted to hospital with bloody diarrhoea. Both her parents and her three siblings are well. They have apparently all eaten the same food during the last week except on a single occasion when the patient ate a beefburger cooked at a local fête. The mother remembers that it looked rather raw inside. The girl had eaten chicken at least three times during the previous week.

She looked slightly dehydrated and had a temperature of 37.8°C. Her abdomen was soft but generally tender, bowel sounds were increased.

**Remember**

Most laboratories now routinely look for E.coli 0157
Abdominal X-rays and sigmoidoscopy may also be required if inflammatory bowel disease is considered a likely diagnosis.

### What is the differential diagnosis in this patient?

Infectious gastroenteritis with bloody diarrhoea due to:

• *Campylobacter* spp (chicken the likely source)

• *E.coli* 0157 (beef the likely source)

• *Shigella* spp

• *Salmonella* spp

• Onset of inflammatory bowel disease

## Investigations

Should include:
• full blood count,
• urea and electrolytes (*E.coli* 0157 can cause haemolytic uraemic syndrome),
• stools for microscopy culture and sensitivity.

Full clinical details should be put on the form accompanying the stool.

## Information
## Haemolytic uraemic syndrome

Features
– Intravascular haemolysis with red cell fragmentation (microangiopathic haemolysis)
– Thrombocytopaenia
– Acute renal failure

Mortality high in elderly

Treatment – ? plasma exchange.

## What would your initial management be?

The patient should be admitted and put into excretion-secretion isolation (assuming a probable infective aetiology). Ensure adequate hydration. Oral/IV antibiotics may have a place in treating severe infections due to *Salmonella spp, Campylobacter spp* and *Shigella spp.* There is controversy about their use in the treatment of infections due to *E.coli* 0157. The disease should be notified to the CCDC both by telephone immediately and in writing, when the diagnosis is made.

This patient with *E.coli* 0157 made an uneventful recovery.

## Beware

• *E.coli* can cause diarrhoea by several mechanisms. Strains causing diarrhoea may be:
  • Enterotoxigenic
  • Enteropathogenic
  • Enteroadherent
  • Enteroinvasive
  • Enterohaemorrhagic

*(see Kumar and Clark 4th Ed, 1998, p34)*

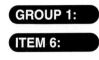

**GROUP 1:**

**ITEM 6:**

# Infectious diseases
# Typhoid

## CASE HISTORY

A 35-year-old Asian male presents with a one-week history of fever, headache, a dry cough and constipation. He is resident in the UK but has just returned from a six week holiday in Bangladesh where he was visiting relatives. He works as a chef in one of your local restaurants. While he was away one of the relatives he was staying with had severe fever and diarrhoea.

The patient has a fever of 39.5°C but his pulse is only 85/minute

Examination of the cardiovascular, respiratory and central nervous systems is unremarkable

Abdomen is slightly tender but examination of it is otherwise unremarkable

The patient has a full blood count, routine chemistry, CXR and blood cultures taken

The full blood count shows a slight leucopenia. Gram-negative rods are seen in a film of the blood cultures taken after 24-hour incubation.

### What is the most likely diagnosis?

*Salmonella typhi* (This was later confirmed as being the definitive diagnosis).

### How would you manage this patient?

The patient should be nursed in a side room with excretion-secretion precautions used (Consult your local infection control manual). The control of infection officer should be alerted as should your local CCDC as soon as a definite diagnosis is made. Your CCDC should be alerted immediately by phone and also via the formal notification book, which should be available on every ward. This is especially important as the patient is a food worker. If the patient subsequently develops diarrhoea it is important to ensure that he is adequately hydrated. Pending antibiotic sensitivity testing the patient should be commenced on ciprofloxacin 500-750mg x2 daily for ten days.

The patient will need follow-up to ensure that he does not become a carrier of *S.typhi*. He must remain away from his job as a food handler until he is known to be carriage-free of *S.typhi*.

Cefuroxime, although frequently used for treating Gram-negative sepsis, is not effective against *S.typhi* which is an intracellular pathogen.

**Remember**

Ciprofloxacin is extremely well absorbed and so may be given by the oral route as long as the patient is not vomiting. It is important to realise that, although after starting ciprofloxacin the patient may start to feel better very quickly, it may take three to six days for the temperature to settle.

## Infectious diseases
## Returning traveller

GROUP 1:

ITEM 7:

### Information

**Causes**

- *Salmonella typhi* or *S.paratyphi*
- Dysentery
- Malaria
- Respiratory tract infections
- Urinary tract infections
- *Mycobacterium tuberculosis*
- Viral hepatitis
- Dengue fever
- Brucellosis
- Leishmaniasis
- Sexually-transmitted diseases
- In travellers returning from parts of Africa, Lassa fever should be excluded.

### Investigations

- Full blood count
- Routine blood chemistry
- Urine analysis
- Blood cultures
- Stool cultures
- CXR
- Thick and thin blood films for malarial parasites.
- Store blood for serology and take a second sample two weeks later

### ⚠ Remember

You can always get advice from National Reference Centres e.g. Hospital for Tropical Diseases London, Liverpool School of Tropical Medicine

### CASE HISTORY

A 20-year-old student returns from a six-week backpacking tour of Africa. Two weeks after his return he goes to A&E complaining of fever, headache and malaise of seven days duration.

The patient is thin and febrile with a temperature of 38°C. Clinical examination is otherwise unremarkable.

### What further questions do you want to ask this man?

It is essential, as always to take a full detailed history. Particular note should be taken as to exactly where the patient has travelled, what vaccinations he had prior to his trip, whether or not he took anti-malarial prophylaxis regularly and, if so, what he took. Did he remember being bitten by any insects? Did he have close contact with anyone who was obviously unwell? What sort of food did he eat? Did he have unprotected sex with any strangers while travelling?

### Beware

Just because someone has come from abroad it does not mean that they can't have a "UK type of infection" such as influenza, a common cold or a sexually-transmitted disease. Some people lose many of their inhibitions when on holiday and are more likely to pick up an STD.

Start with simple, cheap and relatively non-invasive investigations whenever possible. Perform other investigations as appropriate, depending on symptoms, signs and results of initial investigations, e.g. imaging – CT scan, ultrasound or MRI – aspiration or needle biopsy, etc.

Thick and thin blood films showed that the patient had malaria with a 5% parasitaemia. His malaria was due to P. falciparum.

### How would you manage the patient?

*P.falciparum* is frequently resistant to chloroquine and therefore patients with this disease should generally be commenced on quinine sulphate 600mg x 3 daily for seven days followed by a single dose in adults of 75mg pyrimethamine and 1.5g sulfadoxine (Fansidar). Tetracycline 250mg x 4 daily for seven days can be used as an alternative to pyrimethamine and sulfadoxine. As this patient has a relatively high parasitaemia he should initially have intravenous quinine (see British National Formulary for details on dose and also for malaria treatment and prophylaxis helplines). Intravenous quinine may potentiate hypoglycaemia and patients on it should have their blood sugar monitored regularly. Ideally they should also be on cardiac monitors.

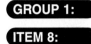

# Infectious diseases
# Shingles

### CASE HISTORY

A 75-year-old man presents to his GP with severe right-sided chest pains of two days duration. In the past 24 hours, he has noted a rash on the right side of his chest, in the distribution of T5-T6.

### What do you think the likely diagnosis is?
Shingles

### What question would you like to ask the patient?
Have you had chickenpox?

### Beware
Not everyone who has antibodies to Varicella zoster virus remembers having the disease.

### What investigations might you perform?
The disease is recognised clinically. It can be confirmed by examination of the vesicular fluid under an electron microscope to look for Herpes virus. Serology can also be performed.

**Remember**

Modification of the dose may be required if the patient has renal impairment

Patients should be prevailed upon not to scratch their lesions as this may predispose to secondary infection.

Calamine lotion may help. They are likely to require analgesia

### How would you manage the patient?
If the patient requires admission to hospital, he should be nursed in a side room and only by nurses who are known to have antibodies against Varicella zoster virus. If at home he should avoid contact with people who have no history of having had chickenpox.

As the patient has had the rash for less than three days, he should be commenced on aciclovir or an alternative anti-viral agent active against Varicella zoster virus – famciclovir or valaciclovir. The usual adult dose of aciclovir for treatment of shingles is 800 mg five times per day by mouth or 5mg/kg three times per day if given intravenously.

The patient is admitted to hospital, as he lives on his own at home,

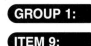

### Information

*Ophthalmic herpes* is infection of the 1st division of the Vth nerve and can lead to corneal scarring and secondary panophthalmitis

*Ramsay Hunt syndrome* is due to herpes infection of the geniculate ganglia. It causes a facial palsy with vesicles on the pinna of the ear

*Post-herpetic neuralgia* is a burning continuous pain in the area of the previous eruption. It is common in the elderly and accompanied by depression. It is difficult to treat

and started on aciclovir. Twenty-four hours later, the patient is found to have a high fever. The House Officer notes that one of the lesions has an inflamed area about it.

### What do you think has happened? How would you manage the patient?

Secondary infection of the shingles lesions has occurred. The most likely pathogens to cause this are *Streptococcus pyogenes* and *Staphylococcus aureus*. Swabs should be taken and sent to Microbiology for microscopy, culture and sensitivity and blood cultures should also be taken. The patient should be commenced on an antibiotic regime such as IV benzyl penicillin (active against *S.pyogenes*) and IV flucloxacillin (active against *S.aureus*).

**GROUP 1:**

**ITEM 9:**

# Infectious diseases
# Epstein-Barr virus

## CASE HISTORY

A 19-year-old college student presents to his GP with a one week history of severe sore throat, fever and extreme fatigue.

### On examination:

The patient is found to have a fever of 38.8°C, and cervical, axillary and inguinal lymphadenopathy

Tonsils appear enlarged and his pharynx erythematous with palatal petechiae present

Spleen is just palpable

### What is the differential diagnosis in this patient?

The most likely diagnosis in a person of this age with a short history of fever, malaise, general lymphadenopathy and severe sore throat is glandular fever – an infection caused by the Epstein-Barr virus.

Streptococcal sore throats may mimic infectious mononucleosis clinically although hepatosplenomegaly and inguinal and axillary lymphadenopathy will be absent.

Cytomegalovirus infections and toxoplasmosis may also present in a similar fashion although the sore throat is usually less severe. Viral hepatitis may also sometimes present with fever, lymphadenopathy, malaise and an atypical lymphocytosis. HIV seroconversion can also present as a glandular fever like illness. Lymphomas and leukaemia may occasionally present in this way.

## How would you confirm the diagnosis?

A full blood count should be performed. In over two-thirds of patients this will show a mononuclear lymphocytosis with atypical lymphocytes present. A mild neutropenia is frequently present and platelet counts are commonly slightly decreased. Serum aminotransferases are usually raised.

Heterophile antibodies that agglutinate sheep red blood cells (the Paul Bunnell test) usually become positive during the second week of infection.

### Remember

If a patient with infectious mononucleosis is given ampicillin he/she will develop a rash in about 90% of cases.

The Monospot test (a rapid screening test) will be positive in glandular fever in 85% of cases. In addition, EBV specific antibodies can be looked for in Paul Bunnell negative "glandular fever" or in atypical cases, but these are generally not performed. Ask your local virology laboratory for further details, if required.

## Treatment

Generally supportive. Contact sports should be avoided while splenomegaly is present. Aspirin may help relieve the sore throat and reduce fever. Occasionally the tonsils may be so swollen that airway obstruction seems imminent: in these cases a short course of steroids is helpful, usually commencing with approx 60mg prednisolone/day in individual cases and stopping within one to two weeks. Corticosteroids are also indicated in cases with marked thrombocytopenia, haemolysis or central nervous system involvement.

If the diagnosis is unclear, and if it is suspected that the patient may perhaps have a sore throat due to *S.pyogenes* or if a secondary streptococcal infection is suspected, the patient should be commenced on intravenous benzylpenicillin (if in hospital) pending culture and serology results. If the patient is not admitted high dose oral penicillin is an alternative.

# Notes

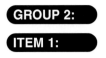

## STDs

## HIV/Aids

### CASE HISTORY

A 35-year-old man, known to be HIV infected, presents with a persistent cough which has developed and worsened over the preceding two weeks. He has a temperature of 39°C, pulse of 100/min and a respiratory rate of 20/min. He is on no regular medication. You are the medical SHO on acute take.

### What are the likely diagnoses and the immediate management?

*Pneumocystis carinii pneumonia* (PCP) commonly has an insidious onset, often with worsening shortness of breath and deteriorating exercise tolerance. The cough is usually non-productive. Examination of the chest may yield few signs other than tachypnoea and tachycardia. Fine inspiratory crackles may be heard. The chest X-ray may be normal or show little, although bilateral perihilar interstitial shadowing with a bat wing appearance is the characteristic abnormality. High resolution CT of the lungs shows a characteristic ground glass appearance, even if there is little radiological change on CXR. Oxygen saturation characteristically falls on exercise. Arterial blood gas analysis may show hypoxia with a normal carbon dioxide and pH. The diagnosis is made on broncho-alveolar lavage.

PCP occurs most frequently in those who are significantly immunosuppressed with a CD4 count below 200cells/mm³. Those who are aware of their HIV status are recommended to use primary prophylaxis (cotrimoxazole is first line) once their CD4 count falls into this range. This intervention alone has reduced the incidence of PCP in HIV infected populations and a further significant decline has been seen over the past two years with the introduction of potent antiretroviral drugs. PCP is an AIDS defining diagnosis.

### How would you treat this case?

Cotrimoxazole IV (trimethoprim 15 mg/kg/day + sulpha-methoxazole 75mg/kg/day) is the preferred first line although a significant proportion of patients will develop allergy. Pentamidine or dapsone plus trimethoprim are alternatives. Treatment is given for three weeks. Systemic corticosteroids (IV methylprednisolone 40mg x4 daily for five days) are added in severe cases (po₂ less than 8kpa). Since the organism is not cleared by treatment secondary prophylaxis (usually cotrimoxazole) is recommended for all those who have had *Pneumocystis carinii* pneumonia to prevent recurrence.

Patients with PCP may develop respiratory failure and require ventilatory support. Pneumothorax is a further complication of pneumocystis development.

## What other chest conditions do you see with HIV?

### TUBERCULOSIS (MTB)

As an organism of high pathogenicity MTB can develop relatively early in the course of HIV infection. Pulmonary infection may present with a cough (usually productive) and chest pain but presentation is often insidious and non-specific with fever, sweats, malaise and weight loss. Patients who have spent time in areas of the world where TB is endemic or who have had a previous episode are at particular risk. History of contact with TB should always be sought plus details of any previous antituberculous therapy. In such patients there may be a risk of multidrug resistant TB (MDRTB). There may be generalised lymph node involvement or hepatomegaly in addition to signs in the chest. The radiological changes may be few. Those that occur are frequently atypical with lower zone changes, without cavitation. Other finding may include hilar lymphadenopathy, pleural effusion or lobar consolidation.

In patients with HIV the usual immunological reactions to MTB may be blunted or absent, making diagnosis more difficult. Mantoux tests are rarely helpful since immunosuppressed patients do not produce a normal delayed hypersensitivity reaction. Granuloma formation may be compromised leading to atypical histological changes. Sputum smears may be negative in up to 50% of those with culture proven TB. Diagnosis relies heavily on clinical suspicion backed by positive cultures from sputum, bronchiolar lavage, blood, bone marrow, lymph nodes etc. as appropriate.

Patients with HIV and pulmonary TB should be managed in single rooms. If smear positive, such patients ideally should be isolated in negative pressure facilities if there is any suspicion of risk factors for MDRTB. Care must be taken in units where there are other immunosuppressed patients as nosocomial clusters of MDRTB have been reported both from the USA and UK in these patients. Treatment regimens should include at least four drugs (isoniazid, rifampicin, ethambutol and pyrizinamide) until full sensitivities are known. There are important interactions between rifampicin derivatives and the protease class of antiretroviral medications leading to an increase in rifampicin toxicity and reduced protease efficacy. This situation requires input from a specialist physician.

**Remember**

Any patient in whom the suspicion of TB is great enough to start antituberculous therapy MUST be notified to the local consultant in Communicable Disease Control.

## BACTERIAL CHEST INFECTION

A range of bacterial respiratory infections are more common in patients with HIV infection, in particular *Streptococcus pneumoniae, Haemophilus influenzae* and *Moraxella catarrhalis*. Onset is usually rapid with a productive cough. Signs of consolidation may occur and radiological changes of consolidation or infiltration may be present. Diagnosis is based on sputum and blood cultures and management is with broad spectrum antibiotics.

## KAPOSI'S SARCOMA

This vascular tumour is thought to be caused by Human Herpes virus type 8 (HHV-8). Although most commonly found on the skin, KS can infiltrate the lungs leading to cough and shortness of breath. On examination other KS lesions are usually found on the skin or in the mouth but in rare cases the lungs alone may be involved. Radiological changes are of diffuse infiltration, often with a nodular appearance. Pleural effusion may be present. Lesions may be visualised on bronchoscopy. Treatment is with systemic chemotherapy.

### How would you manage a HIV case with chest problems?

**Assessment**

Full history and examination including details of travel, previous infections, previous or existing HIV related pathology. Assess degree of respiratory distress

Assess degree of immunosuppression by looking for clinical signs such as oral candida infections, hairy oral leukoplakia, and seborrhoeic dermatitis. Look for pathology in all systems

Chest X-ray, exercise oximetry, blood gases, blood cultures, sputum examination for acid-fast-bacilli (AFB) and microscopy, culture and sensitivity. Full blood count, liver and renal function

Initiate plans for bronchoscopy/high resolution CT scan

DO NOT do a CD4 count when the patient is acutely unwell – it will be inaccurate and misleading

**Treatment**

If the patient is clinically immunosuppressed or has a previous AIDS defining illness or is known to have a CD4 count below 200/mm$^3$ AND has chest X-ray abnormalities or desaturates on exercise or has a hypoxic blood gas picture suggestive of PCP, institute PCP therapy pending bronchoscopy. Organisms will still be found on lavage up to 4 days into treatment.

**Remember**

In HIV infected patients:
- Common conditions may have unusual presentations
- Uncommon conditions occur more frequently
- Many different conditions can present in similar ways clinically and radiologically
- Those standard investigations that depend on an intact immune system will not be useful
- A tissue or culture diagnosis is frequently required

Pathology in HIV infected patients is related to:
- Their degree of immunosuppression
- The virulence of the organism
- The microbiological repertoire to which an individual has been exposed
- The multiple pathology that is frequently encountered

**Beware**
- Drug allergies
- Marrow suppression with high dose cotrimoxazole
- Hypotension/hypoglycaemia with IV pentamidine

If the patient has a history of or exposure to TB or has clinical and radiological findings consistent with TB, isolate and investigate. Do not initiate empirical antituberculous therapy without an expert opinion as this will have long-lasting and far-reaching consequences for the patient and his future management.

If the patient has a sputum smear positive for AFB or has culture positive TB, isolate and start antituberculous therapy with four drugs. Notify, seek expert opinion.

If the patient has clinical or radiological signs of bacterial infection, institute therapy with broad spectrum antibiotics e.g. amoxicillin or azithromycin.

**Remember**
- If the patient does not respond as detailed
- RECONSIDER THE DIAGNOSIS
- SUSPECT MULTIPLE PATHOLOGY

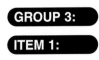

**GROUP 3:**

**ITEM 1:**

# Nutrition
## Feeding the patient

*(see Kumar and Clark, Clinical Medicine, 4th Ed, p210-213)*

### CASE HISTORY

A surgical colleague phones you to ask about parenteral nutrition for a 70-year-old man who had had an oesophago-gastrectomy five days previously. Postoperative care had been straight forward and no prior provision for parenteral nutrition had been made. It now seemed likely that he has an anastomotic leak.

### What should you advise?

Parenteral nutrition is never an emergency therapy. It can always wait until expert advice is available next day. You say that you will bring your consultant along the following morning.

### How do you assess the nutritional state?

This can be done simply by looking at the patient! Does he look malnourished?

Other parameters that can help are:

• Weight loss >10%

• Serum albumin <35g/l

• Serum transferrin <1.5g/l

### Nutrition will be necessary for

• All severely malnourished patients on admission to hospital

• Moderately malnourished patients who are not expected to eat for three to five days because of their illness

• Normally nourished patients not expected to eat for seven to ten days

**Always feed enterally rather than parentally if possible.**

### Methods of enterally feeding

• By mouth

• By fine bore naso-gastric tube

• Percutaneous endoscopic gastrostomy (PEG)
  (refer to gastroenterologists to insert) for prolonged period - more than 30 days)

**Remember**

• It is better to predict (if possible) whether some form of supplementary nutrition is likely to be required before an event

• Over 10% of patients in hospital are said to be malnourished

---

**Standard enteric diet providing 12,000 kJ per day (2000 to 3000 kcal)**

**Energy:**
Carbohydrate as glucose polymers (49 - 53% of total energy)
Fat as triglycerides (30-35% of total energy)
**Nitrogen:**
Whole protein (6-7 g of nitrogen/l)

Additional electrolytes, vitamins and trace elements.

This provides:
Ratio of energy to nitrogen kJ: g = 620:1 (kcal : g = 150:1)
Osmolality = 285 - 300 mosmol/kg

*See current British National Formulary for ready-made formulations.*

---

**Remember**

Remember to monitor carefully with:
• Daily plasma electrolytes
• Daily glucose
• Weekly assessments of nutritional status

This patient would not be suitable for enteral nutrition because of his GI surgery and parenteral nutrition is appropriate.

Peripheral nutrition is the initial preferred option. Each catheter will last five days and the procedure has fewer complications than a central venous catheter which has to be inserted in theatre.

Most hospitals now have nutrition teams who will advise on the nutritional regimens that are required.

**GROUP 4:**

**ITEM 1:**

# Gastroenterology
# Vomiting

This is a common symptom often due to dietary (or alcohol!) indiscretion. It can be a symptom of general ill health. It is associated with neurological, psychological, metabolic, renal as well as gastrointestinal disease.

The history is normally the best indication of the cause.

### Duration

**Acute** <48 hours – alcohol, toxins, etc., acute infective disease, medication, acute neurological disease e.g. vertigo, acute abdominal disease e.g. appendicitis, gall stones.

**Chronic** >48 hours think of gastrointestinal obstruction. Remember psychological (usually in young women), endocrine (Addison's) and metabolic disease (renal failure) Neurological (raised intracranial pressure) can also cause vomiting.

**Frequency and relationship to food** (Differentiate from regurgitation). Vomiting occasionally eases the pain of peptic ulcer disease.

### Content

Haematemesis (see haematemesis/melaena – Group 5, Item 5), faeculent (intestinal obstruction), semi-digested food, (evidence of gastric retention).

### Associated symptoms

Abdominal pain, weight loss, constipation, diarrhoea

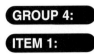

**Investigations**

Haematological
– FBC, ESR
Radiological
– Abdominal X-ray
– Chest X-ray
Biochemical
– Electrolytes
– Urea
– LFTs
– Calcium
– Amylase

### CASE HISTORY

A 70-year-old man was admitted with a two week history of repeated vomiting. He had lost more than one stone in weight and has recently developed upper abdominal discomfort.

His abdomen is distended and he is tender in the epigastrium

Remember non-gastro-intestinal causes – therefore full examination is necessary. Note, look at the fundi for papilloedema.

### Chest X-ray

Look for evidence of air under the diaphragm (perforation), signs of pneumonia, hilar mass (tumour).

### Abdominal X-ray

**Normal**

With a history of this length a normal X-Ray suggests that large or small bowel obstruction is unlikely. High obstruction in G.I. tract (oesophagus or stomach) is possible. Investigate for non-GI causes (metabolic, neurological – exclude brain stem lesion), occasionally severe depression.

**Abnormal**

May show evidence of small or large bowel obstruction or gastric distension. In this patient the AXR showed small bowel obstruction.

**Fig 4.1.1 Small bowel obstruction**

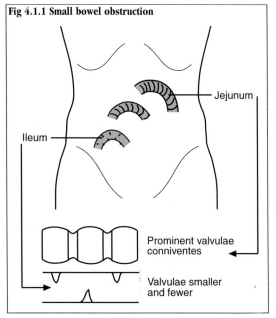

Jejunum

Ileum

Prominent valvulae conniventes

Valvulae smaller and fewer

### Action

Ultimate goal is to relieve obstruction but

**Interim management**

- Infuse dextrose/saline to maintain electrolyte balance (may need additional K+)
- Insert nasogastric tube (on continuous drainage)
- Contact surgeons, await instruction as to further investigations (such as Ba studies or CT scan to localise obstructive lesion).

**GROUP 4:**

**ITEM 2:**

# Gastroenterology
# Weight loss

Weight loss is often a perceived symptom by patients but does need to be verified. However it is a general symptom which may reflect disease in any part of the body.

It is essential first to ascertain whether the patient has a sufficient calorie intake for his/her requirements. Bear in mind the amount of exercise taken. In a young female think of anorexia nervosa.

Reduced calorie intake is usually due to anorexia, which is another symptom of generalised disease.

## CASE HISTORY

A 40-year-old man has been admitted with a fever, tremor and two stone weight loss. He has previously been counselled for alcohol abuse.

### What should you do?

You need to consider a number of diagnoses and may be helped by additional history and examination. The following should be considered:

Thyrotoxicosis – check for signs of toxicity (Group 14 Item 11)

Alcoholic liver disease (Group 5, items .4, 5, 6, 7)

Check for malnutrition by asking his family, perhaps there is a psychiatric history

Consider underlying cancer, particularly lung, bowel and pancreas

Biochemical investigations may well help determine underlying metabolic or renal disease

Malabsorption often causes anorexia which contributes to weight loss.

**Our patient** had no major signs of chronic liver disease but did admit to recurrent episodes of upper abdominal pain radiating through to his back. These particularly occurred on Monday following his weekend binges. This suggests pancreatic disease resulting from his heavy alcohol intake.

### What initial investigations are appropriate?

FBC, LFTs, calcium, blood alcohol

Plain X-ray of the abdomen for pancreatic calcification

Abdominal ultrasound to assess the pancreas for cysts and potential masses.

### Investigations

CT scanning of the pancreas
* MRCP (see Group 5, Item 2) this is non invasive and increasingly recognised for its value in assessment of the pancreas and biliary tree
* ERCP to deliniate the biliary and pancreatic ducts
* Endoscopic ultrasound may help define pancreatic cysts and masses

### Remember

Our patient has been admitted in a malnourished, hyperdynamic state

Consider acute alcohol withdrawal symptoms (see group 5, Item 7). Treat this initially and investigate the pancreas later.

**GROUP 4:**

**ITEM 3:**

# Gastroenterology
# Hiccups

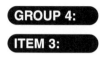

### Information

Hiccups are due to involuntary diaphragmatic contractions with closure of the glottis. They are very common and usually not sinister – even if persistent.

## CASE HISTORY

You are called by the surgical SHO because he is concerned that a 70-year-old man has had continuous hiccups for 48 hours. Ten days ago he had been admitted with intestinal obstruction (see 4.1.1) and a laparotomy for a carcinoma of the ascending colon had been performed. This is a classic situation of a subphrenic abscess occurring post-surgery in an elderly person.

### How would you investigate?

Check Hb, WBC and liver biochemistry. An urgent ultrasound. This will confirm the diagnosis. If febrile – blood cultures should be taken.

### Treatment

With drainage under ultrasound control and antibiotics. Hiccups can be controlled with chlorpromazine 50mg or diazepam 5mg as necessary.

### Other causes

• Metabolic e.g. uraemia
• Neurological e.g. brain stem tumour
• Other abdominal pathology
• No pathological cause

**GROUP 4:**

**ITEM 4:**

# Gastroenterology
# Dysphagia

### CASE HISTORY

A 55-year-old patient has been admitted because of acute dysphagia. She gave a history of reflux for years and increasing dysphagia for six months. She had been eating an orange which became lodged in her gullet and all efforts to vomit it were unsuccessful. The underlying diagnosis is likely to be food bolus obstruction on an already present oesophageal stricture.

### What should you do?

The correct investigation is an urgent endoscopy. Food can often be removed and the patient's symptoms relieved.

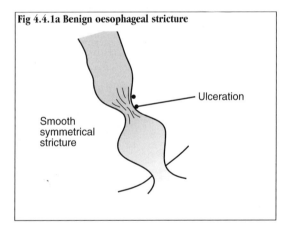

**Fig 4.4.1a Benign oesophageal stricture**

Ulceration

Smooth symmetrical stricture

Endoscopy may be normal in a motility disorder e.g. achalasia.

This lady is thought to have a benign stricture, the barium swallow appearances are shown in fig 4.4.1a. This is treated with a proton pump inhibitor and a dilatation is performed.

Compare fig 4.4.1a with fig 4.4.1b which shows a typical malignant stricture.

**Fig 4.4.1b Malignant oesophageal stricture**

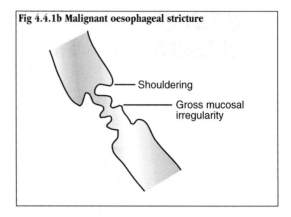

- Shouldering
- Gross mucosal irregularity

Unfortunately this lady developed severe chest pain immediately after the dilatation and surgical emphysema could be felt in her neck. Clinically, an oesophageal tear is suspected.

A CXR and Gastrograffin swallow confirmed an oesophageal rupture.

The underlying diagnosis is more likely to be oesophageal cancer as careful dilatation of benign lesions rarely causes a tear. Biopsies now confirm a carcinoma.

**Initial management**
- Nil by mouth
- IV infusion
- Antibiotic prophylaxis
- Surgical referral

**Remember**
Submucosal cancer can look like a benign lesion.

Small tears may resolve on conservative management, but large tears generally need surgery in a dedicated thoracic unit. Endoscopic stenting can be used for tears in malignant lesions.

This patient has cancer, management will include assessment for surgery with:
- Blood count, liver biochemistry
- CXR
- ECG
- Respiratory function tests
- Abdominal US, CT scan to assess operability
- Endoscopic ultrasound is the most accurate way of staging lesion.

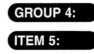

# Gastroenterology
# Constipation

### CASE HISTORY

Your house officer asks you what he should prescribe for an elderly man who hasn't opened his bowels for five days. The patient who was previously well and active had been admitted a week ago with a chest infection. Rectal examination revealed a loaded colon with no local lesion.

### Should this patient be investigated?

Not initially as it seems likely that constipation is due to immobility. A barium enema may be necessary if no improvement

### Treatment

• Initially he will require a laxative to "get things moving"! Glycerine suppositories are useful. Magnesium sulphate, an osmotic purgative, is effective and cheaper than the more usually prescribed osmotic laxative lactulose

• Do not use stimulant laxatives

• Stop "constipating" drugs if possible

• Faecal impaction may require digital extraction followed by small volume phosphate enemas

• Advise patient regarding high fibre diets and fluid intake.

---

## Information

**Causes**
• Simple/idiopathic
• Intestinal obstruction
• Colonic disease e.g. carcinoma
• Painful anal conditions
• Drugs e.g. codeine, iron, verapamil
• Hypothyroidism, hypercalcaemia
• Depression
• Immobility

---

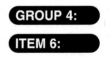

# Gastroenterology
# Diarrhoea

Increased frequency of defecation can, even in a previously fit patient, produce dehydration and SEVERE electrolyte depletion. Diarrhoea can also be a recurrent problem in patients with established gastrointestinal disease *(see Kumar and Clark, 4th Ed, p276)*.

### What should you do in a case of diarrhoea presenting in A&E?

In the history ascertain whether the patient has eaten suspect food or travelled abroad. Check for drug history, e.g. antibiotics. Ask about accompanying symptoms e.g. abdominal pain, weight loss.

It is essential to:

- Establish history of onset
- Determine frequency, consistency, content of stool, presence of blood
- Determine the state of hydration and electrolyte balance
- Send stool for culture, parasites (ova or cysts) and C. difficile toxin
- Do a rectal examination. Sigmoidoscopy (if bloody diarrhoea)
- Do blood cultures in severe cases with a temperature
- Do a plain abdominal X-ray

---

**Likely pathogens causing diarrhoea:**

Bacteria – 50%
- E-Coli
- Campylobacter
- Salmonella
- Shigella

Viruses – 10% (but seldom produce severe diarrhoea in adults)
- Rotavirus
- Norwalk

Protozoa – 5%
- Giardia
- Entamoeba histolytica
- Cryptosporidium

Helminths e.g. Strongyloides          No pathogens/Multiple pathogens – 20-50%

---

**Management:** This will depend on the case scenario (see below) but most diarrhoeal illnesses are self-limiting and short lived. One to ten per cent may persist for a month. Identification of the pathogen will determine specific therapy. (See also Group 1, Item 5)

**Information**

Causes
- Giardiasis
- Cryptosporidiosis
- Amoeblasis
- Tropical Sprue (SE Asia, Caribbean)
- Schistosomiasis
- Strongyloidiasis

### CASE HISTORY 1

A 24-year-old returns from travelling for three months, during which he passed through several countries. He has had severe diarrhoea for two weeks. He could have been exposed to all sorts of infective agents.

On admission he is dehydrated and has lost over one stone in weight.

**What immediate action would you take?**

- FBC, U&Es, LFTs
- Send stools for culture x3
- Rehydration may require large amounts of balanced infusion fluids but often glucose/electrolytes solutions orally are sufficient

- Vomiting may need to be treated with an anti-emetic, (metoclopramide 10mg x3/day)
- Evidence of anaemia will need correction and further investigation e.g. folate deficiency in Tropical Sprue, in which no organism can be isolated.

**Giardiasis** is very likely and treatment is with metronidazole 2gm a day for three successive days. If bacterial, many will settle without antibiotics. Ciprofloxacin, will shorten the clinical course.

## CASE HISTORY 2

A 30-year-old female patient presents with a two week history of six to ten motions a day. She has felt tired and has lost about one stone in weight.

On admission she is not dehydrated but has a fever and is lethargic.

### Action

- Consider infective diarrhoea and screen (as above)
- Consider first presentation of inflammatory bowel disease (most likely in this lady). Check plain abdominal film
- Consider possibility of steatorrhoea and diseases of small bowel and pancreas

### Inflammatory bowel disease

In any case of diarrhoea presenting in A&E, either ulcerative colitis or Crohn's Disease should be considered as possible causes. There may be a previous history of chronic diarrhoea or abdominal pain which will lead you to this possibility.

### Action

**General**

- Determine general biochemical and haematological status as above.
- Check plain abdominal X-ray for presence of stool, mucosal oedema, bowel dilatation or perforation.
- Sigmoidoscopy. The presence of inflammation, ulceration and exudation should make you consider inflammatory bowel diseases. Take a rectal biopsy.

Acute colitis may be associated with diarrhoea, abdominal pain, fever and systemic disturbance. There is usually blood in the stools.

To assess severity – check factors shown in the box.

Always consider the :

- Presence of toxic dilatation (colon: > 5cms diameter and mucosal islands on plain abdominal X-ray – Fig 4.6.1)
- Presence of perforation (on abdominal X-ray)

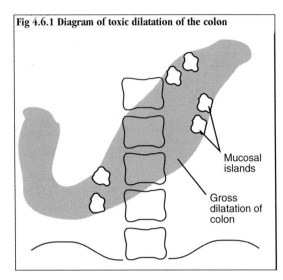

**Fig 4.6.1 Diagram of toxic dilatation of the colon**

Mucosal islands

Gross dilatation of colon

**ACUTE COLITIS – assessment of severity**

| | | |
|---|---|---|
| Hb | ↓ | <10 g/dL |
| Alb | ↓ | <30g/l |
| Fever | ↑ | >37.5C |
| Stool frequency | ↑ | >6/day |
| ESR | ↑ | >30mm per hour |
| Pulse rate | ↑ | >90 bpm |
| Platelets | ↑ | |
| WBC | ↑ | |

## Information

**CROHN'S DISEASE**
- Affects any part of GIT from mouth to anus
- Seventy per cent of cases affect the terminal ileum
- Can be controlled but not cured

**ULCERATIVE COLITIS**
- Confined to colon
- Cured by colectomy
- Can affect the:
  Rectum alone (proctitis)
  Sigmoid and descending colon (left-sided colitis)
  Whole colon (total colitis)

**Action:**

If acute inflammatory disease of the bowel is the likely diagnosis a sigmoidoscopic biopsy should be taken to determine whether Crohn's or ulcerative colitis. It will also be necessary later to do a colonoscopy to determine extent of disease. This should be done after the patient has improved.

**How would you manage this acute situation?**
- Intravenous fluids
- I.V. therapy with steroids (Hydrocortisone I.V. 100mg x4/day) followed by oral therapy (enteric coated Prednisolone 40mg per day) if patient improves
- I.V. Antibiotics (metronidazole/cephalosporin) if infection is suspected
- Further management – refer to gastroenterologists; consult GI surgeons

**Has this lady got Crohn's disease or**

### ulcerative colitis?

Both can produce an acute colitis. The differentiation is by colonoscopy and histological appearance (see below).

| Histological findings | Crohn's | U.C. |
|---|---|---|
| Inflammation | Deep (transmural), patchy | Superficial (mucosal) continuous |
| Granulomas | ++ | rare |
| Goblet cells | present | depleted |
| Crypt abscesses | + | ++ |

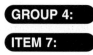

# Gastroenterology
## Abdominal pain

Most diseases of the gastrointestinal tract are associated with abdominal pain, but pain may be referred to the chest or back. The characteristics of the pain may help in the diagnosis.

### CASE HISTORY

A 40-year-old man presented with epigastric and central abdominal cramping pain. For 48 hours it had become continuous, severe and associated with vomiting. He has no alteration of bowel habit and no loss of weight.

### What should you do?

**Assess** severity of pain and associated symptoms

• Duration
• Frequency/characteristics/exacerbating or relieving factors
• Site and referral of pain
• Examine patient; fever, tachycardia, abdominal tenderness, bowel sounds

**Assess** degree of systemic effects

• Haematological – Hb, WCC, ESR
• Biochemical – U&Es, liver biochemistry
• Radiological – initial AXR, for obstruction. CXR, in acute pain, for perforation

**Develop** the management plan to include:

• Symptomatic relief
• Establish disease specific therapy
• Information for patient and relatives
• Further investigations (endoscopy, ultrasound, CT and MRI to exclude perforation, obstruction, stones, calcification, cancer and ascites)
• Consultation with colleagues in surgery and other disciplines

Abdominal pain situated in the epigastrium and central abdomen of the severity in the case described would usually be associated with pathology, but since abdominal pain is so common you should always consider irritable bowel syndrome (IBS) as a possible cause. Some pathological problems are considered here but always remember an acute surgical cause, e.g. aortic aneurysm or appendicitis.

### Features of IBS

• Pain – often cramping and intermittent, and at different sites. Relieved by defaecation
• Alternating diarrhoea/constipation
• Feeling of incomplete emptying on defaecation
• Wind and abdominal bloating
• Unassociated with pathological findings
These symptoms have usually been present for some time tending to fluctuate

### Features of dyspepsia

(See Group 4, Item 8)

### Features of acute pancreatitis

• Severe pain
• Often associated with alcohol abuse, gallstones, viral infection (e.g. mumps)
• ↑Serum amylase (>5x normal)
• Gastric retention and vomiting
• Ultrasonographic changes and contrast enhanced dynamic CT (best investigation) show pancreatic swelling, necrosis and peripancreatic fluid collection.

**Remember**
ACUTE PANCREATITIS
Assessment of severity and poor prognosis (First 48 hours)
• Age > 55 y
• Blood glucose > 10 mmol/l
• S urea > 16 mmol/l
• S calcium < 2mmol/l
• S LDH > 600u/l
• PaO$_2$ < 8kPa
• WCC > 15 x 10$^9$/l

### Features of gall stone disease

**Biliary pain**

• Pain usually continuous in the right hypochondrium lasting up to two hours (not colicky)
• Often associated with abnormal LFTs
• Often previous similar episodes but well in between episodes

**Acute Cholecystitis**

• Severe, continuous pain in epigastrium and right hypochondrium
• Ultrasound shows gallstones, distension of gall bladder, gall bladder wall thickening, sonographic Murphy's Sign

### Features of cancer

• Cancer of pancreas, bowel, stomach, ovary, kidney can present as abdominal pain
• There are usually associated symptoms of weight loss, debility and organ failure dependent on site
• There may also be additional biochemical and haematological abnormalities specific to the organ involved
• Radiology, ultrasonography and MRI are vital in the diagnosis, localisation and detection of spread of disease

**Remember**

- Gallstones and upper abdominal symptoms are both common. Great care must be taken to establish that the two are related.
- Fair, Fat, Fertile Females of Forty have the same chance of having gallstones as the rest of the population!

### Symptom relief

Symptom relief is dependent on diagnosis. Use antispasmodics (hyoscine 20-40mg x4/day). Minor analgesics (paracetamol) may help. NSAIDs useful in some cases. Caution should be used when prescribing opiates (morphine, codeine) since they can increase constipation and spasm in the sphincter of Oddi. Antiemetics (metoclopramide 10mg x2/day or prochlorperazine 5mg x2/day).

### Patient information

This depends on diagnosis but should be delivered to both patients and relatives sensitively and with an understanding of underlying pathology.

**GROUP 4:**

**ITEM 8:**

# Gastroenterology
# Dyspepsia

Dyspepsia is a common condition accounting for seven per cent of all GP consultations. It is a vague term that encompasses epigastric and substernal pain and discomfort. It is usually related to food intake.

### CASE HISTORY

A 45-year-old man was admitted with severe epigastric pain radiating up into his chest. He thought he had had a heart attack (see Group 10, Item 6).

**Investigations**

- FBC, liver biochemistry, serum amylase
- ECG
- CXR
- Cardiac enzymes

### What investigations would you do on admission?

It is critical to consider life threatening conditions such as myocardial infarction, pulmonary embolism, pneumothorax before labelling such pain as dyspepsia.

In this patient the ECG, CXR and enzymes were normal.

Additional features in the history included:

- Long history of reflux (GORD)
- Burning nature of the pain
- Flatulence
- A relationship of the present pain to previous similar pain
- A food related element
- Exacerbation of pain with drinking hot liquids

**Investigations**

- Endoscopy looking for peptic ulcer or gastric cancer, or the presence of oesophagitis
- Ultrasound looking for gallstones or pancreatic disease if endoscopy negative and pain epigastric
- Ba Swallow and meal looking for reflux (not a reliable test)

**Remember**

- Reflux can be difficult to diagnose and although it is often associated with an hiatus hernia, more formal investigation may be necessary e.g. oesophageal pH and pressure monitoring.
- The possibility of significant disease in this patient should always be considered and the presence of alarm features would demand urgent endoscopy.

**Remember**

ALARM FEATURES
- Weight loss
- Anaemia
- Dysphagia
- Vomiting
- Continuing severe pain

In the absence of alarm features it is reasonable to try a proton pump inhibitor if history suggestive of reflux, e.g. heartburn worse on bending

*Features of gastro-oesophageal reflux:*

- Burning pain produced by bending, stooping or lying down
- Pain seldom radiates to the arms
- Pain precipitated by drinking hot liquids or alcohol
- Pain relieved by antacids

*Features of Myocardial ischaemia:*

- Gripping or crushing pain
- Pain radiates into neck, shoulders and both arms
- Pain produced by exercise
- Accompanied by dyspnoea

Diagnosis of GORD strongly suggested if patient responds to acid suppression therapy.

Testing for the presence of Helicobacter Pylori (see below) is necessary in peptic ulcer disease, and perhaps in the case of reflux if one is considering the long term use of acid suppressing agents.

**Fig 4.8.1 Urea breath test**
Tagged urea ($^{13}$C or $^{14}$C) given orally is metabolised by urease, produced by H.pylori, into ammonia and $CO_2$. The latter is measured in the breath.

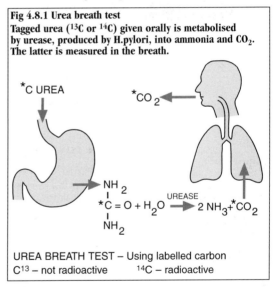

UREA BREATH TEST – Using labelled carbon
$C^{13}$ – not radioactive     $^{14}$C – radioactive

### Tests for Helicobacter Pylori

- Serological (useful in community – but does not distinguish between past or current infections)
- Urea breath tests measuring $^{13}$C or $^{14}CO_2$ (for current infections) (see fig 4.8.1)
- Antral biopsy – either for histology or for CLO (urease) testing (for current infections)
- Stool assay becoming available.

### Treatment

Patients with peptic ulcer disease who are H Pylori +ve should be given combination eradication therapy e.g.

• Clarithromycin 500mg twice daily
• Amoxicillin 1gm twice daily
• Omeprazole 20mg twice daily

**CASE HISTORY**

**GROUP 4:**

**ITEM 9:**

## Gastroenterology

## Peptic ulcer disease

You are asked by the cardiologists to see a man with epigastric pain. He has been admitted for a coronary angioplasty. He is already on aspirin 75 mg daily. He has had many similar episodes of pain over the years. In 1988 he had an endoscopy and was told that he had an ulcer and was given Zantac. He points with one finger to his epigastrium as the site of his pain.

This is a classical story of Duodenal Ulcer disease.

### What should you do?

As the angioplasty is tomorrow you recommend he is given a proton pump inhibitor e.g. omeprazole 20 mg x2 daily and is referred to gastroenterology outpatients.

The cardiology SpR would like to put him on anticoagulants and is worried that he has an ulcer. This is a problem of balancing the risks. If the angioplasty is urgent they will have to go ahead with anticoagulants. If his pain was not characteristic, an endoscopy to ascertain if he has an ulcer should be performed prior to angioplasty. The ideal situation for this man would be to heal his ulcer prior to angioplasty.

**Remember**

• HP serology remains positive even after successful eradication of HP
• Current H.pylori infection can only be detected by the urea breath test (see fig 4.8.1) or on endoscopy (urease test, histology or culture)

### How do you investigate a patient with a suspected ulcer in the community?

*Less than 45 years:* H. pylori serology If positive Eradication therapy (see Group 4, Item 8). If negative Treat symptomatically.

*Greater than 45 years:* Patients with new dyspepsia and those with alarm symptoms (e.g. anorexia, weight loss) should be referred for endoscopy

**GROUP 4:**

**ITEM 10:**

# Gastroenterology
# Iron deficiency anaemia

## CASE HISTORY

A 40-year-old female, globe trotting managing director was found at routine screening to have a Haemoglobin of 8.0g/dl with an iron deficient appearance on the film.

She admitted to some ankle swelling and increased breathlessness of recent onset. Examination was unhelpful. FBC, film and low serum ferritin confirmed iron deficiency.

Exclude all obvious causes of bleeding:

• Heavy periods
• Rectal bleeding
• Haematuria
• Recurrent nose bleeds

It is rare for the last two to cause severe iron deficiency anaemia.

If no obvious cause, assume the anaemia is due to gastrointestinal disease:

Malabsorption – Coeliac disease is very underdiagnosed

The patient travels a lot abroad and could have a bowel infestation. Remember hookworm is the commonest cause of iron deficiency anaemia world-wide

Occult bleeding from the gastrointestinal tract is common and can be confirmed by haemoccult testing. This is however totally unnecessary in a patient with iron deficiency because if there is no history of blood loss blood can then only be lost from the GI tract

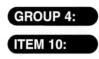

**Information**

Faecal Occult Bloods

• Of no use in males or post-menopausal females with iron deficiency anaemia and no other cause for bleeding
• Possibly useful for screening populations

### What additional investigations are appropriate?

Rectal examination is mandatory to exclude rectal cancer. Proctoscopy to exclude piles

Gastroscopy – peptic ulcer, gastric cancer and GORD can certainly occur in this age group. Also do duodenal biopsy for coeliac disease

If gastroscopy is unhelpful, full colonic assessment is necessary. This can be achieved with barium enema and flexible sigmoidoscopy (the rectum is poorly visualised on barium enema). Note, the best investigation is colonoscopy which will allow full assessment of the colon when biopsy, polypectomy, laser treatment of angiodysplasia can be performed as appropriate

If the above investigations are negative you have a problem. A small minority of patients fall into this category and a host of differential diagnoses exist.

Further investigations performed with advice from the G.I. unit include:

- Small bowel follow through
- Enteroscopy
- Meckel's scan
- Angiography – preferably performed when a patient is bleeding and in this patient unlikely to be helpful
- Laparotomy with possibly simultaneous on-table endoscopy at the time

**Remember**

COELIAC DISEASE

A history of steatorrhoea can be missed unless a detailed stool history is taken (Note, many patients do not have steatorrhoea)

Coeliac disease is increasingly recognised world-wide and has an incidence of less than one in 1000 in the UK. Certain areas of the world are said to have a higher incidence e.g. Ireland and Italy

Malabsorption of iron as well as increased iron loss can occur

There may be other deficiencies as well e.g. calcium and folic acid

Diagnosis is made by biopsy of duodenal/jejunal mucosa. However anti-reticulin and anti-endomysial antibodies are simple to perform and have high specificities and sensitivities. Tissue transglutaminase (the target antigen for the endomyseal antibody) is now available, and should be more specific.

**Fig 4.10.1 Small Intestinal mucosa showing normal villi with normal columnar cells compared to coeliac mucosa showing subtotal villus atrophy, crypt hyperplasia, lamina propia inflammation and an increase in intra-epithelial lymphocytes.**

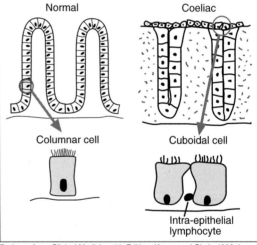

Redrawn from *Clinical Medicine*, 4th Edition, Kumar and Clark, 1998, by permission of the publisher WB Saunders

This lady turned out to have menorrhagia due to fibroids.

**Remember**

Iron Deficiency Anaemia

A post-menopausal female or any male with no obvious cause of blood loss **must have a G.I. cause for the anaemia.**

**GROUP 4:**

**ITEM 11:**

# Gastroenterology
# Rectal bleeding

Rectal bleeding is characterised by the passage of fresh blood rectally as opposed to either occult loss when blood can only be acknowledged by laboratory testing or melaena (see Group 5, Item 5).

## CASE HISTORY

An 80-year-old lady was admitted in a shocked state after having passed "a great deal" of fresh blood from her rectum. She gave no other history and prior to the incident had just returned on her bicycle from doing the shopping! Abdominal examination was normal.

### How would you manage her initially?
- Establish IVI and give colloids
- Check Hb and U&Es
- Insert CVP line
- Transfuse blood

Patient stabilised and had no further bleeding.

### Additional investigations on the ward must include a rectal examination, proctoscopy and sigmoidoscopy.

**Proctoscopy** will allow the diagnosis of haemorrhoids and an anal fissure. These are the commonest causes of rectal bleeding, but rarely cause torrential blood loss.

Features of bleeding from the anus:
- Passage of blood after a motion, and not mixed with it
- Blood dripping into the pan
- Blood just on the paper
- Anal pain particularly with anal fissure

**Sigmoidoscopy** will determine the presence of a colitis and may show a lesion e.g. carcinoma

### If local ano-rectal disease excluded, other causes include
- Cancer
- Diverticular disease
- Colitis
- Angiodysplasia

**Remember**

Even in the presence of severe diverticular disease, a polyp and carcinoma can be the cause of the bleeding and must be excluded by colonoscopy.

• Polyps
• Ischaemia

In this lady sigmoidoscopy showed that the blood was coming from above the limit of the scope. Colonoscopy showed a bleeding polyp.

**GROUP 4:**

**ITEM 12:**

# Gastroenterology
# Family history of colon cancer

### CASE HISTORY

A GP phones to discuss a possible referral to the gastroenterology clinic. He has just seen a 32-year-old anxious lady whose mother has recently died of colonic cancer. The patient has just discovered that her maternal aunt died of a similar complaint. The GP emphasises that the patient herself has no GI symptoms.

**Remember**

RISKS FOR DEVELOPMENT OF COLON CANCER
Normal 1 : 50
With a 1st degree relative 1 : 17
With an elderly 1st degree relative 1 : 30

### What should you advise?

The patient needs to be seen by a gastroenterologist with a view to having a colonoscopy.

There are two family cancer syndromes:

**Familial adenomatous polyposis**

Multiple polyps are found throughout the colon and upper small bowel. All patients should be screened after age 12 years as ALL patients will develop colon cancer unless the colon is removed.

**Hereditary non-polyposis cancer of the colon (HNPCC)**

This accounts for 5-10 % of colon cancers. the average age of diagnosis is 45 years. Cancers are mainly in the right-hand side of the colon.

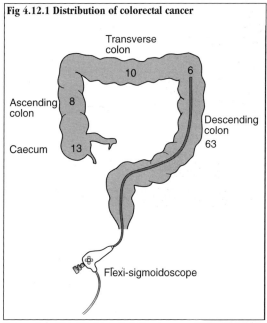

**Fig 4.12.1 Distribution of colorectal cancer**

Transverse colon
10
6
Ascending colon 8
Descending colon 63
Caecum 13
Flexi-sigmoidoscope

Redrawn from *Clinical Medicine*, 4th Edition, Kumar and Clark, 1998, by permission of the publisher WB Saunders

A flexible sigmoidoscope can reach 60-70 cm up the colon – where approximately 70% of cancers occur.

The gastroenterologist advises a colonoscopy.

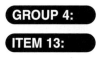

**GROUP 4:**

**ITEM 13:**

# Gastroenterology
# Functional bowel disease

A 30-year-old woman is in the A&E department with severe lower abdominal pain. She is rolling around in agony but the surgical registrar has found no evidence of serious disease. He has already fully examined her and investigated her with routine blood tests and an abdominal X-ray, all of which are normal. Her boyfriend is aggressive and insisting that something must be done! The casualty officer is looking for help.

### What do you do?

• Re-take the history with the possibility of this being the irritable bowel syndrome (IBS).

**Information**

**ACUTE ABDOMINAL PAIN**

*Sudden onset*
- Perforation e.g. of D U
- Rupture e.g. aneurysm
- Torsion e.g. ovarian cyst

*Gradual onset*
Inflammatory conditions, e.g.
appendicitis + back pain

*Think of*
- Pancreatitis
- Ruptured aortic aneurysm
- Renal tract disease

- Re-examine the abdomen – think of all the causes of an acute abdomen again (see box)
- Review the investigations

The history strongly supports the diagnosis of IBS (see Group 4, Item 7). Remember the pain can be very severe and real to the patient even though stress related i.e. "not in the mind".

**Management**

This can be very difficult particularly as relatives often feel unable to cope. The situation needs to be calmed down with strong reassurance and pain relief (e.g. NSAID and antispasmodics). Refer to gastroenterology outpatients.

## Notes

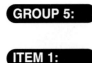

**GROUP 5:** **Liver, biliary and pancreatic disorders**

**ITEM 1:** **Abnormal liver function tests**

### CASE HISTORY 1

A GP telephones you to ask whether a hospital referral is necessary. She has recently seen a 55-year-old patient for a medical insurance examination for an American bank. She had found no problems with the patient at the time of the examination but the results of the liver function tests have come back abnormal.

Tests showed:

- Serum bilirubin          14 µmols/l
- Serum alkaline phosphatase   134 IU/l
- AST                70 IU/l
- ALT                90 IU/l

### What should she do?

These tests suggest intrahepatic disease and you politely enquire about the alcohol history. Answer is no alcohol. You suggest that she could arrange the following tests while waiting for an OP appointment:

- Repeat LFTs
- Viral markers
- Serum autoantibodies
- Serum ferritin

These tests will yield a diagnosis in most cases.

### The GP asks: Would an ultrasound be helpful?

No. This is not the pattern of biliary or pancreatic disease.

You arrange to see the patient with your consultant in outpatients.

At outpatients the history again is unhelpful

No history of:

- Blood transfusions
- Previous hepatitis
- IV drug abuse
- Sexual promiscuity

On examination you notice a few spider naevi

The results of the tests performed by the GP are now available (see box).

| Results | | |
|---|---|---|
| Repeat LFTs | similar to above | |
| Hepatitis A | IgG positive } | i.e. patient has been infected with HAV |
| | IgM negative } | in the past. It does NOT cause chronic liver disease. |
| HB$_s$Ag | negative | |
| HCV antibodies | positive | (see below) |
| Autoantibody screen | negative | (positive titres usually found in autoimmune hepatitis) |
| Serum ferritin | 110 µg/l | This excludes haemochromatosis. |

HCV antibodies indicate HCV infection (chronic hepatitis) and the patient will require HCV RNA, liver biopsy and possible treatment with anti-viral therapy *(see Kumar and Clark, 4th Ed, p312)*.

Armed with the HCV result you confidentially discuss IV drug abuse with your patient who then admits to the very occasional use of IV drugs in the "Swinging Sixties"!

Although this patient did not have HBV, you need to know the significance of HBV markers – see table 5.1.1

**Table 5.1.1**

**Significance of viral markers in Hepatitis B**

**Antigens**

| | |
|---|---|
| Hb$_s$Ag | Acute or chronic infection |
| HbeAg | Acute hepatitis B |
| | Persistence implies: |
| | Continuos infectious state |
| | Development of chronicity |
| | Increased severity of disease |
| HBV DNA | Implies viral replication |
| | (Found in serum and liver; also rarely positive in HbsAg-negative patients) |

**Antibodies**

| | |
|---|---|
| Anti-HBs | Immunity to HBV; previous exposure |
| Anti-HBe | Seroconversion |
| Anti-HBc IgM | Acute hepatitis B (high titre) |
| | Chronic hepatitis B (low titre) IgG |
| | Past exposure to hepatitis B (HbsAg-negative) |

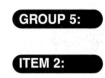

**GROUP 5:** # Liver, biliary and pancreatic disorders

**ITEM 2:** ## Jaundice

---

**Investigations**

- Blood count, liver biochemistry
- Liver function ( INR and albumin)
- Abdominal ultrasound
- Viral markers to exclude hepatitis causing intrahepatic cholestasis

---

### CASE HISTORY 1

A 45-year-old woman has been admitted with deep jaundice. Abdominal examination is unhelpful, there are no signs of chronic liver disease.

Ultrasound in extrahepatic obstruction can show:
- Dilatation of the intra hepatic biliary tree
- Dilatation of the common bile duct
- Gallstones in the gall bladder
- Gallstones in the biliary tree
- A pancreatic mass
- Metastatic liver disease

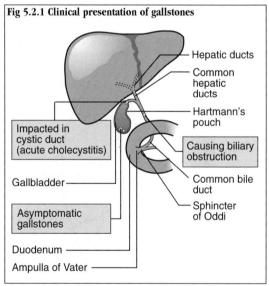

**Fig 5.2.1 Clinical presentation of gallstones**

Hepatic ducts
Common hepatic ducts
Hartmann's pouch
Impacted in cystic duct (acute cholecystitis)
Causing biliary obstruction
Gallbladder
Common bile duct
Asymptomatic gallstones
Sphincter of Oddi
Duodenum
Ampulla of Vater

Redrawn from *Clinical Medicine*, 4th Edition, Kumar and Clark, 1998, by permission of the publisher WB Saunders

---

**Remember**

Cholangitis is a common accompaniment with gallstones obstructing the biliary tree. This will be more common after intervention, and a drainage procedure should always be performed. Antibiotics will be necessary if the system has not been fully cleared. In this patient the initial management would include clearance of the common bile duct followed by a laparoscopic cholecystectomy.

---

In this patient, the ultrasound shows gallstones in the gall bladder and a dilated common bile duct. Provided this patient's clotting is satisfactory, the next investigation should be an ERCP (but see below). This would enable a better visualisation of the system, and would allow a gallstone that is causing the obstruction in the common bile duct to be removed. A sphincterotomy would need to be performed beforehand, and the stone could be removed with a basket or a balloon. If the stone is very large, the options would be to crush the stone and remove the debris, or alternatively surgery with a cholecystectomy and exploration of the common bile duct. In an elderly patient stent insertion to maintain drainage is an option.

Many surgeons now prefer to go directly to laparoscopic cholecystectomy (following the ultrasound) with intraoperative cholangiography and removal of duct stones, if present.

## CASE HISTORY 2

A 78-year-old man is admitted with marked jaundice. He was previously fit and well but the ultrasound showed a dilated biliary system with the probability of a pancreatic mass.

An endoscopic ultrasound and/or CT scan should be performed to assess the vague possibility of operability. An ERCP with placement of a stent through the stricture would enable drainage and is the usual treatment. This would make the patient feel a lot better as well as relieving the jaundice.

Both patients (**cases 1 and 2**) presented with jaundice without pain. This is quite common with carcinoma of the pancreas but with gallstones there is often a history of biliary pain accompanying the jaundice.

A similar obstruction could equally well be related to an obstruction higher up in the duct system, perhaps due to a cholangiocarcinoma. This could arise in pre-existing sclerosing cholangitis although this would occur at a younger age.

### Complications of ERCP sphincterotomy (complication rate 8-12%)

• Bleeding (severe in 2%)
• Perforation
• Acute Pancreatitis (5%)
• Cholangitis

An alternative investigation in these patients is **MRCP** (Magnetic Resonance Cholangio Pancreatography). This non invasive procedure is available and does show good definition of the biliary tree and pancreatic tree. However it must be remembered that there are a number of false positives, and indeed false negatives, and it may not remove the requirement of therapeutic ERCP.

## CASE HISTORY 3

A 20-year-old woman is admitted in a confused state and deeply jaundiced. She had recently returned from India where she had been trekking. She had had a major argument with her boyfriend, and subconjunctival haemorrhage was noticed on examination.

**Investigations**
- Haemoglobin
- Clotting studies and albumin
- Liver enzymes
- Blood sugar
- U&E

**Remember**

Hepatic encephalopathy should be treated with a low protein diet and lactulose

This patient is potentially critically ill with fulminant hepatic failure, and it is essential to stabilise her as soon as possible. She will need a central venous line and, if her haemoglobin is low then she may well need colloid support. The clotting studies will give an indication of the degree of damage to her liver, and will be useful for daily follow up. It is also necessary to make sure that the patient's potassium and blood sugar are satisfactory and clearly replacements may be necessary.

**Further management**

This patient is liable to infection and intravenous antibiotics are required after having taken blood cultures

It is essential to try to establish a cause of this patient's jaundice. This may be:

a) hepatitis A

b) hepatitis E

– both are endemic causes of hepatitis in India, and often follow a respiratory type of illness initially. They rarely cause fulminant liver damage but can occasionally do so.

c) paracetamol overdose is the **diagnosis in this case**

Markers for these causes, also paracetamol levels, must be obtained urgently. Further investigations would include the following if no cause has been found:

- Autoantibodies
- Copper studies
- Alpha 1 antitrypsin levels

The patient may well stabilise at this stage but a close eye will need to be kept on her for potential infections, particularly with opportunistic organisms. It is reasonable to give N-acetyl cysteine in the initial management of these patients whether or not they have had a paracetamol overdose.

This patient's clinical condition deteriorated and urgent advice was sought from the nearest liver unit.

In specialised units 70% of patients with paracetamol overdose and Grade IV encephalopathy survive. Factors which indicate a poor prognosis without transplantation are:

- arterial pH < 7.3
- serum creatinine > 300 µmol/l
- prothrombin time > 100 sec
- Grade III – IV encephalopathy

**GROUP 5:**

# Liver, biliary and pancreatic disorders

**ITEM 3:**

## Acute liver disease

### CASE HISTORY 1

A medical student turns up in A&E with jaundice. He is very worried that he may have gallstones and may need surgery! He has never seen jaundice outside a surgical ward.

### How do you approach this situation?

Firstly you point out that gallstones are rare in a young person and that a viral hepatitis is, by far and away, the most likely diagnosis. You quickly ascertain that he has an immune status to hepatitis B and only drinks beer after rugby. He denies IV drug abuse. Your thoughts now turn to how he acquired hepatitis A.

There is no clue from the history:

- No contacts with jaundice
- No prodromal features
- No travel abroad

On examination, apart from jaundice, there are no other abnormal signs.

Take blood for:

- Liver biochemistry
- HAV Ig M

You tell him to go back to his student flat, be careful with his personal hygiene and return in two days for his results.

| Results: | | |
|---|---|---|
| S Bilirubin | 70 µmol/l | |
| AST | 300 iu/l | compatible with acute hepatitis |
| ALT | 280 iu/l | |
| ALP | 140 iu/l | |
| HAV IgM surprisingly is **negative**! | | |

OOPS! You realise that although hepatitis A is very, very common in this situation there are other causes. You had forgotten to take a careful drug history in someone you knew – remembering ecstasy! He turned out to have glandular fever which can rarely present with jaundice.

**GROUP 5:**

# Liver, biliary and pancreatic disorders

**ITEM 4:**

## Ascites

### CASE HISTORY

A 45-year-old woman presents with ascites gradually increasing over two weeks. Examination shows no abnormality outside the abdomen. The determination of the cause is essential to develop a management plan.

### Ascitic Fluid

High protein >25g/l suggests tumour or infection.

If malignant cells are present, then further imaging with ultrasound, abdominal and pelvic, or CT, will be necessary to determine tumour site. Subsequent treatment will depend on malignancy demonstrated. In this patient, the age, sex and absence of signs of chronic liver disease suggests malignancy (probably ovarian).

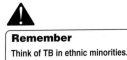

**Investigations**

- Liver biochemistry
- FBC
- PT and albumin
- Ascitic tap – for white cell count, culture, protein, malignant cells

### CASE HISTORY 2

A 45-year-old man has attended his GP on many occasions with alcohol related problems. He is sent up to A&E with a swollen abdomen. He admits to drinking 60 to 80 units per week for 20 years. On examination he is not jaundiced, has spider naevi, liver palms, Dupuytren's contractures and testicular atrophy. He has gross ascites and pitting ankle oedema.

### What should you do?

Immediate investigations as above. The ascitic tap is necessary to rule out infection and malignancy even though he has chronic liver disease.

### Findings

- A transudate in ascitic fluid (<25g/l) indicates cirrhosis without complication
- In a patient with known liver disease a high white cell count and high protein suggests infection (spontaneous bacterial peritonitis)

Ultrasound of the liver and spleen is now performed and shows splenomegaly which indicates portal hypertension.

**Remember**

Think of TB in ethnic minorities.

### Immediate management

- Bed rest
- Salt restriction
- Daily weights
- Start diuretics – spironolactone 100-400mg/day to obtain a weight loss of 500 gms/day
- If inadequate response to above then introduce – frusemide 40-120 mg/day

Refer to gastroenterologists for follow-up. He must STOP DRINKING. Give thiamine 25-50mg.

### Subsequent management

It may be necessary to undertake liver biopsy to confirm cause of cirrhosis only after ascites removed. If it is impossible to do percutaneous liver biopsy (ascites, prolonged clotting), then biopsy can be undertaken through the jugular vein under X-ray control. He should be referred to the Alcohol Dependency Unit. He may be suitable for liver transplantation.

**Remember**

Liver disease with few cutaneous or other signs of failure can occur particularly in chronic hepatitis C.

---

**GROUP 5:**

**ITEM 5:**

# Liver, biliary and pancreatic disorders

# Haematemesis and melaena

### CASE HISTORY

A 70-year-old man has been admitted with a haematemesis and melaena.

The initial assessment must include:

- Pulse rate
- Blood pressure (standing and lying)
- Haemoglobin
- Urea and electrolytes
- Clotting

### RESUSCITATE

- IV access
- CVP assessment
- Fluid replacement (initially with colloid e.g. Haemaccel)
- Blood transfusion

Inform gastroenterologists and surgical team.

**Remember**

Hb < 10, Urea↑, Postural hypotension present. Pulse rate 110/min. This patient is severely compromised and needs urgent treatment.

Further history and examination of this man may help elucidate the underlying diagnosis i.e.

- History of alcohol abuse and signs of chronic liver disease (Group 5 Item 4)
- History of long term dyspepsia – (Group 4 Item 8)

### The potential diagnoses are:

- Oesophageal varices
- Peptic ulcer
- Gastric cancer
- Gastric erosions

### Management

If signs of chronic liver disease present then immediate endoscopy will confirm diagnosis and allow injection or banding of oesophageal varices.

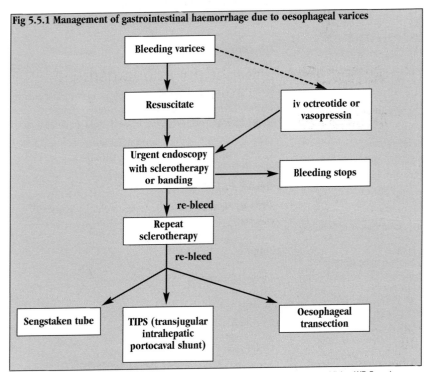

**Fig 5.5.1 Management of gastrointestinal haemorrhage due to oesophageal varices**

Redrawn from *Clinical Medicine*, 4th Edition, Kumar and Clark, 1998, by permission of the publisher WB Saunders

of octreotide 50µg/hour should be started. This may be less effective than Terlipressin (synthetic vasopressin) given by bolus injection (2mg/6 hourly) until bleeding stops followed by 1mg 6 hourly for a further 24 hours. Octreotide has fewer side-effects.

**Remember**

Stigmata of a recent bleed from an ulcer on endoscopy:
• Spurting vessel
• Prominent vessel
• Fresh adherent clot

**Remember**

Erosions can bleed torrentially and be very difficult to control

Balloon tamponade with a Sengstaken-Blakemore tube can be used if the bleeding continues. Initially use the gastric balloon only but if the bleeding is not controlled, inflate the oesophageal balloon, remembering that continuous inflation leads to oesophageal damage. It has serious complications and should only be left in situ for 24 hours.

If these measures fail then TIPS (Transjugular intrahepatic portosystemic shunt) may be required and is often considered the treatment of choice for gastric varices.

**If no signs of chronic liver disease** and **not** actively bleeding then endoscopy should be performed within 24 hours.

If a **bleeding ulcer** is seen on endoscopy this should be injected with epinephrine 1:10,000. Repeat if rebleeding occurs. A heater probe can also be used. Occasionally surgery is required.

A bleeding ulcer may have certain stigmata that suggest rebleeding is likely to recur.

Gastric cancer does not usually cause an acute GI bleed; it is more likely to produce anaemia from chronic blood loss.

### Discharge policy

The patient's age, diagnosis on endoscopy, co-morbidity and the presence or absence of shock should be taken into consideration. In general, patients under the age of 60, as well as older patients who are haemodynamically stable and have no stigmata of recent haemorrhage on endoscopy can be discharged within 24 hours.

Note, all shocked patients need careful observation in hospital. **CHECK YOUR OWN HOSPITAL'S GUIDELINES.**

### Causes of bleeding

These are shown in Fig 5.5.2.

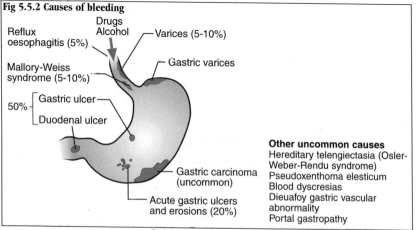

**Fig 5.5.2 Causes of bleeding**

Reflux oesophagitis (5%)

Drugs Alcohol

Varices (5-10%)

Gastric varices

Mallory-Weiss syndrome (5-10%)

50% { Gastric ulcer / Duodenal ulcer

Gastric carcinoma (uncommon)

Acute gastric ulcers and erosions (20%)

**Other uncommon causes**
Hereditary telengiectasia (Osler-Weber-Rendu syndrome)
Pseudoxenthoma elesticum
Blood dyscresias
Dieuafoy gastric vascular abnormality
Portal gastropathy

Redrawn from *Clinical Medicine*, 4th Edition, Kumar and Clark, 1998, by permission of the publisher WB Saunders

**GROUP 5:**

# Liver, biliary and pancreatic disorders

**ITEM 6:**

# Liver failure

### CASE HISTORY

A 60-year-old female has been a known abuser of alcohol for the past 20 years. She is admitted because of deterioration in her health with confusion and the development of ascites.

Further history indicates that she has stopped drinking some three months ago, and suffered no withdrawal symptoms.

On examination you wonder whether she has liver failure.

### What are the signs that indicate liver failure?
• Jaundice
• Ascites/portal hypertension (splenomegaly)
• Hepatic encephalopathy
 – hepatic flap
 – foetor hepaticus
 – constructional apraxia
• Signs of chronic liver disease e.g.
 – spider naevi
 – gynaecomastia
 – Dupuytren's contracture
 – liver palms

### Information

**Porto-systemic encephalopathy (PSE)**

This is a neuropsychiatric syndrome that occurs in cirrhosis. The blood by-passes the liver via collaterals allowing "toxic" metabolites to pass directly to the brain. The nature of these "toxins" is unclear but appears to be related to ammonia. Treatment is aimed at reducing protein breakdown in the gut.

If no risk of bleeding, then concentrate on determining level of encephalopathy: Early signs should be demonstrated by asking patient to copy a five pointed star.

| Grades of Encephalopathy | 1 disorientated |
| --- | --- |
| | 2 confused |
| | 3 comatose |
| | 4 unconscious |

### Immediate management
• Measure electrolytes and blood sugar, liver function and liver biochemistry.
• Low protein and low salt diet
• Establish infusion of 5% dextrose (10% if BS low)
• Diuretic therapy (see ascites)

• Use purgatives – lactulose 10-20ml x3/day to produce two to three stools a day
• Determine presence of infection both in ascites (ascitic tap) and systemically (blood culture) and treat

### Further management
**(Monitor daily)**

• Weight (see ascites)
• Conscious level measurement
• Liver function tests and coagulation
• Electrolytes and blood sugar
• Consider further intervention (transplantation referral) if no improvement

**GROUP 5:**

# Liver, biliary and pancreatic disorders

**ITEM 7:**

# Alcohol abuse

*i*

### Information

• Epilepsy occurs in 3-10% of patients who have alcohol dependence associated with:
• Alcohol intoxication
• Alcohol withdrawal
• Hypoglycaemia
• Full history and examination must be undertaken to exclude:
Neurological damage (central, peripheral)
Hepatic damage/signs of liver failure
Use of other drugs

### CASE HISTORY

A 45-year-old man presents with a history of excessive alcohol intake for ten years since his marriage failed. He had sought help from counselling services but had been unable to remain sober. His presenting symptoms were of collapses in the street and home – the most recent collapse was witnessed and reported as epileptic.

Saturate with vitamins (Parental Vitamin B and C should be used in first three days). Thiamine 100mg x3 day given orally throughout admission

| Neurological findings | |
| --- | --- |
| **Central** | |
| Nystagmus | These are the features of the Wernicke |
| Confusion | Korsakoff syndrome and this needs |
| Ataxia | urgent treatment with parenteral thiamine. With early treatment these features can be reversible. |
| **Peripheral** | |
| Loss of light touch | These are due to the longer effect of |
| Pin prick and vibration | alcohol abuse and are not usually reversible on withdrawal. |

## Treatment

- Withdraw all alcohol
- Sedate – use Benzodiazepines in adequate doses to produce sedation but beware of respiratory depression
- Keep under supervision
- Do not mix sedatives
- Reduce Diazepam slowly over next five days observing resolution of signs of withdrawal:
  - sweating
  - shaking
  - vomiting
  - agitation
  - hallucination
- Do not use antiepileptics

## Further management

Seek help from agencies dealing with alcohol and drug abuse in area for assessment and further management. Following abstinence give acamprosate 2gm daily. This drug acts by enhancing GABAergic inhibition.

Lesser degrees of damage than in the above case can occur in any area of function and are commonly hidden and should be sought in non-judgemental interviewing style.

Additional biochemical tests can help to determine physical damage produced by alcohol( MCV, triglycerides, uric acid, $\gamma$GT).

**Remember**

It is important to recognise that there are many initiating factors for alcohol abuse. It produces damage in many areas of function – financial, social, psychological and physical – and all need addressing.

## GROUP 5:
# Liver, biliary and pancreatic disorders

## ITEM 8:
# Cholecystitis

### CASE HISTORY

A 28-year-old man presents with right hypochondrial pain in A&E. He is seen by the A&E officer and surgical registrar who find little apart from right hypochondrial tenderness. In view of his age and general good health he is sent home with paracetamol to be followed by his GP.

Two days later a rather concerned GP phones to say that the patient's pain has persisted and the tenderness is marked. You ask him to send him back to A&E. In A&E you confirm the GP's findings. He has a temperature of 37.8°C.

### What should you do now?

In view of the persistence of pain and second referral by GP, admit the patient. Do blood tests in box.

One hour later your HP phones you to say his WCC is 19,000. Clearly he has an infection and you tell the HP to organise an urgent ultrasound while you call the surgical registrar. The surgical SpR recognises the patient he discharged two days ago. You discuss possible diagnoses.

### The U/S shows:

• Gallstones in the gall bladder
• Sonographic Murphy's sign
• Gall bladder wall thickening
• Peri-cholecystic fluid

### Diagnosis
**Acute cholecystitis**

The surgical SpR starts antibiotics (a cephalosporin e.g. cefuroxime) nil by mouth and IV fluids. He books him for a laparoscopic cholecystectomy in two days time.

### Investigations
• FBC, U+Es
• Liver biochemistry
• Serum amylase
• Blood culture in view of pyrexia

### Remember
• Acute appendicitis – but the site of pain is a bit high
• Acute cholecystitis – but 28 years old and a man – surely not!
• A localised perforation and other mischief run through your mind.

### Remember
GALLSTONES can occur at any age and not necessarily in fat females! Always think of appendicitis in a young patient with acute pain. US/CT are invaluable.

**GROUP 6:**

**ITEM 1:**

# Haematology and Oncology
# Microcytic and macrocytic anaemia

### Remember
- An accurate result depends on a correctly taken blood sample

  Avoid prolonged venous occlusion

  Don't take the sample from an arm with an I.V. infusion
- If the haemoglobin concentration doesn't fit the clinical picture take another sample

### Investigations
The classification of anaemia is based on the mean red cell volume (MCV; NR 80-96 fl). Further investigation is determined by whether the anaemia is microcytic, (< 80fl) macrocytic (>96fl) or normocytic.

### Definition
This is based upon the haemoglobin concentration; the normal range varies at different ages and between men (13 – 18 g/dl) and women (11.5 – 15.5 g/dl).

### Assessment
The impact of anaemia on an individual is variable and will depend on:

- The speed of onset
- Age
- Cardiovascular reserve

Symptoms are non-specific and clinical signs easily overlooked:

- Tiredness, lack of energy
- Shortness of breath on exercise
- Palpitations
- Ischaemic pain

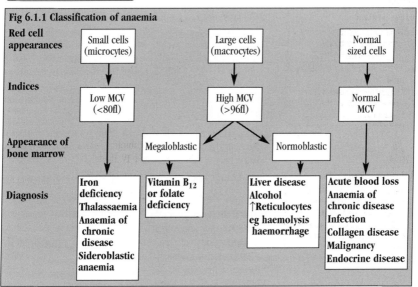

**Fig 6.1.1 Classification of anaemia**

| Red cell appearances | Small cells (microcytes) | | Large cells (macrocytes) | | Normal sized cells |
|---|---|---|---|---|---|
| Indices | Low MCV (<80fl) | | High MCV (>96fl) | | Normal MCV |
| Appearance of bone marrow | | Megaloblastic | | Normoblastic | |
| Diagnosis | Iron deficiency Thalassaemia Anaemia of chronic disease Sideroblastic anaemia | Vitamin B$_{12}$ or folate deficiency | Liver disease Alcohol ↑Reticulocytes eg haemolysis haemorrhage | | Acute blood loss Anaemia of chronic disease Infection Collagen disease Malignancy Endocrine disease |

Reprinted from *Clinical Medicine*, 4th Edition, Kumar and Clark, 1998, by permission of the publisher WB Saunders

## CASE HISTORY 1

A 45-year-old Afro-Caribbean woman presents to the A&E Department with chest pain which is thought to reflect cardiac ischaemia. She is found to have a microcytic anaemia.

| Blood count: | Blood film: |
|---|---|
| Hb 9.9 g/dl | anisopoikilocytosis + |
| MCV 59fl | target cells ++ |
| WBC 6.4 x$10^9$/l | |
| Platelets 309 x$10^9$/l | |
| ESR 10 mm/hr | |

**Remember**

* Ferritin is an acute phase protein. Iron deficiency can therefore be difficult to diagnose in the presence of inflammatory disease and tissue iron stores may need to be examined directly by bone marrow aspiration

• Serum transferrin receptor assay does differentiate – see Group 6 Item 14

### What is the reason for this and is it relevant to her presentation?

The most important cause to exclude is iron deficiency, commonly due to uterine or gastrointestinal bleeding. Iron deficiency is unlikely in this patient:

• Very low MCV with only moderate anaemia
• Minimal variation in red cell size and shape

The serum ferritin (30µg/l) was normal indicating normal tissue stores of iron. The anaemia of chronic disorder, a form of functional iron deficiency, is also unlikely without an obvious underlying illness and a normal ESR.

A common cause of a microcytic anaemia in patients of the right ethnic group is ß-thalassaemia trait. Common in people from Africa, the Mediterranean, Middle East, India and S.E. Asia. ß-thalassaemia trait is diagnosed by measuring HBA$_2$ which is normally < 3.4% of total haemoglobin. The HBA$_2$ in this patient was 5.2% confirming a diagnosis of ß-thalassaemia trait. α-thalassaemia trait is a diagnosis of exclusion in patients from the right ethnic group.

Characteristically ß-thalassaemia trait results in a marked microcytosis with only a moderate anaemia as shown in this patient.

Patients are asymptomatic and require no treatment. The anaemia is not contributory to this patient's cardiac ischaemia.

**Iron deficiency anaemia** (see Group 4, Item 10) responds to treatment with oral iron supplements – ferrous sulphate 200mg x3 daily (or all in one dose) for six months – it is essential to give a full course of treatment. Lower the dose if GI symptoms occur. Parenteral therapy is only rarely required. The cause of iron deficiency is almost always blood loss and the cause must always be determined. Don't forget uncommon causes:

**Remember**

The anaemia of thalassaemia trait is:
• Life-long
• Stable

- Pulmonary haemosiderosis
- Paroxysmal nocturnal haemoglobinuria
- Fragmentation haemolysis

## CASE HISTORY 2

An 81-year-old woman presents to the A&E Department with recent onset congestive cardiac failure. She is mildly jaundiced, with a severe macrocytic anaemia and moderate neutropenia and thrombocytopenia.

| Blood count: | Blood film: |
|---|---|
| Hb 3.2g/dl | Anisopoikilocytosis +++ |
| MCV 121fl | Hypersegmented neutrophils present |
| WBC 1.5 x10$^9$/l | |
| Platelets 64 x10$^9$/l | |

Vitamin $B_{12}$ or folate deficiency impairs DNA synthesis and affects all rapidly dividing cells particularly in the bone marrow, resulting in pancytopenia when severe. The anaemia is slow to develop and elderly patients, in particular, may not present until very late. *Avoid blood transfusion*, if at all possible, as there is a risk of volume overload and acute left ventricular failure. If really unavoidable:

- Transfuse slowly; each unit over four to six hours
- Give only one or two units
- Give IV frusemide
- Consider exchange transfusion

It is important to make a precise diagnosis by:

Measuring serum vitamin $B_{12}$, serum and red cell folate

- In $B_{12}$ deficiency the serum vitamin $B_{12}$ concentration is always reduced and in folate deficiency the red cell folate concentration is always reduced
- Severe vitamin $B_{12}$ deficiency may be associated with a low red cell folate and a normal or high serum folate. Vitamin $B_{12}$ is required to polyglutamate folate without which folic acid cannot be retained within cells.

Bone marrow aspiration (not necessary in an obvious case with low $B_{12}$ levels)

- Confirms megaloblastic erythropoiesis
- Documents pre-treatment iron stores
- Excludes other conditions – myelodysplasia, acute leukaemia and aplastic anaemia which may all present with a macrocytosis and pancytopenia

## Causes

Nutritional deficiency is almost always a factor in any cause of folate deficiency whether this be due to increased requirements (e.g. myelofibrosis, haemolysis) or with alcohol abuse. In malabsorption e.g. coeliac disease there is also poor dietary intake of folate.

Most cases of $B_{12}$ deficiency are due to malabsorption, either gastric, due to intrinsic factor deficiency, or intestinal.

### Remember

- Drugs and rare metabolic defects can result in megaloblastic anaemia with normal vitamin levels:
- Methotrexate induces functional folate deficiency
- Transcobalamin II deficiency results in intracellular vitamin B12 deficiency

## Consider

- Intrinsic factor antibody assay (positive in 50% of patients with pernicious anaemia)
- Barium meal and follow through (to exclude small bowel disease e.g. Crohn's
- Endomysial antibody and/or Jejunal biopsy (to exclude coeliac disease)
- Schilling test when patient is vitamin $B_{12}$ replete (to delineate site of $B_{12}$ malabsorption). This is only performed in the difficult case

Many patients with moderate vitamin $B_{12}$ or folate deficiency have a normal blood count although many have a raised MCV. Also consider vitamin assays if the clinical scenario is suggestive of a deficiency picture:

- Gastrointestinal disease or surgery including glossitis, malabsorption or diarrhoea
- neurological disease, including visual loss, a peripheral neuropathy or evidence of demyelination
- Psychiatric disorders including dementia, confusion or depression
- Malabsorption or restricted diets, including vegans and anorexia nervosa
- Alcohol abuse
- Infertility
- Autoimmune endocrine disease
- Family history of pernicious anaemia
- Drug therapy, particularly anticonvulsants

### Diagnosis

This patient had megaloblastic anaemia (see investigations below) secondary to severe vitamin $B_{12}$ deficiency.

### Management

Whenever possible treat with one haematinic only. In this patient treat with hydroxocobalamin 1000µg IM x1. If assay results are unavailable or ambiguous treat with hydroxocobalamin 1000µg IM and folic acid 5 mg orally daily.

| serum $B_{12}$ 25ng/l | (NR 160-960ng/l) |
|---|---|
| serum folate 14.6µg/l | (NR 4.0-18.0µg/l) |
| red cell folate 86µg/l | (NR 160-640µg/l) |

Full blood counts + reticulocytes and urea and electrolytes initially daily (in a severely anaemic patient-as in this case) to look for:

Hypokalaemia which may occasionally develop one to two days post therapy

Reticulocyte count which starts to increase two to three days after treatment and reaches a peak on days five to seven days

The haemoglobin concentration which often falls further prior to starting to rise

Stay calm!

Avoid blood transfusion

⚠️

**Remember**

Pernicious anaemia is an auto immune disease, one to two per cent of patients will also develop thyroid disease

Failure of the reticulocyte count and haemoglobin to rise in the predicted manner may be due to:

Incorrect diagnosis and/or treatment – review laboratory data

Co-existent iron deficiency – check iron stores on bone marrow aspirate

Intercurrent infection – review patient, chest infection? urinary tract infection?

Co-existent hypothyroidism

The majority of patients with vitamin $B_{12}$ deficiency have vitamin $B_{12}$ malabsorption and require life-long treatment with vitamin $B_{12}$

Hydroxocobalamin 1000µg 1M every three months is usually given but high doses of $B_{12}$(5mgs) daily by mouth are also effective

Nutritional deficiency of vitamin $B_{12}$ is rare and confined to vegans.

### Anaemia due to folic acid deficiency

These patients need six months treatment with folic acid 5mg daily after the cause has been defined and treated e.g. coeliac disease. Folic acid is, however, ineffective in the treatment of methotrexate toxicity where folinic acid 15 mg iv daily is given.

| GROUP 6: |
| ITEM 2: |

# Haematology and Oncology
# Haemolytic anaemia

### CASE HISTORY I

A 60-year-old presents feeling tired and exhausted for the last week. She is clinically jaundiced, with cervical lymphadenopathy and a just palpable spleen. She has a normocytic anaemia with a raised white cell count and a reticulocytosis (see box).

A normocytic anaemia may be due to:

• Acute blood loss
• Erythropoietin lack – chronic renal failure
• Bone marrow infiltration – carcinoma
• Haemolysis

The patient described is anaemic, jaundiced with splenomegaly suggesting a haemolytic anaemia. To confirm this you need to demonstrate:

• Increased red cell production
• A reduced red cell lifespan

### Increased red cell production

• Reticulocytosis:
  Reticulocytes are immature red cells newly released from the bone marrow
  They are larger than mature red cells
  They contain mRNA and appear polychromatic on standard blood films
• Bone marrow aspiration:
  Erythroid hyperplasia

### Reduced red cell lifespan

• Acholuric jaundice:
  Unconjugated hyperbilirubinaemia
  Urobilinogen but no bilirubin in the urine

• Abnormal red cell morphology:
  This may also indicate the specific cause of the haemolytic anaemia (see below)

• Directly by radioactive isotope studies:
  Reduced survival of 51Cr labelled autologous red cells

---

**Investigations**

BLOOD COUNT
• Hb 6.8 g/dl
• MCV 90fl
• WBC 30 x10$^9$/l
• Platelets 172 x10$^9$/l
• Reticulocytes 18.8%

BLOOD FILM
• Anisopoikilocytosis ++
• Polychromasia ++
• Spherocytes present
• Lymphocytosis with smear cells

**Remember**

Cortisol, androgens and thyroxine are all required for optimal erythropoiesis. Consider endocrine gland failure.

---

There are many specific causes of haemolysis. The diagnosis can often be made by review of the blood film. Speak to the Haematology Medical Staff.

## Features of haemolysis on blood film:

- Spherocytes – Autoimmune haemolytic anaemia, Hereditary spherocytosis, Clostridium welchii septicaemia, Extensive burns
- Red cell fragments – Leaking mechanical heart valve, Disseminated malignancy
- Sickled cells – Sickle cell anaemia, Sickle cell – HbC disease
- Bitten out red cells – G6PD deficiency, Unstable haemoglobin, Oxidative drug therapy e.g. dapsone
- Malaria parasites

This patient had a strongly positive DAGT with anti-lg G (see Fig 6.12.1, page 120). The antibody eluted from her red cells was also present free in her serum and did not have any easily definable antigen specificity. She therefore has *autoimmune haemolytic anaemia (AIHA)* due to an IgG red cell autoantibody active at 37°. AIHA may be primary or secondary. This patient had lymphadenopathy and a lymphocytosis with small, mature lymphocytes. Her AIHA is secondary to underlying chronic lymphocytic leukaemia (CLL). Ten to 15% of patients with CLL develop AIHA.

## Management

- Start oral prednisolone 60mg/day
- Consider blood transfusion if the haemoglobin continues to fall. Compatibility testing is complex; the laboratory may carry out autoabsorption studies to exclude additional alloantibodies. Transfuse slowly
- Consider high dose I.V. immunoglobulin to decrease splenic destruction of red cells

### Investigations

- Antibody screen and direct antiglobulin test (DAGT):
  In autoimmune haemolytic anaemia auto-antibodies to red cell membrane antigens are present in serum and on the red cell surface
- Urinary haemosiderin:
  Positive in chronic intravascular haemolysis such as Paroxysmal nocturnal haemoglobinuria (PNH) and leaking mechanical heart valves
- Ham's test:
  Positive in PNH due to increased sensitivity of red cells to complement mediated lysis
- Glucose-6-phosphate dehydrogenase assay:
  Common enzyme deficiency in the right ethnic groups African, Mediterranean, S.E. Asian

### Remember

AIHA can develop acutely with a rapid fall in haemoglobin. This patient has a short history. Check the haemoglobin concentration at least once a day.

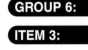

**GROUP 6:**

**ITEM 3:**

# Haematology and Oncology
## Sickle cell crisis

### CASE HISTORY 1

An 18-year-old Afro-Caribbean female came to A&E with severe pains in her right leg, left hip and back. She was well known to many of the staff as she had attended on many occasions with painful sickle crises. She had been at an all-night rave club!

The examination should initially be brief until adequate pain control has been achieved.

Important points to check are:

### Investigations

- Performed in A&E, aimed at assessing the severity of the crisis and determining any treatable cause.
- FBC + reticulocytes
- Urea and electrolytes
- Liver biochemistry.
  Compare values with normal steady state values
  Many nucleated red cells may result in an erroneously high WBC count
- MSU
- Blood cultures
  Infection is a frequent precipitant of a painful crisis
- O2 saturation on air
- Group and save

### Information

A low $O_2$ saturation may reflect acute lung pathology e.g. pneumonia or the acute chest syndrome or chronic sickle cell related lung damage.

CXR and arterial gases are only indicated if:

- rib, sternal and thoracic vertebral pain
- signs of consolidation
- tachypnoea (>25/minute)
- $O_2$ saturation < 80% on air or <95% on maximal supplementary $O_2$

### Distribution of pain? Any bone tenderness?
- Lumbar back pain can be particularly severe
- Rib, sternal or thoracic vertebral pain may impair respiratory effort and pre-dispose to the acute chest syndrome.

### Any precipitating factors?
- Exposure to cold/skin chilling ⎱ Both may apply
- Dehydration ⎰ to this patient
- Hypoxia
- Infection

### Any fever?
- Fever +/-leucocytosis may indicate an underlying infection but is also compatible with ischaemic tissue necrosis secondary to intravascular sickling alone

### Any hepatosplenomegaly?
- Splenomegaly is unusual in adults with HbSS or HbS-beta (0) thalassaemia
- A larger spleen than normal for the patient (ask the patient or parents/consult medical notes) may indicate acute splenic sequestration

### Compliance with hyposplenic prophylaxis?
- Patients with HbSS and HbS-beta (0) thalassaemia have severe hyposplenism and are susceptible to overwhelming sepsis particularly with Streptococcus pneumoniae
- Prophylaxis includes penicillin V 250 mg x2 daily and vaccination with Pneumovax and the Hib vaccines.

## Treatment

### Pain Relief

Most patients will have tried a variety of oral analgesics and once having presented to A & E will require parenteral opiates.

Reassurance and sympathy will do much to alleviate associated anxiety and fear.

A suggested regime for adults and adolescents would be:

- Diamorphine 5 mg SC + cyclizine 50mg SC
- Reassess pain 20 minutes later
- Repeat dose if pain unrelieved or halve dose if pain partially relieved
- Reassess pain 20 minutes later and repeat analgesia
- Once pain control achieved transfer to PCA system using SC diamorphine given as a variable bolus dose with a fixed lockout time.

When using diamorphine or other parenteral opiates the following parameters must be monitored regularly on an hourly basis:

- Pain score
- Respiratory rate
- $O_2$ saturation on air
- Analgesia consumption

Supplementary analgesia may be provided by:

- Regular oral dihydrocodeine and/or NSAIDs
- TENS
- Acupuncture
- Massage with analgesic rub

### Supportive Measures

- Keep warm/use heat pads
- Hydration – aim for 3.0 l/24 hours – orally if possible
- Venous access is often very difficult in these patients; in order to conserve peripheral veins the repeated insertion of IV lines should be avoided.
- IV hydration is indicated if:
  Nausea/vomiting is uncontrolled
  The patient is sedated
  The urea/creatinine are rising
- Oxygenation – aim for $O_2$ saturation 95%
- Monitor the haemoglobin concentration daily and consider blood transfusion if it falls to < 5.0 g/dl

**Remember**

- To determine appropriate bolus dose:
- Review amount of diamorphine required to achieve pain control
- Ask patient about usual dose
- Consult medical notes and previous discharge summaries

**Remember**

- Failure to maintain oxygenation may:
  Exacerbate the painful crisis
  Indicate the development of the acute chest syndrome

### The Acute Chest Syndrome

Most painful sickle cell crises resolve without complications within seven to 10 days. The development of the acute chest syndrome is the commonest cause of death in adults with SCD.

The syndrome is characterised by:

- Rib, sternal and/or thoracic vertebral pain
- Bilateral basal chest signs with new infiltrates on CXR
- Tachypnoea
- Deteriorating oxygenation
- Falling haemoglobin concentration
- Fever and leucocytosis

*Pathophysiology of Acute Chest Syndrome*
- Infection
- Fat embolism from necrotic bone marrow
- Pulmonary infarction due to sequestration of sickled red cells.

### Treatment

- Exchange blood transfusion to reduce the amount of HbS to < 20%
- Maintenance of oxygenation – this may include, for example, CPAP or IPPV
- Aggressive pain relief
- Intravenous antibiotic therapy

The majority of patients with a sickle cell crisis present with severe, acute bone pain secondary to ischaemic bone marrow necrosis. Beware the patient with sickle cell disease (SCD) who presents unwell but without pain, they may have other, less common, complications of SCD which may progress very rapidly.

### Types of Sickle Cell Disease

- Sickle cell anaemia HbSS
- Sickle cell – haemoglobin C disease HbSC
- Sickle cell – beta thalassaemia
- Rare compound heterozygotes e.g. HbSD

**Remember**
- Pneumococcal septicaemia
- Splenic sequestration
- Parvovirus infection associated with marrow aplasia
- Acute folate deficiency

**Fig 6.3.1 Patterns of haemoglobin electrophoresis**

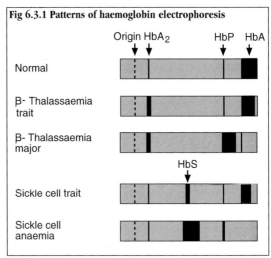

Redrawn from *Clinical Medicine*, 4th Edition, Kumar and Clark, 1998, by permission of the publisher WB Saunders

## Diagnosis in A&E:

- Information from patient
- UK Haemoglobinopathy card
- Blood count and reticulocyte count and blood film review
- Serum bilirubin
- Sickle solubility test

Later:

- Haemoglobin electrophoresis (see Fig 6.3.1) on cellulose acetate membrane (CAM) at alkaline PH or
- High pressure liquid chromatography (HPLC)

Typically the patient will be anaemic with evidence of haemolysis (elevated bilirubin and reticulocyte count). The blood film will show sickled red cells in variable numbers. The sickle solubility test will be positive and CAM electophoresis or HPLC will confirm the presence of HbS +/- HbC or HbD with no HbA (except in HbS-beta (+) thalassaemia.

## Beware

- In HbSC and HbS-beta (+) thalassaemia the haemoglobin concentration, reticulocyte count and serum bilirubin may be virtually normal
- The sickle solubility test is a qualitative test only and will be positive in any individual where the amount of HbS is > 10%. This will include both sickle cell trait and sickle cell disease

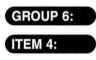

# Haematology and Oncology
# Elevated haemoglobin (polycythaemia)

**GROUP 6:**

**ITEM 4:**

## CASE HISTORY 1

On your medical take you admitted a 70-year-old man with breathlessness, wheeze, fever and cough productive of sputum. Initial investigations have shown Hb 23g/dl, and PCV 0.62 a mild neutrophilia and platelets 200 x10⁹/l. As a long-standing smoker he suffers bouts of bronchitis, but is otherwise in reasonable health.

## CASE HISTORY 2

In the next bed a 54-year-old man has been admitted with chest pain and a suspected myocardial infarct. His general health is reasonable but he has developed severe night sweats and has lost 7kg over the last three months. He denies smoking cigarettes and does not have any previous history of chest problems. His Hb was found to be 22g/dl with PCV 0.58, WBC 20 x10⁹/l and plts 600 x10⁹/l.

### These two cases both have elevated Hb, but is their cause the same?

Haemoglobin (in red blood cells) is required for oxygen transport, and like most things, too much Hb has serious consequences and needs appropriate management.

How to visualise the Hb level:

• Hb is expressed as a concentration i.e. grams/dl blood
• But blood = plasma + solids (RBCs mainly)

### Preliminary management

• Ensure no hyperviscosity symptoms or signs i.e.
  – Confusion
  – Visual disturbance
  – Peripheral circulatory disturbance
• Patient adequately hydrated
• Infection (if present) treated
• Identify correctable causes e.g. chronic hypoxia

Having made sure your patient is stable, the next step is to determine the cause of the high Hb concentration. Before carrying out extensive investigation, it is sensible to contact the

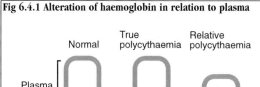

### Fig 6.4.1 Alteration of haemoglobin in relation to plasma

|  | Normal | True polycythaemia | Relative polycythaemia |
|---|---|---|---|

Plasma ~55%

RBC ~45%

≡PCV 0.45

Increased RBC mass eg Polycythaemia vera 2° polycythaemia

RBC mass normal but plasma volume is reduced with effect that Hb concentration increases eg dehydration

---

$i$

## Information

Hb may be high in:

- Primary proliferative polycythaemia (polycythaemia vera, PV)
- Secondary to underlying hypoxic state – ↑Hb serves a purpose
  - Chronic lung disease
  - Cyanotic heart disease
- Inappropriately high level of erythropoietin production – ↑Hb serves no purpose
  - Renal cell carcinoma
  - Uterine tumours
  - Cerebellar haemangioblastoma
- Relative/spurious/pseudo
  - Where the plasma component is reduced with effect that Hb concentration rises
  - Dehydration, associated with obesity, hypertension, diuretics, smoking

---

haematology team who will either advise on further tests or take over the patient's care.

The haematology registrar advises you to arrange some tests

### Investigations

- Repeat FBC (to check the result is correct and perhaps with some oral/I.V. fluid the Hb has normalised)
- Biochemistry screen – renal function – is it normal? Uric acid – may be high in some types of polycythaemia
- Blood film – these patients had elevated platelets and WBC – make sure these are normal peripheral blood cells, with no evidence of leukaemia
- Whole blood viscosity – hyperviscosity may result from extremely high Hb/PCV
- Blood gases or pulse oximetry (latter is painless and quite adequate to exclude hypoxia only)
- Chest radiograph – emphysema, other lung pathologies
- Abdominal ultrasound – is the spleen enlarged? Remember renal and uterine causes of polycythaemia
- Bone marrow – not diagnostic in isolation but gives additional information
- Red cell volume studies – is there a true increase in red cells or has the plasma component become smaller?

### Classical features of

**PV:**

- Weight loss, sweats, pruritus
- High Hb and may be ↑WBC + platelets
- Splenomegaly ±hepatomegaly

- Other causes (e.g. hypoxia) excluded
- ↑Red cell mass
- Plasma volume normal

**2° Polycythaemia:**

- As above, generally with no hepatosplenomegaly, no thrombocytosis,
- Usually 2° cause found, such as cyanotic heart disease, lung disease

**Spurious:**

- Red cell mass normal
- Reduced plasma volume
- No hepatosplenomegaly

## Management

This is where knowledge of the underlying cause becomes crucial.

**1) Your first patient has 2° polycythaemia due to lung disease:**

This is a physiological rise in Hb. If we reduce the Hb to normal this may have serious consequences.

The initial aim is to reduce the Hb to a safe level. Generally this is achieved by venesection (removal of ~ 400-500ml blood) every two days. In males the PCV is reduced to < 0.5 and in females to < 0.45.

Other causes of 2° polycythaemia should be treated with venesection and treatment of the underlying cause if possible.

**2) Your second patient has polycythaemia vera:**

- Venesect initially
- Then control marrow activity with hydroxyurea (or $^{32}P$ in elderly→ reserved for this group since it induces 2° leukaemias five to ten years later)

**3) Spurious polycythaemia**

- Correct dehydration
- Lose weight (if obese)
- Stop smoking
- Encourage exercise
- Venesection less often required

## Long-term complications

Ten to 15% patients with PV will develop intense marrow fibrosis (less often they may develop acute myeloid leukaemia). The other polycythaemias do not transform.

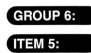

**GROUP 6:**

**ITEM 5:**

# Haematology and Oncology
# Elevated white blood cell count

There are many causes of this and there is overlap with haematological malignancies, many of which present with WBC elevation. As a non-specialist confronted with a patient who has an elevated WBC the key question is: does this elevation represent a haematological malignancy or is it reflecting some other process?

---

## HIGH WHITE BLOOD CELL COUNTS

**Patients with haematological malignancies likely to have high WBC:**

- Acute myeloid leukaemia
- Acute lymphoblastic leukaemia
- Chronic lymphocytic leukaemia
- Chronic myeloid leukaemia
- Lymphoma
- Other infiltrations – myeloma, myelofibrosis

**Situations where reactive WBC occurs:**

- Infection
- Corticosteroid therapy
- Brisk GIT bleeding
- "Stress" eg post-operative
- Post-splenectomy

---

A thorough history and examination will usually allow you to determine the cause of the elevated WBC

"Alert" features suggesting a possible malignant cause include:

- Ill patients
- Those with bleeding/bruising
- Fever
- Enlargement of liver or spleen or lymphadenopathy
- Weight loss
- Lymphocytes or bizarre/abnormal cells on blood film

### Is it glandular fever or acute leukaemia?

The atypical lymphocytes seen in infectious mononucleosis are often confused with leukaemic blasts, since the lymphocytes are large, often have nucleoli and resemble lymphoblasts. Specific tests such as 'Monospot' may help confirm the diagnosis. In general the haematology department will advise on further investigation e.g. cell marker analysis to exclude leukaemia.

**Remember**

If in doubt – contact the haematology staff. Early intervention in a patient with acute leukaemia is advised, and if you are not confident that the WBC rise is "benign" – seek expert help.

There is less urgency if:

- Patient obviously well
- Isolated WBC only (Hb/platelets normal)
- Obvious infection, post-operative patient etc.
- Simple neutrophilia

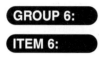

GROUP 6:

ITEM 6:

# Haematology and Oncology
# Elevated platelet count

## CASE HISTORY

A 75-year-old woman was admitted with acute ischaemia of the toes in both feet. On examination she was found to have dusky skin on both feet, with evidence of early gangrene in the toes. FBC showed normal Hb, WBC of 18 x10$^9$/l (neutrophilia) and platelet count 1500 x10$^9$/l.

Other significant features in this patient:

• Evidence of weight loss
• Splenomegaly 4cm below the costal margin

You need to decide whether the marked elevation of the platelet count is likely to be REACTIVE to some underlying process/ disorder, or whether she has a PRIMARY marrow disorder as the management is dictated by the underlying cause.

### Why does the platelet count rise in a reactive manner?

In simplistic terms, any acute stress (bleeding, operative surgery, severe infection) causes intense marrow activity with elevation of white cells and platelets in a non-specific way.

Reactive thrombocytosis does not usually exceed 1000 x10$^9$/l whereas primary thrombocytosis often > 1000 x10$^9$/l but do not rely on platelet count alone.

### Immediate action

• Contact haematologist
• Check end organs – are they threatened?
 – look at fundi? (vascular occlusion)
 – extremities (too late at this point as there is vascular damage to feet in this patient)
 – renal function
• Is there a secondary (reactive) cause?
 – infection
 – bleeding
 – malignancy (breast, lung, bowel)
 – connective tissue disorder (e.g. rheumatoid)

If none obvious – check again for splenomegaly as was found in this case

If platelets + splenomegaly likely myeloproliferative disorder

**This patient** has a myeloproliferative disorder.

These disorders are discussed elsewhere (Group 6 Item 13).

### Is there a test that will confirm a primary bone marrow pathology?

Unfortunately not. Bone marrow trephine may help since increases in megakaryocyte numbers (these cells make platelets) with clustering favours a diagnosis of essential thrombocythaemia but often it is a diagnosis of exclusion. Blood film examination may show marked variation in size and shape of the platelets (platelet anisocytosis) in primary thrombocythaemia – but this is not diagnostic.

### Management

- Consider low dose aspirin 75-300mg/day (or dipyridamole if aspirin contraindicated)
- Plateletpheresis (using cell separator) if organ function threatened and need rapid reduction in platelet count
- Reactive elevation of platelet count will resolve once underlying disorder treated
- If features suggest primary thrombocythaemia commence oral hydroxyurea to suppress bone marrow production of platelets (but beware neutropenia if dose too high). Suggested regimen: 10-30mg/kg/day or $^{32}$P in elderly (beware 2° leukaemias)

### Complications

Reactive thrombocytosis – depends on underlying disorder

Primary thrombocythaemia – generally indolent course but may transform to myelofibrosis in ~ 5% (occasionally transforms to acute myeloid leukaemia)

**Information**

Myeloproliferative disorders associated with thrombocytosis
- Primary (essential) thrombocythaemia
- Polycythaemia vera
- Chronic myeloid leukaemia
- Myelofibrosis

**Remember**

Seek specialist advice before prescribing cytotoxics or administration of $^{32}$P.

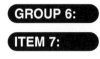

**GROUP 6:**

**ITEM 7:**

# Haematology and Oncology
# Glucose-6-phosphate dehydrogenase deficiency

### Remember

- G6PD deficiency will be present in all males who carry an affected X chromosome
- Heterozygous females will have a dual population of red cells; because X chromosome inactivation is random some heterozygous females will demonstrate clinical G6PD deficiency

### Definition

G6PD is an enzyme in the Hexose-monophosphate pathway responsible for generating NADPH. In the red cell NADPH is a major source of reducing potential required to maintain the iron atoms of haemoglobin in the ferrous state and to prevent membrane lipid peroxidation.

Deficiency of G6PD arises from a large number of different mutations in the G6PD gene, the majority of which are point mutations resulting in single amino acid substitutions. G6PD deficiency is widespread in many tropical and subtropical populations where malaria was, or is, endemic. Frequencies of 20% of the population in Southern Europe and Africa and 40% in S.E. Asia and the Middle East have been reported.

G6PD deficiency may present as:

- Neonatal jaundice
- Chronic haemolytic anaemia
- Acute haemolytic anaemia

An acute haemolytic crisis is the commonest presentation and most affected individuals are asymptomatic until this happens. Acute haemolysis occurs when an exogenous factor imposes an extra oxidative stress which overwhelms the red cells' limited supply of NADPH. Acute haemolysis may be precipitated by:

- Infection
- Drugs
- Fava beans

Many drugs have been implicated in attacks of acute haemolysis in susceptible individuals. the following drugs are generally considered the most common culprits.

**Antimalarials**
- Primaquine
- Pamaquine

**Sulfonamides**
- Sulfanilamide
- Sulfadimidine
- Sulfalpyridine
- Sulfasalazine

- Dapsone
- Co-trimoxazole

**Other antibiotics**
- Nitrofurantoin
- Nalidixic acid
- Quinolones eg ciprofloxacin

**Analgesics**
- Aspirin
- Phenacetin

**Antihelminthics**
- Beta-napthol
- Stibophan (not used now)
- Niridazol

**Miscellaneous**
- Vitamin K analogues
- Naphthalene
- Probenecid
- Dimercaprol

**FAVISM** is a form of severe, acute, intravascular haemolysis, often with massive haemoglobinuria, precipitated by exposure to fava beans (Vicia faba) in individuals with G6PD deficiency. It is commonest in children following the ingestion of fresh, raw beans. Haemolysis is probably precipitated by divicine, a glucoside constituent in fava beans, which generates free oxygen radicals when oxidised.

## Diagnosis

### Clinical features

- Sudden onset
- Severe malaise and pallor often with fever and abdominal pain
- Dark urine
- Jaundice

### Laboratory features

- Blood count:
- Normocytic anaemia
- Reticulocytosis
- Bitten out and irregularly contracted red cells.

The spleen "bites out" Heinz bodies which are aggregates of oxidised methaemoglobin, from affected red cells.

**Remember**
- Some drugs e.g. primaquine, aspirin and vitamin K can be safely given in reduced doses
- Some agents e.g. dapsone and naphthalene in sufficient amounts will cause haemolysis in individuals with normal levels of G6PD

**Remember**
- The jaundice of haemolysis is pre-hepatic and the bilirubin is unconjugated and therefore does not appear in the urine
- The dark urine is partly due to haemoglobinuria and partly to increased urobilinogen which oxidises and darkens on standing

### Features of intravascular haemolysis

- Decreased haptoglobins
- Increased LDH
- Haemoglobinaemia
- Haemoglobinuria
- Positive Schumm's test due to methaemalbumin

Particularly in adults haemoglobinuria may result in acute renal failure – monitor urine output, urea and creatinine.

### Remember

- Old red cells have less G6PD than young red cells and are destroyed first during a haemolytic attack
- Newly formed reticulocytes have relatively high concentrations of G6PD
- As a result of these two factors the concentration of G6PD in an affected individual may rise during an acute haemolytic episode to within the normal range
- If in doubt retest one month later

### Assessment of G6PD activity

- Qualitative screening test e.g. cresyl blue decolourisation test
- Quantitative enzyme assay by spectrophotometry

### Treatment

- Stop any drug which may have precipitated the acute haemolysis
- Search for and treat any infection
- Monitor haemoglobin concentration twice daily until stable.
- Bed rest; urgent blood transfusion may be required in severe cases
- Patient education
  - issue G6PD deficiency card and information leaflet
  - discuss avoidance of specific drugs and fava beans
  - offer family screening

### CASE HISTORY 1

A 30-year-old Nigerian man was brought to A&E having collapsed in the street. He had returned from a three month holiday in Nigeria six days previously. Two days before admission he had developed central colicky abdominal pain and diarrhoea; one day before admission he began to feel weak and noticed his urine was discoloured red. On examination he was pyrexial (37.8°C), anaemic and jaundiced. There was no hepatosplenomegaly. Dip stix testing of urine was negative for bilirubin but positive for urobilinogen and blood. Urine microscopy revealed no red cells.

| The haematology on admission showed: | |
|---|---|
| Hb | 5.4 g/dl |
| MCV | 91 fl |
| WBC | 15.8 x10⁹/l |
| platelets | 249 x10⁹/l |
| reticulocytes | 11.61% |
| Blood film | • Polychromasia |
| | • Irregularly contracted and bitten out red cells |
| | • No malaria parasites |
| | • No Heinz bodies |

The patient has a normocytic anaemia with a reticulocytosis suggesting acute haemolysis or haemorrhage.

Polychromasia refers to the appearance of reticulocytes, or immature red cells, when stained by May-Grunwald Giemsa.

The appearance of the red cells is compatible with oxidative red cell damage. It is unusual to see Heinz bodies when patients have a functional spleen.

Malaria is a common cause of haemolysis in patients returning from the tropics

| There was other evidence to suggest acute intravascular haemolysis: | |
|---|---|
| serum bilirubin | 65 μmols/l |
| serum haptoglobins | undetectable |
| serum LDH | 587 iu/l |
| Schumm's test | positive |

One of the isoenzymes of lactate dehydrogenase (LDH) is found in high concentrations in red cells and is released in red cell damage.

Rapid depletion of haptoglobin with the formation of methaemalbumin is typical of intravascular haemolysis. In the absence of other scavenging serum proteins excess haem binds to albumin and the ferrous iron is subsequently oxidised to ferric iron to give methaemalbumin and a positive Schumm's test.

| The cause of the intravascular haemolysis was established by further tests: | |
|---|---|
| Haemoglobin electrophoresis | HbA + HbS |
| Direct antiglobulin test (DAT) | negative |
| Isopropanol stability test | negative |
| G6PD assay | 1.9 iu/gHb |

Hb electrophoresis on cellulose acetate membrane (CAM) and agar gel demonstrated sickle cell trait but no other structural haemoglobin variant. Sickle cell trait does not result in a haemolytic anaemia.

The negative isopropanol stability test excludes an inherited, unstable haemoglobin variant.

The negative DAT or Coomb's Test excludes immune mediated red cell destruction.

G6PD was assayed by two methods which confirmed G6PD deficiency; the commonest G6PD variant in individuals of African descent is G6PD A-.

### What had precipitated a haemolytic crisis in this man with G6PD deficiency?

This was initially obscure. He denied any drug ingestion but, on repeated questioning, admitted drinking approximately 50ml of oily liquid. He had obtained this from his church in Nigeria where it was used for anointing the faithful. When he produced the bottle it smelt strongly of mothballs and ultraviolet spectrophotometry confirmed the presence of naphthalene. Naphthalene is well known to cause acute haemolysis, first described in the 19th Century following the introduction of beta naphthol to treat hookworm infestations. Many cases of affected infants have been described where the naphthalene was used as a moth repellant in clothes. The presence of G6PD deficiency greatly increases sensitivity to the oxidative red cell damage mediated by naphthalene.

The patients' haemoglobin concentration did not fall any further but rose slowly reaching 9.2g/dl seven days later. The reticulocyte count peaked at 17.4% on the fifth day, and the jaundice had resolved by 14 days. Re-assay six weeks later confirmed G6PD deficiency.

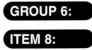

**GROUP 6:**

**ITEM 8:**

# Haematology and Oncology
# Bleeding disorders

It is important to identify bleeding that arises from a coagulation disorder rather than disease itself.

### CASE HISTORY 1

You are phoned by a surgical specialist registrar to ask for your advice. He has just finished a bilateral hernia repair on a 50 year old man and the right side is bleeding excessively. He has had to transfuse two units in the last 30 mins. He tells you that the APTT is 2 seconds prolonged and wants you to sort out his clotting.

### What do you think?

This patient is most likely to be bleeding from a surgical cause – two units in 30 mins is far in excess of what you would expect to give in a patient with a clotting disorder, and he is only bleeding from one of the repair sites, not both. Best to advise him to find the bleeding vessel!

This may seem like a somewhat silly example, but it shows the point that not all bleeding is due to abnormal clotting. Look at the whole picture before jumping in with fresh frozen plasma (FFP).

⚠️

**Remember**

Management of inherited disorders is complex – always seek specialist support

## Inherited bleeding disorders

You are far more likely to see acquired bleeding disorders than inherited. Inherited disorders are uncommon, but must be identified.

### How can I identify the inherited disorders?

Most inherited disorders of any severity present in childhood and hence most, if not all patients, will tell you about their problem. They should carry a medical card with them, identifying their problem and their haematology consultant. It should be easy to sort out these patients and get in touch with the appropriate specialist for this. Always take any suggestion of an inherited bleeding disorder seriously.

### How can I identify milder forms?

Milder inherited disorders may not present until later life and usually do so after surgery or other interventions. They can be identified by following the plan given later.

## Acquired bleeding disorders

As mentioned, these are far more common than inherited problems and are usually seen in particular clinical settings. These common scenarios will be outlined later. Most acquired disorders involve multiple and complex defects of coagulation.

## Investigation of a suspected bleeding disorder

**Should I check the clotting on everyone who bleeds?**

Probably this isn't absolutely necessary but have a low threshold. A normal set of results might help you be more secure that you aren't overlooking something. Remember, however, always take a full history and family history to try to identify any underlying inherited coagulation defect. For example, if a patient had:

• Excessive bleeding after a previous haemostatic challenge
  – operation
  – dental extraction
  – trauma
• Needed a previous blood transfusion for bleeding
• Family history of bleeding
• Epistaxis, easy bruising

**Remember**

Even a two second prolongation may indicate an inherited clotting problem of significance and should be investigated more fully

## What should I request?

You request a basic coagulation screen:

- Full blood count to check platelet number
- PT (prothrombin time)
- APTT (activated partial thromboplastin time)

These are the minimum tests. If you really want to check that a clotting disorder doesn't exist, the following should also be performed:

- Fibrinogen level
- Thrombin time (TT)
- Bleeding time – assesses global haemostasis and platelet function. It will be long if platelet count is less that 100 and/or Hb less than 10g/dl. Use only if you suspect an inherited platelet disorder or renal disease.

These tests form your baseline investigations or screening tests.

Acquired disorders are relatively easy as clotting times are usually notably prolonged.

There are a whole range of specialist investigations for the complete study of a coagulation disorder – best to seek specialist advice.

## CASE HISTORY 2

You are called to see a patient on the ward who is bleeding excessively. What should you think about as you walk over? What are the common causes?

### Causes

- Liver disease
- Vitamin K deficiency
- Renal disease
- Disseminated intravascular coagulation (DIC)
- Anticoagulants
- Surgical

**Less common**

- Undiagnosed inherited defect
- Weird and wonderful acquired defects

### Liver disease

This causes widespread coagulation and bleeding problems. Always be aware that significant liver dysfunction means a potentially severe bleeding disorder. The components of liver related bleeding are listed below.

- Reduced synthesis of coagulation factors – the liver is the source of all coagulation factors
- Associated vitamin K deficiency – coagulation proteins may be synthesised but will not be active because of vitamin K deficiency
- Thrombocytopenia – frequently secondary to splenomegaly from portal hypertension
- Chronic low grade DIC – see later
- Abnormal fibrinogen synthesis – in liver disease excess sialic acid residues are added to fibrinogen and hence an acquired dysfibrinogenaemia occurs

The classical lab defects would be:

- PT prolonged due to Factor II, V, VII or X decrease
- APTT prolonged due to decrease in all factors
- TT prolonged due to abnormal fibrinogen
- Fibrinogen degradation products (FDPs) increased (due to failure to remove from circulation +/- chronic DIC)

## Management

(via replacement therapy and vitamin K)

- Give 10mg vitamin K daily I.V. for three days
- For acute bleeding give 10-20ml/kg FFP to replace all coagulation proteins
- If the fibrinogen level is low or TT prolonged give cryoprecipitate to supply fibrinogen

In extreme degrees of liver failure it may be very difficult to correct the defect. Remember, the aim is to control bleeding rather than to aim for complete correction of *in vitro* tests.

### Vitamin K deficiency

This is probably more common than you think. Be aware of it.

It's easy to diagnose – check the PT as this will reflect Factor VII levels which are most susceptible to vitamin K depletion. The APTT may also be long if the deficiency has led to low IX, X or XI.

## Treatment

Obvious, vitamin K is given parenterally or orally dependent on the cause and severity.

### Renal Disease

Anyone with significantly impaired renal function may also have an acquired bleeding disorder. The major cause is toxic metabolites impairing platelet function.

**Information**

Causes of vitamin K deficiency
- Biliary obstruction
- Oral anticoagulants
- Liver disease
- Malabsorption states
- Inflammatory bowel diseases (with ileal resection)

### Is the APTT or PT abnormal in renal disease?

NO. As mentioned above the major defect is an acquired platelet disorder. The clotting times are usually normal. The give away test is a prolonged bleeding time.

### Should the bleeding time be regularly measured on patients with renal failure?

This isn't usually done, but remember that renal disease is a cause of an acquired bleeding disorder. If you're planning surgery on these patients, remember that they may have a bleeding problem, and make sure that everyone appreciates this. Seek senior advice.

### What can we do in renal failure?

There are a range of approaches to treatment but sorting out the renal problem first is the best option. Dialysis will improve platelet function; that is why few stable dialysed/controlled patients actually bleed. The real risk group are those with a very high creatinine/urea.

Other treatments include:

• DDAVP
• Cryoprecipitate
• Platelet transfusion

It is always best to seek senior advice.

### Disseminated Intravascular coagulation (DIC)

This is the most complex of the acquired bleeding disorders.

### What is DIC?

DIC is inappropriate and continued activation of coagulation that leads ultimately to both bleeding and thrombosis.

The initial phase of DIC is thrombosis. This is why DIC is associated with end organ damage leading to multiorgan failure.

Bleeding arises as a secondary phenomena due to consumption of coagulation factors and platelets (due to continued activation of clotting) and the activation of fibrinolysis (breaking down any fibrin that gets laid down).

**Remember**
DIC is always secondary to some other major clinical problem

### Action

• Always think about DIC in a bleeding patient
• Try to make the diagnosis
• If you find they have DIC then look/think about the associated cause

### Causes

• Infection

- Obstetric complications
- Surgical
- Trauma
- Malignancy
- Liver disease
- Transfusion reactions

If someone is bleeding and you always think about DIC you won't go wrong. In many ways the long list of causes is academic when you first see the patient – but if they have got DIC it is important to identify the cause.

### How do I make the diagnosis?

Send off all the screening tests and fibrinogen degradation products (FDPs)

| The pattern is: | |
|---|---|
| | Reason: |
| Platelets low | consumption |
| PT prolonged | consumption |
| APTT prolonged | consumption |
| TT prolonged | consumption of fibrinogen and FDPs |
| Fibrinogen low | consumption |
| FDPs high | breakdown of fibrin |

### Why are FDPs important?

FDPs tell you that fibrin is being broken down. The most specific test is the D-dimer which tells you that cross linked fibrinogen has formed and has then been broken down.

### How do I manage DIC?

- Treat the underlying disorder
- Treat the underlying disorder!
- Treat the underlying disorder!
- Support with FFP, cryoprecipitate and platelets

You must aim to treat the underlying disorder! DIC is always secondary. As mentioned earlier it is due to inappropriate and continued activation of clotting. Until you stop this by treating the underlying problem it won't get better.

Blood component therapy is purely supportive. Give:

- 10-20ml/kg FFP + cryoprecipitate
- Platelets
- Blood as required

**Remember**

People die from their underlying disorder rather than the DIC per se.

Aim to get the fibrinogen concentration to normal and the PT/APTT to within 4 secs of normal.

Always ask for specialist advice! This will save a lot of heartache when you are trying to get platelets, FFP and cryoprecipitate from blood bank.

## CASE HISTORY 3

Has this patient got DIC? He is 50-years-old with carcinoma of the lung with a prolonged PT, APTT, TT, low fibrinogen and platelet count and high FDPs but he isn't bleeding.

This is the picture of sub-clinical DIC – laboratory abnormalities but no bleeding. It is seen in chronic DIC in eg liver disease, malignancy. DIC ranges from florid bleeding to laboratory only abnormalities.

### Anticoagulant overdosage

An obvious cause of bleeding. Don't forget to look for warfarin/heparin usage.

### Action:

Confirm this by finding a prolonged PT or APTT

Treatment of bleeding: Depends on problem but in essence:

**Remember**

High prothrombin time (due to warfarin) without bleeding usually requires no treatment apart from stopping warfarin

| | |
|---|---|
| **If due to Warfarin** | STOP WARFARIN |
| Minor bleeding | • INR>6.0 Restart warfarin when INR<5.0; check INR daily |
| | • INR>8.0 give vitamin K 2.5mg oral or 0.5mg IV. |
| Major bleeding | • Give prothrombin complex concentrate 50 units/kg or FFP 15 mls/kg |
| | • Give vitamin K 5 mg IV |
| **If due to heparin** | STOP HEPARIN |
| | If bleeding excessive or uncontrolled: |
| | Protamine reversal (1mg IV neutralises 100u heparin – maximum dose 40mg) |
| | Seek advice |
| | Heparin excess will correct in a few hours |

**Surgical**

Suspect if rapid blood loss at operation. Don't underestimate the number of times this is forgotten and people end up chasing a medical cause for bleeding when a vessel has a hole in it.

If you have a hole in a vessel it won't stop unless it's fixed, however good the coagulation system is.

Remember surgical and medical bleeding may co-exist. If you correct the coagulation and the patient is still bleeding think surgical whatever the surgeon says!

**Undiagnosed inherited disorder**

This often presents as prolonged persistent bleeding rather than florid, acute blood loss. Suspect if:

- Isolated defect of APTT or PT or normal APTT/PT and continuing non-surgical bleeding
- History of previous or family bleeding

Plan: Refer on to specialist

**Rare causes**

If recent onset bruising or bleeding and prolonged APTT and no surgery, think rare cause eg acquired factor VIII inhibitor refer to specialist

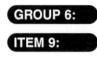

## Haematology and Oncology
## Platelet disorders

**Remember**

Meningococcal septicaemia has a purpuric rash and/or petechiae

### CASE HISTORY 1

You are asked to see a 24-year-old woman who is in A&E. She has presented with petechiae. The casualty officer has found that she has a platelet count of 10 x10$^9$/l.

There are multiple causes of thrombocytopenia (see below). Thrombocytopenia may be the presentation of another disorder rather than a primary platelet disorder. All patients with severe thrombocytopenia require admission for investigation/ treatment.

### Causes
**Failure of platelet production**

• Marrow aplasia
• Metabolic defects:
– B12/folate deficiency
– Uraemia
– Alcohol excess
– Liver disease
• Drugs:
– Chemotherapy ± radiation
• Marrow infiltration:
– Leukaemia
– Lymphoma
– Myeloma
– Myelofibrosis
– Carcinoma

**Decreased platelet survival**

• Immune:
– Idiopathic thrombocytopenic purpura (ITP)
– Systemic lupus erythematosus (SLE)
– Chronic lymphatic leukaemia (CLL)
– Hodgkin's disease
– Drug related
• Infection:
– Malaria
– Virus Infection
• Consumption:
– DIC
– Extracorporeal circulation

– Thrombotic thrombocytopenic purpura (TTP)
- Loss from circulation:
  – Splenomegaly
  – Massive transfusion

## Questions that need to be answered immediately are:

- Does she have ITP?
- Does she have acute leukaemia?
- Does she have aplastic anaemia?

## What further information do you need?

You need to know:

- If she is systemically unwell
- Has she any lymphadenopathy/splenomegaly
- Is the rest of the FBC normal?
- Has the count been repeated and film examined to exclude artifactual decreased platelets (pseudothrombocytopenia), technical error or blood clot in initial sample.

Information from the FBC and clinical examination should help exclude/confirm ITP/acute leukaemia/aplasia.

| | |
|---|---|
| • ITP | normal Hb, normal WCC, no hepatosplenomegaly or lymphadenopathy |
| • Acute Leukaemia | see Group 6 item 13 high WCC, abnormal white cells on film |
| | Lymphadenopathy, hepatosplenomegaly (possibly) |
| • Aplastic Anaemia | low Hb, low WCC, no L/Ns, no hepatosplenomegaly |

While considering the diagnosis you are called back to see the patient who has had a massive haematemesis. You think the diagnosis is ITP as there are no other features to make you think it is aplastic anaemia or acute leukaemia.

Major bleeding in ITP is not common but can be a serious complication. Treatment approaches should be decided by a haematologist.

## Approaches to management would include

- Adequate and secure IV access
- ABO and Rh (D) group and crossmatch 6 units of blood
- Fluid and blood replacement as appropriate

**Remember**

This list of causes is not comprehensive and excludes inherited thrombocytopenia or causes that would present in childhood.

- Start high dose IV imunoglobulin infusion 0.4 g/kg/24 hours
- Platelet transfusion – two units asap
- Oral prednisolone 1mg/kg daily

### Learning Points

- High dose immunoglobulin elevates the platelet count by Fc-receptor blockade of the reticulo-endothelial system. Endogenous platelets usually rise after 24-48 hours; the survival of exogenous platelets is improved
- Platelet transfusion is usually contraindicated in ITP except in the situation of life threatening haemorrhage
- Seventy-five per cent of patients respond to oral steroids but the full therapeutic effect may take several weeks to develop

### CASE HISTORY 2

You are asked to see a 50-year-old man on a surgical ward who has come into hospital for an elective hernia repair. He is found on a routine pre-op FBC to have a platelet count of 90 x10⁹/l. His Hb and WCC count are normal.

This chronic presentation of mild thrombocytopenia is reasonably common. To establish the cause you should systematically go through the causes of thrombocytopenia from initially a clinical history and examination.

#### Can he go ahead and have his hernia repair?

It may take a while to get to the bottom of his thrombocytopenia. Elective surgery can be performed if the platelet count is greater than 75 x10⁹/l.

Avoid any NSAIDs as post op analgesia; check whether aspirin taken within last ten days.

### CASE HISTORY 3

A 28-year-old lady has had a D and C for long-standing menorrhagia. She is now five days after the procedure and still bleeding. She has been back in theatre and no local defect is found. She says she had problems in the past with bleeding after dental extractions. Her PT and APTT and platelet count are normal.

This is the typical picture of a possible inherited platelet disorder. Severe platelet function disorders present in childhood, but milder versions usually do not present until surgery in adulthood. Clues here are bleeding after dental extraction and long-standing menorrhagia.

#### Management:

Assess extent of bleeding

- Treatment options include:

---

⚠️

**Remember**

ITP may become chronic and may require long term treatment +/- splenectomy.

---

**Investigation**

Platelet function studies (organise through haematologist)

if platelet transfusion has been given, delay until at least two weeks post infusion

---

– tranexamic acid 1g 4 x daily if mild bleeding
– platelet transfusion if severe bleeding

In a classic platelet function disorder the bleeding time is prolonged, but this test is difficult to perform. If you suspect a platelet function disorder organise platelet function studies.

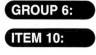

# Haematology and Oncology
# Thrombosis

### CASE HISTORY

You are asked to see a 24-year-old woman who has had a life threatening pulmonary embolus. She wants to know why she has developed a pulmonary embolus. She has a family history of DVT. Are investigations indicated?

Thrombosis is common but relatively rare under the age of 45 years. In such patients with a family history, about 50% have a definable underlying prothrombotic state. It is well worth formally investigating her for a prothrombotic state.

Attempt to identify any precipitating event, such as:

• Combined oral contraceptive pill
• Immobility and/or recent surgery/fracture/injury
• Long-haul flight
• Obesity
• Malignancy

### Should she be investigated now or later?

If on anticoagulants these can interfere with thrombotic investigations. Identifying an underlying thrombotic state acutely will not change immediate management.

She could be investigated now if she is:

• Not on any anticoagulants
• On heparin alone she can only be partially investigated

If she is on warfarin, formal studies must be delayed.

If she cannot be investigated now refer her on to a specialist for follow up and investigation.

**Remember**
• An abnormal result after an acute thrombosis does not mean an abnormality genuinely exists
• It must be rechecked
• However – a normal result is normal

## What investigations should be requested?

*(Clinical Medicine, Kumar & Clark, 4th Ed, p410)*

These are many and listed in the box. They are aimed at looking for an inherited deficiency of natural anticoagulants, mutations leading to increased thrombin generation or acquired causes of a prothrombotic state.

These investigations are the essential collection.

If a defect is identified, refer on to a specialist for long-term follow up and counselling and family studies.

### Investigations

- Lupus anticoagulant
- Antiphospholipid antibody
- Protein C deficiency
- Protein S deficiency
- Antithrombin deficiency
- Factor V Leiden
- 3' Prothrombin UTR variant

## CASE HISTORY 2

You are asked to see a 70-year-old man who had a DVT post knee replacement. He has no family history.

### Should he be investigated for thrombophilia?

It is likely that at this age a DVT in this setting has been precipitated by the surgery. The pick up rate for a thrombotic disorder of significance is very low in this setting. When asked to assess the thrombotic status, balance the likelihood of finding a defect against the value of identifying the exact defect.

## CASE HISTORY 3

You are called to see a 45-year-old man who is being anti-coagulated for acute ileo-femoral vein thrombosis with heparin. His APTT remains normal on 28000 units heparin per 24 hours. His dose has been progressively increased over the last three days and his leg swelling is worse.

### You are asked to advise.

The target APTT for heparin for an acute thrombosis is 1.5 – 2.5 times the mid point of the normal range. The commonest reasons for failure are:

- Under monitoring
- Under dosing
- Not actually receiving dose prescribed

### Action

- Ensure prescribed dose is being given
- Increase dose by 10% per 24 hours
- Recheck APTT in four hours
- If still low, repeat 10% increase and recheck at four-hourly intervals.

Heparin monitoring is notoriously bad in most hospitals. If I.V. heparin is being used it should be monitored as follows:

**Remember**

- Outcome is dependant on the effectiveness of anticoagulation within the first 48 hours
- Heparin resistance is rare. Poor heparin control is very common.

- Check APTT every four hours until target reached
- Increase dose in 10% increments
- Once target APTT reached repeat at four hours
- If stable APTT repeat 12-hourly

## How long should a patient with venous thromboembolic disease be anticoagulated with warfarin for?

The duration and target INRs for various thrombotic conditions are listed below:

| | Duration | INR target |
|---|---|---|
| Uncomplicated DVT | 6 months | 2.5 |
| Complex DVT | 6 months | 2.5 |
| Pulmonary Embolus | 6 months | 2.5 |
| Recurrent venous thrombo-embolism (VTED) | indefinite | 2.5 – if the recurrent event occurs whilst taking warfarin the intensity of anti-coagulation is increased, target 3.5 |
| TIAs, Arterial thrombosis, AF | indefinite | 2.5 |
| Mechanical heart valves | indefinite | 3.5 |

Recurrent VTED is essentially two or more events. The more events the greater the likelihood of recurrence.

Long-term anticoagulation carries risks – major haemorrhage (4% per annum) and death (~ 0.5%). These must be balanced against recurrence prevention. Complications are far more common in the older patient.

Recurrence is much higher in patients anticoagulated for six weeks rather than six months.

**Remember**

- Drug interactions with warfarin
- Need to amend dosage in patients undergoing invasive procedures
- Regular anticoagulant clinic follow up

## CASE HISTORY 4

You are asked to see a 36-year old-woman with an acutely swollen calf. Clinical diagnosis is a distal DVT. She has no complicating problems.

### How should she be treated?

Initially the diagnosis should be confirmed by Doppler US/duplex or venogram. An acutely swollen leg has a range of causes.

### Causes

- DVT
- Ruptured Baker's Cyst
- Rupture of head of gastrocnemius
- Acute knee injury
- Haematoma

• Infection (eg. cellulitis)

**Action**

A Confirmed DVT (if limited) give:

• S/C Low Molecular Weight (LMW) heparin e.g. Dalteparium 200units/kg/24 hours
• Warfarinise

This can be managed in out patients with good nursing and laboratory support

DVT (complex, ileo-femoral):

• Admit
• I.V. unfractionated heparin
• Warfarinise

There is an increasing move to outpatient management of VTED. This is likely to increase over the ensuing years.

## CASE HISTORY 5

You are phoned about a 36-year-old man with an acute arterial thrombosis who has a family history of thrombosis. The houseman has sent off a standard thrombophilia screen. He asks if this is all that you need.

Arterial and venous thrombosis have many common features but differ in some respects. Inherited/acquired defects predisposing to arterial disease are somewhat different to venous. In addition to the standard screen (see Investigation box in Case History 1) the following should be requested:

• Plasma homocysteine
• Lipid profile
• Plasminogen activator inhibitor

Finding a cause in arterial disease is less likely than in venous thrombosis.

## CASE HISTORY 6

You are asked to see a 60-year-old woman with a right leg DVT on heparin. She has been in hospital for five days. She has now developed a cold painful leg on the left that is pulseless. You are told her platelet count has been falling since admission.

What is the most important diagnosis to consider?

This would be a good picture for heparin induced thrombo-cytopenia with thrombosis (HITT). The classic features here are progressive platelet decline and new thrombosis. HITT is a clinical diagnosis and should be identified and considered in any patient on heparin whose platelet count falls significantly.

**Action**

• Stop heparin – ALL heparin
• Contact Haematologist
• Alternate forms of anticoagulation may be required

HITT is due to an immune reaction against the heparin/platelet complex. There is usually a previous history of heparin exposure.

It is important to identify: be aware that fatal thrombosis both venous and arterial can arise if heparin not stopped and alternate treatments instituted.

HITT can occur after SC heparin use. Be aware. It is increasingly common with the widespread use of heparin prophylaxis.

Management of pulmonary embolus (see Group 11, Item 13).

# Haematology and Oncology
# Splenomegaly, splenectomy and hyposplenism

Spleen size may be assessed by abdominal palpation or by radiographic imaging. The most useful techniques are:

• Ultrasound
• CT
• MRI

The functional size of the spleen may be assessed by scanning with a scintillation counter following the injection of radio labelled (99mTc), heat damaged, autologous red cells. These cells are removed from the circulation solely by the spleen.

The causes of splenomegaly are legion, with the most frequent causes showing geographical variation. In the West, malignant blood diseases, portal hypertension, haemolytic anaemias and infective endocarditis account for most cases, whereas in tropical countries malaria, leishmaniasis and the haemoglobinopathies are prevalent.

### Causes
- **Malignant haematological disease**
  e.g. acute or chronic leukaemia
  malignant lymphoma
- **Myeloproliferative disorders**
  e.g. polycythaemia vera
  myelofibrosis (often massive)
- **Haemoglobinopathies**
  e.g. beta-thalassaemia major, haemoglobin
  H, SC, or E disease

- **Haemolytic Anaemias**
  e.g. hereditary spherocytosis
- **Congestive splenomegaly**
  e.g. portal hypertension (cirrhosis)
- **Inborn errors of metabolism**
  e.g. Gaucher's disease
- **Collagen disease**
  e.g. SLE, rheumatoid arthritis (= Felty's syndrome)
- **Infections**
  (i) Viral e.g. infectious mononucleosis
  (ii) Bacterial – any bacteria occasionally
       remember infective endocarditis
  (iii) Protozoal
       e.g. malaria, kala azar
- **Miscellaneous (rare)**
  e.g. amyloid, tropical splenomegaly

Enlargement of the spleen from any cause may be complicated by hypersplenism. This is characterised by:

- Splenomegaly
- Pancytopaenia
- Normal or hypercellular bone marrow

### Pathophysiology of Hypersplenism
Mature red cells, neutrophils and platelets "pool", or are trapped, in the sinusoids of the large spleen and prematurely destroyed.

### Surgical splenectomy may be carried out because of:
- Trauma
- As an aid to diagnosis (note, in the past but not now) e.g. Hodgkin's disease/malignant lymphoma
- Treatment e.g. hereditary sphecocytosis/immune

thrombocytopenic purpura/myelofibrosis

Long-term complications of splenectomy are also found in patients who have functional hyposplenism i.e. patients who retain an anatomical non-functional spleen.

## Hyposplenism may be due to:

- Congenital absence
- Splenectomy
  - surgical or by irradiation
- Splenic atrophy
  - e.g. coeliac disease, chronic inflammatory bowel disease
- Splenic infarction
  - e.g. sickle cell anaemia (HbSS)
- Splenic infiltration

## Splenic function can be assessed by:

- Peripheral blood film – look for abnormal red cells
  - Acanthocytes
  - Target cells
  - Pappenheimer bodies
  - Howell-Jolly bodies
- Differential interference microscopy of blood
  - increased pitted red cell count
- Radioactive spleen scan (see above)

## CASE HISTORY

A six-month-old baby boy of Nigerian parents was admitted to A&E, collapsed and unconscious. The family were travelling to Heathrow by taxi and diverted the car to hospital when the baby became suddenly unwell. Twelve hours before admission the child had been seen at a different casualty department with a short history of poor feeding, irritability and diarrhoea. He was noted to be febrile but not thought to be seriously unwell. On review the child was noted to be pale and febrile with a firm spleen extending to below the umbilicus. Shortly afterwards the child had a cardio-repiratory arrest and could not be resuscitated.

## A blood count taken before death showed

- Hb — 2.4 g/dl
- MCV — 76 fl
- WBC — 30.5 x10$^9$/l
- Platelets — 27 x10$^9$/l
- Reticulocytes — 7.0%

> ⚠ **Remember**
> Acanthocytes
>   = spikey red cells
> Target cells
>   = like an archery target
> Pappenheimer bodies
>   = iron granules
> Howell-Jolly bodies
>   = nuclear DNA fragments
> Pitted cells
>   = red cells with submembrane vacuoles.

**Blood film review showed**

- Polychromasia
- Very reduced platelets
- Nucleated red cells
- Occasional elongated sickle cells
- Diplococci both within neutrophils and macrophages and free in the plasma.

**Remember**

Prevention of pneumococcal sepsis in babies with sickle cell anaemia is dependent on:

- Maternal antenatal haemoglobinopathy Screening and identification of pregnancy at risk
- Haemoglobinopathy screening of cord blood samples
- Institution of penicillin prophylaxis by eight weeks of age.

**Subsequent investigations demonstrated**

- Streptococcus pneumoniae on blood culture
- Haemoglobin electrophoresis showed:

Hb S      90%
Hb F      8%
Hb A2     1.8%

A West-African baby presented moribund with splenomegaly, severe anaemia and thrombocytopenia. The reticulocytosis/polychromasia and nucleated red cells suggested a haemolytic anaemia. Haemoglobin electrophoresis subsequently confirmed sickle cell anaemia (HbSS). The sickle cell mutation affects the beta-globin gene and only assumes clinical importance four months after birth when gamma-globin gene activity is suppressed and the beta-globin gene activated.

Death was due to overwhelming infection with Streptococcus pneumoniae, which was present in enormous numbers in the blood stream. The thrombocytopenia was almost certainly related to DIC secondary to the bacterial infection. Severe hyposplenism is a characteristic feature of sickle cell anaemia and is established by four to six months. Pneumococcal sepsis secondary to hyposplenism is a common cause of death in children less than three years old with sickle cell anaemia.

**Remember**

- The greatest risk of OPSI following splenectomy is in the first two years but there remains an increased risk lifelong.
- The mortality rate with OPSI due to Streptococcus pneumoniae is 50% despite treatment.

The gross splenomegaly and severe anaemia was due to acute splenic sequestration of sickled red cells within the spleen and often accompanies pneumococcal sepsis in this age group.

Overwhelming post-splenectomy infection (OPSI) is the most feared complication of hyposplenism.

**Pathophysiology**

- Decreased antibody synthesis
- Decreased phagocytosis of opsonised bacteria

**The major pathogens involved in OPSI are**

- Streptococcus pneumoniae > 80%
- Haemophilus influenzae type B
- Neisseria meningitidis

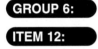

**Remember**

- Following vaccination check adequacy of antibody response.
- Repeat antibody levels at five years post-vaccination and give booster doses if appropriate.

These are all encapsulated bacteria – the spleen is a vital first line of defence against encapsulated organisms. Severe infections in the hyposplenic patient can also occur in malaria and babesiosis ( mosquito and tick bites respectively) and following dog bites with Capnocytophaga carnivorus.

### Prevention of OPSI depends on

- Identification of the patient at risk
- Education of the patient about the risks of infection, dog bites and tropical travel
- Issue of a "Post-splenectomy" card and leaflet to the patient
- Lifelong prophylactic antibiotic therapy e.g. penicillin V 250 mg x 2 daily
- Vaccination with Pneumovax and the Hib vaccine

**GROUP 6:**

**ITEM 12:**

# Haematology and Oncology
# Blood transfusion

The Blood Transfusion Department supplies red cells, platelets and plasma products, such as fresh frozen plasma, cryoprecipitate and human albumin. *(see Kumar & Clark, 4th Ed, Clinical Medicine p395)*

The efficient and safe provision of blood products depends on good communication between you and the laboratory, and accurate patient identification.

### Always

- Provide complete and accurate patient identification on the blood sample and request form
- Tell the Blood Transfusion Department how much of what blood product is required and the urgency of the clinical situation

### Never

- Take blood from more than one patient at a time
- Pre-label the blood sample tube

To provide compatible red cells for transfusion the following procedures are undertaken by the Blood Transfusion laboratory:

### ABO and Rh(D) blood group

– major haemolytic transfusion reactions usually result from the transfusion of ABO incompatible blood

– the Rh(D) antigen is very immunogenic and the development of anti-D must be avoided in women of childbearing age

**Antibody screen**

– excludes the presence of clinically significant red cell alloantibodies in the patient's plasma. These may result in an acute or delayed haemolytic transfusion reaction

**Selection of appropriate donor units**

– wherever possible blood of the same ABO and Rh(D) group as the patient is selected and will be negative for the appropriate antigen if an alloantibody has been identified.

**Cross-match**

– the patient's plasma is reacted with the donor red cells in vitro. Incompatibility is indicated by agglutination or haemolysis

A full compatibility procedure is always completed but this maybe retrospective if the clinical demand for blood is urgent.

## CASE HISTORY 1

You are asked to see a 72-year-old man with myelodysplasia who receives regular blood transfusions. One unit of blood was given uneventfully, but 15 minutes into the second unit he began to shiver, felt unwell and developed a pyrexia and tachycardia.

A febrile transfusion reaction to HLA or granulocyte antigens is common in multi-transfused patients, but cannot be safely distinguished from a haemolytic transfusion reaction due to red cell antibodies without appropriate laboratory tests.

### Action
• Stop the transfusion immediately
  – replace giving set
  – keep IV line open with 0.9% saline
• Check patient identification
  – wrist band
  – compatibility form
  – compatibility label on unit of blood
• Take appropriate samples
  – blood count
  – blood cultures
  – blood transfusion sample
  – urine for haemoglobin
• Take samples + relevant unit of blood to laboratory
• Inform haematology medical staff of the problem
• The laboratory will
  – check laboratory documentation
  – repeat ABO Rh(D) group, antibody screen and cross match on pre- and post-transfusion samples in parallel

**Remember**

• When you request blood always make clear the urgency of the clinical situation.

• Very urgent
  – life threatening haemorrhage
  – blood required in 1-5 minutes
  ACTION: No pre-transfusion compatibility test. The laboratory will issue group 0 Rh(D) negative blood

• Urgent
  – blood required in 5-10 minutes
  ACTION: ABO and Rh(D) group on patient sample. The laboratory will issue ABO and Rh(D) group compatible blood.

• Non-urgent
  – blood required in 30-60 minutes
  ACTION: Full pre-transfusion compatibility test. The laboratory will issue fully compatible blood.

– carry out a direct antiglobulin test (DAGT or Coomb's test, see figure 6.12.1) to exclude the presence of alloantibodies on the patient's red cells

## Outcome

If the above investigations are negative the reaction can be assumed to be a febrile transfusion reaction.

The patient should receive leucocyte depleted blood products in future.

If a red cell alloantibody is identified, the reaction is likely to be a haemolytic transfusion reaction.

Monitor renal function, urine output, haemoglobin concentration and check coagulation screen. Red cells negative for the appropriate antigen must be provided for future transfusions.

If a major ABO incompatibility is identified, the reaction may be life threatening with acute renal failure and disseminated intravascular coagulation:

• Monitor as above
• Insert urinary catheter and monitor urine output
• Give IV fluids to maintain urine output (>1.5ml/hr/kg)
• If urine output inadequate consider CVP line, fluid challenge and diuretics
• Consider referral to renal unit
• Report to SHOT (=Serious Hazards of Blood Transfusion), a confidential enquiry into major blood transfusion errors.

## Other acute complications of blood transfusion may present with

• Breathlessness
  – acute volume overload
  – acute transfusion related lung injury (TRALI)
• Urticaria or anaphylaxis
  – reaction to plasma proteins
• Collapse or hypotension
  major ABO incompatibility
  infected blood product
• Cardiac arrhythmia
  – hypocalcaemia
  – hyperkalaemia
  – rapid transfusion with 'cold' blood

## Management of massive haemorrhage

• Communicate
  – nature and urgency of the situation to the laboratory
• Predict
  – requirements for blood and blood products; always try to think ahead

**Remember**

• There are other longer term complications of blood transfusion including:
• Post transfusion purpura (PTP)
• Viral infection – hepatitis C, hepatitis B, HIV, (N.B. blood in UK checked for these) CMV
• Iron overload
• Graft versus host disease

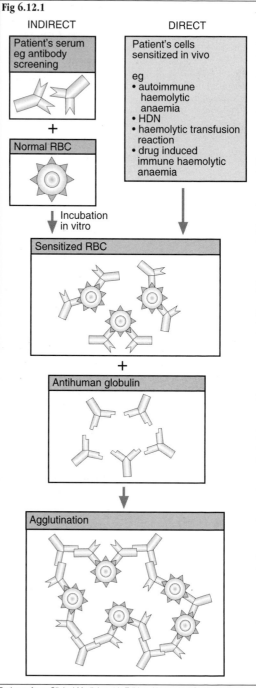

**Fig 6.12.1**

Redrawn from *Clinical Medicine*, 4th Edition, Kumar and Clark, 1998, by permission of the publisher WB Saunders

**Remember**

Give blood through a blood warmer to minimise hyperkalaemia and cardiac arrhythmias

**Investigations**

Anticipate haemostatic failure
Check:
Blood count
PT/INR
APTT
Fibrinogen concentration
Fibrin breakdown products
(FDPs or fibrin D-dimers)

**Remember**

Fresh frozen plasma takes 30 minutes to unfreeze
Platelets may need to be delivered from Regional Transfusion Centres

• Monitor
  – volume replacement
  – haemostatic parameters
  – serum calcium – blood is anticoagulated with EDTA which chelates calcium
• Maintain intravascular volume
• Avoid
  – Hypovolaemia
  – Renal failure
  – DIC
  – cardiac arrhythmias
• Use
  a) Saline/colloid solutions
  b) Group 0 Rh(D) negative blood
  c) ABO Rh(D) group compatible blood until fully compatible blood available

### Check for haemostatic failure

• Initially at beginning of emergency
• Every five units of blood given
• Whenever additional blood products (platelets, FFP, cryo.) are given

### Haemostatic failure may be due to

• DIC
  Secondary to hypovolaemic shock with additional liver failure, infection or tissue trauma
• Dilutional coagulopathy
• Stored blood is depleted of coagulation factors and contains few platelets

### Action

Request platelets – to maintain platelet count > 50 x10$^9$/l or if sequential platelet counts are falling progressively

Request cryoprecipitate (10 units) if fibrinogen concentration <1.0 g/l

Request fresh frozen plasma (10-20 ml/kg) if PT/INR and PTTK prolonged

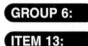

**GROUP 6:**
**ITEM 13:**

# Haematology and Oncology
# Haematological Oncology

This umbrella term covers a huge range of disorders. There are those that present dramatically and require urgent treatment, and at the other end of the spectrum there are diseases that are indolent and chronic, often requiring no therapy. You should be able to recognise the low grade (non urgent) disease and high grade (urgent) disorders and refer to your haematology department (outside normal hours do not be afraid to talk to the haematology registrar/consultant on call).

### What main groups of disease are there?

• Leukaemias
  Can be acute (short duration, serious, rapidly fatal if not treated) or chronic. Generally have elevated WBC and other features (see below). These are marrow/blood based diseases.

• Lymphomas are lymph node based, sometimes involving blood and marrow. Some need urgent treatment and others can be sorted out at leisure.

• Myeloma is a low grade highly destructive disorder of plasma cells, often presenting with for example bone pain, renal failure, hypercalcaemia.

Don't worry about the details of these different disorders for now, they are all discussed in the following clinical cases.

### CASE HISTORY 1

A 63-year-old cleaner is admitted to your ward with pyrexia and cough productive of sputum. Her general health has been reasonable until now. On examination she has chest signs suggestive of pneumonia. In addition she has generalised lymphadenopathy and a three fingerbreadth spleen. A rash over her trunk, she claims, was due to shingles four months earlier.

A full blood count shows mild anaemia (Hb 10.6g/dl), normal platelets, and a WBC elevated at 25 x10⁹/l. The haematology technician phones to say most of the white cells are lymphocytes and there are smear cells on the film.

### You need to establish if

• This is an acute or chronic disease
• Urgent treatment is required
• What steps would you need to take to make a diagnosis?

**Remember**

A smear cell is an artefact induced by making the blood film (the CLL cells are fragile and burst. There are no smear cells actually circulating in the patient's blood).

**The key features here are:**

• Elderly patient
• Fairly well
• Shingles
• Active infection
• Lymphadenopathy/splenomegaly
• High WBC with smear cells

This must be **chronic lymphocytic leukaemia (CLL)**, the commonest leukaemia in adults. It is a slowly progressive disorder and is an incidental finding or presents with an infective complication. (Shingles is a fairly common presenting feature.)

CLL is a disease mainly of B lymphocytes (95%, the rest are T) – determined by checking cell markers. There is a reduction in immunoglobulin synthesis leading to the infective complications.

**Other features**

• May be decreased Hb and platelets (depends on disease stage)
• Haemolytic anaemia (red cell autoantibodies)
• Other autoimmune complications

**Management**

**On day of admission:**

You have already started this with I.V. antibiotics (e.g. cefuroxime 750mg x3, erythromycin 500mg x4), rehydration if necessary. Refer to the haematology department next day. This patient's leukaemia is incurable (almost all chronic leukaemias share this feature) and the aim is to palliate – maintaining good quality of life. The disease may remain stable for several years.

**Long-term treatment:**

Observation, may require oral chemotherapy at later stage (e.g. chlorambucil).

## CASE HISTORY 2

You are called to see a 43-year-old accountant in A&E. This man went to see his GP suffering excessive tiredness. You are presented with an anxious, pale man, who has bruising over his lower limbs and arms. Temperature is 39°C. He is admitted urgently to the ward and examined in detail. Although febrile, no localising signs are present.

**What tests would you arrange?**

• FBC and U&E
• Blood cultures
• MSU
• CXR

The Hb is 6.0 g/dl, WBC 90 x10$^9$/L and platelets are 30 x10$^9$/L. Renal function is normal and CXR shows minimal increased shadowing at the right base.

### Is this an acute or chronic disorder?

A short history in an ill patient with severe anaemia and thrombocytopenia suggests the former.

You must ask what the white cells are, morphologically.

If they are neutrophils (neutrophilia) this may reflect an underlying infection; unlikely with such a high WBC.

However the technician looks at the blood film and tells you they look like blasts.

Blast = primitive white cell Present in bone marrow in small numbers Never seen in peripheral blood in health

This suggests an acute leukaemia. In a patient of this age acute myeloid leukaemia is likeliest. (If he were a child then acute lymphoblastic leukaemia is more likely).

You should only aim to perform the initial treatment steps: I.V. fluids, empirical (blind) therapy of infection (send cultures first) then notify the haematology staff as soon as possible.

### CASE HISTORY 3

A 72-year-old butcher is currently on the orthopaedic ward with collapse of one of his lumbar vertebrae. The orthopaedic SHO is concerned since some results have come back which he wishes to discuss with you.

The patient has mild anaemia with an elevated WBC (26 x10$^9$/L, mainly neutrophils). The ESR is 120mm/hr.

Blood film comment: red cell rouleaux.

There is mild renal impairment and hypercalcaemia (corrected Ca 3.21 mmol/l)

The patient appears quite uncomfortable, and appears to have lower back pain and admits to pain in the left rib cage, right humerus and right thigh. His general health was excellent until about 4 months ago when he developed anorexia and mild weight loss. His wife, who is present, is concerned as he is forgetful and confused at times (this has been much worse over the past one to two weeks).

### What possible diagnoses are there?

Although not in extremis this man is ill.

- An ESR of 120 suggests serious underlying pathology (an ESR of 120 could be due to serious infection, autoimmune disease, rheumatoid, malignancy)
- Red cell rouleaux, renal impairment and hypercalcaemia in a

---

### Remember

Do not wait until the next morning – the patient may succumb before then!

### Investigations

- Specific diagnostic tests (performed by haematology department)
- Peripheral blood film examination (are there Auer* rods? If so, confirms AML; these are actually not all that common)
- Bone marrow aspirate and biopsy
- Cell marker analysis (determines pattern of antigens on white cells)
- Cytogenetic studies on marrow blasts – several karyotypic abnormalities are diagnostic
- Plus other tests e.g. HLA typing
- Condensed granules, pathognomonic of AML

patient with bone disease suggests either a primary bone disorder (such as myeloma) or possible infiltration by malignancy e.g. carcinoma.

If outside working hours there is little else you can request. Your main objective is to treat the symptoms e.g. rehydrate, start antibiotics if you think infection is present, correct the elevated calcium level (see Group 14, Item 19). Alert the haematology team.

## As soon as possible check

- Blood film
- Immunoglobulin levels/serum protein electrophoresis
- Repeat biochemistry to check renal function and calcium level
- Send urine for Bence-Jones protein (free immunoglobulin light chains)
- Blood cultures if febrile
- MSU
- Arrange skeletal survey (plain radiology of skull, spine, pelvis, femora).

## In this case

- Elevated total IgG with reduced IgA and IgM
- Serum IgG M paraprotein
- Bence Jones protein present – kappa Light chains
- Widespread lytic lesions throughout skeleton
- Subsequent bone marrow aspirate showed infiltration by abnormal plasma cells

The diagnosis is multiple myeloma

## CASE HISTORY 4

A 50-year-old bank manager is admitted with weight loss, sweats and splenomegaly. Initial investigations show mild anaemia, WBC 200 x10$^9$/L and platelets 600 x10$^9$/L.

### What further information do you require?

- White cells – are they blasts?
  No – there are neutrophils, eosinophils, basophils and early (= immature) granulocytes eg promyelocytes, myelocytes etc.
- How large is the spleen?
  Palpable to umbilicus
  (ultrasound = 24 cm)

### Biochemical screen

Normal apart from elevated serum uric acid level

Re-examine patient yourself

Are there any other abnormal findings?

There is no lymphadenopathy

Liver edge is palpable

Chest is clear

Fundi – NAD

### What is the underlying diagnosis?

There are several significant findings: e.g. very high WBC, splenomegaly with weight loss and sweats. Could he have an underlying infection/neoplasm producing these features i.e. reactive process? Yes, but it is much more suggestive of an underlying primary blood disorder such as chronic myeloid leukaemia (the white cell count is high with whole spectrum of granulocytic cells present. If the blood picture were "reactive", a neutrophilia would be more likely).

### What single investigation will confirm the diagnosis?

Cytogenetic analysis of peripheral blood white cells or bone marrow white cells.

In most (not all) CML the Philadelphia chromosome will be present (translocation of DNA between chromosomes 9 and 22).

### Does he need urgent referral to the haematology team?

Unless the patient is very unwell or has features of leucostasis (blood sludging due to high WBC) then there is no immediate need for urgent referral, but you should alert the haematology staff who should take over the patient's care next day.

Leucostasis: → 
- Confusion
- Visual disturbance
- Cough and dyspnoea

### Features suggestive of acute leukaemia/high grade lymphoma

- Acute onset
- Unwell
- Dramatic presentation
- Extensive     – infection
                 – bruising
- Gum swelling
- Fundal haemorrhage
- Coagulopathy
- Blasts/immature cells in peripheral blood
- Auer rods

**Remember**

Philadelphia chromosome is present in some acute leukaemias but this patient does not have features of acute leukaemia, and the bone marrow will confirm this.

### Features suggestive of chronic/low grade haematological malignancy

- Less dramatic onset
- Not particularly unwell
- Previous infection (eg chest infection or herpes zoster)
- Absence of blasts in blood
- Abnormal peripheral blood cells: lymphocytes with abnormal morphology or immature granulocytes. Generalised lymphadenopathy present for months

Refer all suspected patients with acute leukaemia to haematology team as soon as possible, for specialist management.

### Remember

The WBC does not have to be high to diagnose acute (or chronic) leukaemia. In many cases acute leukaemia may present with normal or low WBC

Not all patients with acute leukaemia are ill at presentation

### Is it lymphoma or leukaemia? Does it matter?

Leukaemias generally involve bone marrow and blood. Lymph nodes and other organs may be involved.

Lymphomas originate in lymphoid tissue (lymph nodes, spleen), sometimes spill over into blood, may involve marrow (especially low grade lymphomas).

High grade lymphoma and acute lymphoblastic leukaemia are very similar.

Low grade lymphomas and chronic lymphoid leukaemias are similar.

## Summary of suspected haematological malignancy

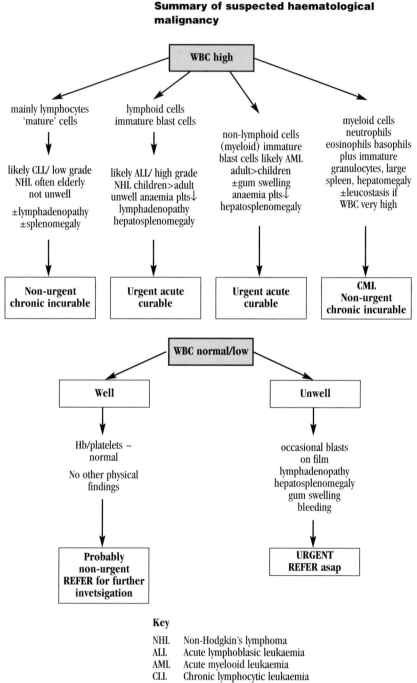

**WBC high**

**mainly lymphocytes 'mature' cells**

likely CLL/ low grade NHL often elderly not unwell

±lymphadenopathy ±splenomegaly

**Non-urgent chronic incurable**

**lymphoid cells immature blast cells**

likely ALL/ high grade NHL children>adult unwell anaemia plts↓ lymphadenopathy hepatosplenomegaly

**Urgent acute curable**

**non-lymphoid cells (myeloid) immature blast cells likely AML** adult>children ±gum swelling anaemia plts↓ hepatosplenomegaly

**Urgent acute curable**

**myeloid cells neutrophils eosinophils basophils plus immature granulocytes, large spleen, hepatomegaly** ±leucostasis if WBC very high

**CML Non-urgent chronic incurable**

**WBC normal/low**

**Well**

Hb/platelets ~ normal

No other physical findings

**Probably non-urgent REFER for further invetsigation**

**Unwell**

occasional blasts on film lymphadenopathy hepatosplenomegaly gum swelling bleeding

**URGENT REFER asap**

Key
NHL   Non-Hodgkin's lymphoma
ALL   Acute lymphoblasic leukaemia
AML   Acute myelooid leukaemia
CLL   Chronic lymphocytic leukaemia
CML   Chronic myeloid leukaemia

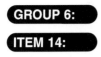

**GROUP 6:**

**ITEM 14:**

# Haematology and Oncology
# Anaemia in rheumatoid arthritis

### CASE HISTORY 1

A 53-year-old woman with rheumatoid arthritis was admitted for investigation of anaemia. Her FBC showed Hb 9.2g/dl, MCV 84 fl, WBC 11.4 x10$^9$/l and platelets 490 x10$^9$/l. Serum B12, folate and ferritin were checked and found to be normal, and the rheumatology SHO has asked for your advice regarding further investigation and management.

The problem here is that there are several possible causes for this patient's anaemia.

- Bleeding (e.g. due to NSAIDs)
  She denies obvious GI bleeding. If she had been bleeding chronically her MCV would probably be reduced (iron deficiency). This woman's MCV is normal, making chronic blood loss unlikely.

- Poor diet
  May induce folate deficiency, but we know her folate level is normal.

- Autoimmune causes
  e.g. pernicious anaemia (she has RA and may possibly have PA, another associated autoimmune disease). Her B$_{12}$ level is normal, excluding PA.

- Felty's syndrome
  RA, splenomegaly and neutropenia. This woman has no features of this disorder.

- Infiltrations, myelodysplasia (MDS)
  Difficult to exclude these in the absence of additional information e.g. bone marrow. In MDS and marrow infiltration due to e.g. carcinoma in the presence of reduced Hb it is likely (though not always the case) that the blood film would show morphological abnormalities such as red cell "tear drop" cells, nucleated red cells, hypogranular neutrophils, immature white cells. This woman's blood film simply showed RBC rouleaux.

- Renal impairment, liver disease
  Again, morphological abnormalities are usually present on the film, and biochemical screen will assess liver and renal function.

- Drug induced anaemia
  Several mechanisms, e.g. haemolysis. There are no features suggesting this. Remember the bone marrow suppressive effect of gold, penicillamine and azathioprine.

This lady's ESR was found to be > 100mm/hour with a high C-reactive protein. Her rheumatoid disease was very active (flare up) and three months prior to admission her Hb was 11.0g/dl. The drop in Hb has coincided with the flare up, a common finding especially in rheumatological patients.

A major diagnostic pitfall in the assessment of anaemia in patients with inflammatory disease is in determination of iron status. Patients may be iron deficient (confirmed by bone marrow aspirate stained for iron, the "gold standard") yet have a normal serum ferritin – an acute phase protein that rises to normal (or > normal) in such patients.

### Assessment of iron status in patients with inflammatory disorders

- Ferritin – likely to be misleading for reasons given above
- Serum iron/TIBC – may show reduction of both in chronic disease
- Bone marrow – will determine iron status, but expensive, painful and to be avoided if possible
- Serum transferrin receptor assay – number of transferrin receptors on red cells rises in iron deficiency but remains normal in secondary anaemia. This test is replacing bone marrow aspirate in diagnosis of iron deficiency in patients such as this.

This woman had normal transferrin receptor levels, confirming anaemia of chronic disease. With appropriate treatment of her RA the ESR and CRP fell and her Hb rose significantly.

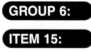

**GROUP 6:**

**ITEM 15:**

# Haematology and Oncology
# Anaemia in chronic renal failure

The kidney is the body's major site of erythropoietin (Epo) production. In renal disease Epo levels fall leading to chronic anaemia.

### Additional factors in development of anaemia in CRF are:

- Reduced RBC lifespan
- Iron deficiency (blood loss in dialysis tubing or GIT blood loss)
- Impaired iron utilisation due to aluminium in dialysis fluid
- Folate loss due to dialysis

## What features should you look for?

- ↓Hb
- Normal MCV
- Reticulocytes normal or reduced. Low Epo reduces RBC production
- Bizarre RBC shape on blood film
  - burr cells

## Management

Generally Epo replacement given at dialysis improves the Hb in these patients (50-100 units/kg 3 x per week SC). May also require additional iron and folic acid.

**GROUP 6:**

**ITEM 16:**

# Haematology and Oncology
# Anaemia in liver disease

Complex and multifactorial.

Patients with chronic liver failure generally have moderate anaemia.

| | |
|---|---|
| Hb | ↓9-10g/dl |
| MCV | normal or raised (100 – 115fl) |
| film | target cells |
| Retics | modestly elevated |
| marrow | hypercellular, erythroid hyperplasia |

## Mechanisms

- Bleeding e.g.varices
- Folate deficiency
- Haemolysis e.g. Zieve's syndrome (jaundice, hypertriglyceridaemia and haemolysis following excessive alcohol intake)
- Direct bone marrow suppression (alcohol)

## GROUP 6:
## ITEM 17:

# Haematology and Oncology
# Cancer

### CASE HISTORY 1

A 55-year-old woman who underwent a right mastectomy ten years earlier, presents with a sub-capsular fracture of the left humerus. This had followed minimal trauma following slipping on the floor in the supermarket. It was thought that she might have disseminated bony metastases.

### What contributory information does the blood count provide?

| Blood count: | | Blood film: |
|---|---|---|
| Hb | 8.6 g/dl | nucleated red cells 4/100 WBCs occasional myelocytes |
| MCV | 78 fl | noted |
| WBC | 14.7 x10⁹/l | rouleaux +platelets clumped ++ |
| platelets | 64 x10⁹/l | |
| reticulocytes | 2.0% | |

> **ⓘ**
>
> **Information**
>
> Rouleaux
>
> The tendency of red cells on the blood film to stack up like a "pile of coins" related to an increase in plasma proteins, particularly fibrinogen, as part of the acute phase response.

She has a microcytic anaemia with rouleaux formation on the blood film. The anaemia of chronic disorder is common in disseminated malignancy and many other inflammatory and infective illnesses.

### Anaemia of Chronic Disorder: pathophysiology
• Functional iron deficiency
• Reduced sensitivity to erythropoietin
• Reduced red cell lifespan

She has a raised total white cell count with nucleated red cells and immature granulocytes seen on the blood film. This is a leucoerythroblastic picture; such cells are normally confined to the bone marrow. Bone marrow infiltration by disseminated malignancy disrupts the normal mechanisms controlling the release of haemopoietic cells.

**Leucoerythroblastic Anaemia** – causes include:

• Acute haemolysis
• Severe infection
• Severe hypoxia
• Bone marrow infiltration
 – carcinoma

- myeloma
- lymphoma
- tuberculosis
- myelofibrosis
- osteopetrosis

**Remember**

Most blood count analysers cannot distinguish nRBCs from white cells, and when nucleated RBCs are present, may give an inappropriately high white cell count. Ask for the blood film to be reviewed.

**Remember**

Before accepting that a patient is thrombocytopenic
- Ask for the blood film to be reviewed
- Repeat the blood count – fibrin formation or a small clot in the sample will result in a low platelet count

The reticulocyte count is not increased and no red cell fragmentation is present on blood film review. Microangiopathic haemolytic anaemia (MAHA) which sometimes complicates disseminated breast, prostate or gastric carcinoma is not likely to be a feature in this patient. MAHA results from mechanical disruption of red cells in small blood vessels and may be complicated by chronic DIC, with a coagulopathy, reduced fibrinogen concentration, elevated fibrin breakdown products and thrombocytopenia.

The patient apparently has moderate thrombocytopenia. The aetiology of thrombocytopenia in disseminated malignancy is complex and may be due to:

- Bone marrow infiltration
- Folate deficiency secondary to anorexia
- Cytotoxic chemotherapy
- Disseminated intravascular coagulation

However, review of the blood film in this patient reveals that the thrombocytopenia is spurious – platelets are clumped on the blood film. Platelet clumping is a common phenomena related to the EDTA anticoagulant that blood is collected into.

**GROUP 6:**

**ITEM 18:**

# Haematology and Oncology
# Infection/sepsis

**Remember**

A neutrophil leukocytosis may reflect processes other than infection:
- Tissue ischaemia:
  - myocardial infarct
  - sickle cell crisis
- Inflammation:
  - rheumatoid arthritis
  - vasculitis
- Endocrine disease:
  - thyrotoxicosis
  - Cushing's disease
- Post-splenectomy

## Bacterial sepsis

This results in a characteristic constellation of changes in the blood which provide confirmatory evidence of sepsis and, in occasional patients with occult infection, may direct appropriate investigations.

- Neutrophil leukocytosis – increased numbers of neutrophils
- Immature granulocytes (= left-shift) – occasional promyelocytes, myelocytes
- Toxic granulation – coarse neutrophil granulation
- Döhle bodies (white cells containing large RNA inclusions – seen in e.g. sepsis, malignancy, pregnancy)

## Uncontrolled sepsis may be accompanied by:

- A falling white cell count/neutropenia
- Granulocyte vacuolation
- Bacteria visible on the blood stained blood film
- Thrombocytopenia
- Disseminated intravascular coagulation (DIC)

Anaemia is common in bacterial sepsis, and is usually related to the acute phase response. Occasionally haemolysis and red cell fragmentation accompanies DIC, and severe haemolysis may complicate Clostridium welchii septicaemia with spherocytosis on the blood film.

**Remember**

If malaria is suspected:
- Ask for thick and thin blood film examination
- Repeat x3-5 if the initial results are negative but clinical suspicion persists

## Malaria

This should be suspected in any individual with a fever from malarial parts of the world. Thrombocytopenia is a frequent accompaniment of malaria infection and haemolytic anaemia may develop, particularly if an individual also has G6PD deficiency.

If malaria is diagnosed:

- Ask for the species of Plasmodium
- If P. falciparum ensure you are given the parasite count, which indicates the severity of infection
  - a high parasite count > 5.0% $\Big\}$ indicate an increased
  - pre-schizont forms $\quad$ risk of cerebral malaria
- Check G6PD assay before treatment with primaquine

## Some features of severe falciparum malaria:

- **CNS**
  - Cerebral malaria (coma, convulsion)
- **Renal**
  - Haemoglobinuria (blackwater fever)
  - Oliguria
  - Uraemia (acute tubular necrosis)
- **Blood**
  - Severe anaemia (haemolysis and dyserythropoiesis)
  - Disseminated intravascular coagulation (DIC – haemorrhage)
- **Respiratory**
  - Acute respiratory distress syndrome
- **Metabolic**
  - Hypoglycaemia (particularly in children)
  - Metabolic acidosis
- **Gastrointestinal/liver**
  - Diarrhoea
  - Jaundice/Splenic rupture
- **Other**
  - Shock – hypotensive
  - Hyperpyrexia

### Beware

The parasite count in falciparum malaria may underestimate the severity of the infection due to parasite sequestration. Always take a diagnosis of falciparum malaria seriously.

### Viral infections

These produce a variety of specific and non-specific effects on the blood which may be helpful diagnostically.

Non-specific – common to many viral illnesses:

- Mild neutropenia and thrombocytopenia
- Occasional reactive lymphoid cells on blood film

Specific:

- Glandular fever is produced by Epstein Barr virus infection (see Group 1, Item 9). Similar features are seen in cytomegalovirus but also in toxoplasmosis. The reactive lymphocytosis must be distinguished from a malignant lymphoid proliferation.

### Remember

Treatment for severe malaria due to falciparum is a MEDICAL EMERGENCY.
- Give - Quinine dihydrochloride 20 mg/kg iv over four hours
  - Then 10 mg/kg.
  - See British National Formulary for details.
  See Group 1, Item 7 for other treatment

### Information

Consider
- Age of patient
- Length of history
- Clinical findings
- Morphology of lymphoid cells
- Monospot or Paul-Bunnell test
- Immunopheno typing

• Parvovirus B19 causes Fifth's disease and specifically infects erythroid progenitor cells resulting in transient erythroid hypoplasia and failure of red cell production. This is of no consequence in otherwise healthy individuals but, in those with chronic haemolytic anaemia, causes a sudden fall in the haemoglobin concentration with absent reticulocytes. Urgent blood transfusion may be life saving.

⚠

**Remember**

Parvovirus B19 is infective, and chronic haemolytic anaemias may be inherited e.g. sickle cell disease. Ask about other family members with haemolysis, "are they well?"

• HIV infection results in anaemia, thrombocytopenia and neutropenia in most patients. The severity of the cytopenia is related to the stage of the disease and is reflected by ineffective haemopoiesis with dysplastic changes in bone marrow precursor cells. It may be exacerbated by intercurrent infection and therapy.

**Anaemia in HIV**
• May respond to erythropoietin
• May be macrocytic following zidovudine

**Thrombocytopenia**
• ITP maybe the presenting manifestation of HIV infection

**Bone marrow biopsy. May be useful in the diagnosis of**
• Histoplasmosis
• Cryptococus neoformans
• Atypical mycobacteria with granuloma formation

# Notes

# Notes

**GROUP 7:**

**ITEM 1:**

# Geriatrics

# Blockout

## CASE HISTORY 1

An 86-year-old woman is brought into A&E with a blackout.

### What should you ascertain from the history?
• Any previous episodes?
• Symptoms preceding blackout
  – chest pain or palpitations, suggests cardiac cause
  – aura, suggests epilepsy

### Epilepsy in the elderly
• Focal fits or a focal origin of generalised seizures are common in the elderly
• Post ictal confusion, headache and focal signs (Todd's paresis) are common
• Fifty to 70% of fits in the elderly are caused by vascular disease
• Twenty per cent of patients with stroke have seizures within the first year
• Elderly are more susceptible to pharmacological causes of fits e.g. neuroleptics, tricyclics, or to drug or alcohol withdrawal
• An EEG can be useful, but a normal or non-diagnostic EEG does not rule out the diagnosis
• Don't forget hypoglycaemia as a cause of fits
• Antiepileptic drugs should be started after the first fit if a vascular or structural cause is suspected.
• Was there a witness?
• Pallor suggests cardiac cause
• Tonic-clonic contractions or incontinence suggests epilepsy
• Was there a history of head turning or tight neckwear – suggests carotid sinus syndrome
• Was there a period of drowsiness after blackout – suggests epilepsy but may occur in cardiac causes

### Cardiovascular causes of blackouts
• **Dysrhythmias** (brady or tachy) can be difficult to diagnose and sometimes require repeated 24 hour tapes or 2-3 week "event recorders". (See Group 10, Item 3).
• **Carotid sinus syndrome** is an underdiagnosed cause of unexplained blackouts. It is caused by an exaggerated response of baroreceptors in the carotid sinus and requires specialist investigation by carotid sinus massage with close observation. Cardioinhibitory variant is diagnosed by > 3 second asystole on massage and vasopressor variant by a 80mmHg drop in blood pressure. Up to $^{1}/_{3}$ cases are mixed.

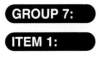

### Investigations
• FBC, U&Es, glucose, TFTs, $Ca^{2+}$
• ECG, plus consider 24 hour tape
• If history suggests epilepsy consider EEG, CT scan and carotid dopplers

### Treatment

As appropriate. In this a dysrhythmia requiring a pacemaker was found.

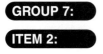

**GROUP 7:**

**ITEM 2:**

# Geriatrics
# Falls in the elderly

### CASE HISTORY 1

A 79-year-old man was brought into A&E following a fall. He had postural hypotension with dizziness. He was taking atenolol 100mg daily, aspirin 75mg daily and bendrofluazide 2.5mg daily.

### What questions should you ask?
- What does he remember about the fall?
- Did he lose consciousness?
- What happened immediately prior to the fall?
- Was there a postural element?
- Did he feel dizzy before the fall?
- Was there a witness?
- Were there physical hazards? (e.g. wet floor, carpet edge)
- Had he fallen before?

These features will help distinguish pathological causes ("Intrinsic") from those with a major external factor ("Extrinsic"), although in practice most falls are a combination of several contributing factors. Falls or "collapse" may be seen as a final common pathway for many diseases common in the elderly.

### Falls – examination
Full physical examination, especially:
- Cardiovascular
  - BP including postural changes
  - Evidence of heart failure or rhythm disturbance
- Musculoskeletal
  - Arthritis – acute or chronic
- Neurological
  - Focal signs, don't forget cerebellar/brainstem
  - Hearing or visual impairment
  - Gait

### Orthostatic hypotension
- Common in elderly – causes up to 30% of falls/syncope

### Investigations
- FBC for evidence of infection, anaemia
- U&Es, creatinine for evidence of dehydration, renal impairment
- Blood glucose for hypo/hyperglycaemia
- Thyroid function tests for subclinical hypothyroidism
- CXR for infection, tumour
- ECG for ischaemia, dysrhythmias, silent M.I.
- MSU and stix testing for infection

- "Physiological" changes in elderly – decreased baroreceptor sensitivity
- "Pathological" changes – e.g. sepsis with vasodilatation; poor L.V. function; neurological disease affecting reflex pathways
- Pharmacological causes – β blockers, vasodilators, antiparkinsonian drugs, sedatives, neuroleptics, diuretics

### Management
- Withdraw exacerbating drugs if possible
- Treat medical factors e.g. sepsis
- Advise – see below
- Plasma volume expansion e.g. fludrocortisone adrenoceptor agonist e.g. midodrine

### Advice for patients
- Get out of bed in stages
- Pause between positional changes
- Wear leg support tights during day – off at night
- Raise head of bed
- Avoid alcohol

---

**GROUP 7:**
**ITEM 3:**

# Geriatrics
# Delirium

### Information
Diagnostic and Statistical Manual (DSM) published by the American Psychiatric Association to provide clear descriptions of diagnostic categories. The 4th edition (DSM IV) was published in 1994

### CASE HISTORY 1

A 76-year-old female is admitted with a three-day history of confusion associated with hallucinations. On examination she has signs of consolidation at the left base. Her temperature and white cell count, however, were within normal limits.

An elderly person presenting with acute confusion associated with disorientation, agitation +/– hallucinations, is a common medical emergency (10 to 20%). In a hospital setting, the elderly may develop delirium whilst receiving treatment for other medical or surgical problems, the reported incidence varying from 25 to 60%.

As a condition (syndrome) it is associated with increased morbidity or mortality.

Diagnosis – use DSM (IV) criteria (see box) or the Confusional Assessment Method (CAM) based on DSM criteria.

**Remember**

- One in four may be hypoactive For diagnosis of confusion you require points one and two, and either three or four.
- While history/questioning may confirm the presence of CAM features, it may be necessary to assess the patient using mental test scores e.g. abbreviated mental test score (AMT) or mini-mental state examination (MMSE).

## Confusional assessment method (CAM) criteria

- Acute onset + fluctuating course – this is usually obtained by a history from the family/carer or from the nurse in charge of a patient already in hospital
- Inattention – is the patient easily distractible or does he or she have difficulty keeping track of what is being said?
- Disorganised thinking – is the patient incoherent? Is the conversation irrelevant?
- Altered level of consciousness – the patient may be hyperactive or lethargic or in a coma.

## What should you do when delirium is suspected/diagnosed?

Identify the cause by taking a medical history and physical examination.

### Medical history

Although illness in old age can present in a non-specific or atypical way, it is important to go through a systematic enquiry to detect symptoms of physical illness, particularly those relating to chest infection and urinary tract infection. The family/carer or GP should also be questioned about recent changes to drug therapy.

### Physical examination

Full physical examination is essential as any physical illness can lead to delirium.

For causes remember the mnemonic DELIRIUM and think of the common conditions.

**Investigations**

Should include:
- FBC
- Urea and electrolytes
- Liver function tests
- Calcium
- Phosphate
- Thyroid function tests
- Chest X-ray
- ECG and MSU

**Remember**

The presentation of illness in the old can be different, e.g. not all patients with pneumonia will have a raised temperature or raised white cell count.

### Causes

**D** Drugs – side-effects, toxicity of drugs such as hypotensives, sedatives etc.

**E** Electrolyte/endocrine disturbance e.g. hyponatraemia, hypernatraemia, hypothyroidism etc.

**L** Lack of drugs – withdrawal of drugs

**I** Infections e.g. pneumonia, cellulitis

**R** Reduced sensory input e.g. visual impairment

**I** Intracranial – TIAs, epilepsy

**U** Urinary retention/faecal impaction

**M** Myocardial – ischaemia/infarct., arrhythmias, CHF

### How would you manage a patient with delirium?

- Treat cause(s) of delirium
- Treat behavioural symptoms – if necessary using small doses of anti-psychotic agents e.g. haloperidol, thioridazine, sulpiride

• General support – fluids/nutrition; bladder/bowel care + environment (nurse in quiet, dimly lit room if possible)

**GROUP 7:**

**ITEM 4:**

# Geriatrics
# Dementia

### CASE HISTORY 1

An 89-year-old man with a six-month history of deteriorating short term memory and increasing confusion is referred to A&E because of self-neglect. He has become even more confused over the previous 24 hours. He was diagnosed as having dementia and referred to the Care of the Elderly team.

Dementia is defined by the Royal College of Physicians as global impairment of higher cortical functions, including memory, the capacity to solve problems of day-to-day living, the performance of learned perceptuomotor skills, the correct use of social skills and the control of emotional reactions in the absence of gross clouding of consciousness. The condition is often irreversible and progressive.

**Remember**

• It is important to distinguish delirium from dementia, but remember that delirium can and does occur commonly in patients with dementia, as in this case

• Incidence: this increases with age: while seven per cent of elderly over 65 years have dementia, the figure reaches 33% in those over 85 years

• Assessment: this is performed using 10 point AMT (Table 7.4.1), or mini mental state examination: MMSE (Table 7.4.2), or clock drawing test (Fig 7.4.1)

• While the screening tests are useful in demonstrating the presence of difficulties/deficits in cognition, they can not be used for diagnosis, which may require imaging (CT or MRI scan), and assessment by a clinical psychologist and/or a psychiatrist. However a history of progressive decline in memory or cognition over four months is important. Initial investigations should include FBC, U&E, random blood glucose, LFTs, TFTs, $B_{12}$, folate and syphilis serology

• Causes: while the common causes of dementia include Alzheimer's disease, multi-infarct dementia, Lewy body dementia, Creutzfeldt-Jakob disease, there are other conditions which may produce a dementia like syndrome (see table 7.4.3)

**Management**

• Alzheimer's disease – although there is no cure for Alzheimer's disease, research on an acetylcholine esterase inhibitor (e.g. donepezil) has shown that in selected patients the decline can

⚠️

**Remember**

• In all types of dementia it may be necessary to use pharmacological agents to control agitation/behaviour, but it must be remembered that patients with Lewy body dementia are very susceptible to the side effects of anti-psychotic drugs

be slowed down. Other agents/drugs that have some benefit to patients with Alzheimer's disease include vitamin E and Gingko-biloba extract

• Multi-infarct dementia – here it is important to treat the risk factors such as hypertension. Aspirin also has a role in preventing further strokes. Gingko-biloba may also help

• As dementia progresses management focus changes to care provision for patients plus support for carers

---

**Table 7.4.1 Abbreviated Mental Test (AMT)**

**Total score ten (one point for each item)**

• Age
• Time (to nearest hour)
• Address for recall
• Year
• Where do you live (town or road)?
• Recognition of two persons
• Date of birth (day and month)
• Year of start of First World War
• Name of present Monarch/Prime Minister
• Count backwards 20-1

**Table 7.4.2**

**Mini Mental State Examination (MMSE)**

**Orientation** – one point for each correct answer

*What is the:*
  time
  date
  day
  month
  year                                                                          **5 points**

*What is the name of this:*
  ward
  hospital
  district
  town
  country                                                                       **5 points**

**Registration**
  Name three objects
  Score one, two or three points according to how many are repeated
  Resubmit list until patient word perfect
  In order to use this for a later test of recall score only first attempt        **3 points**

**Attention and calculation**
  Have the patient subtract seven from 100 and then from the result a total of five times
  Score one point for each correct subtraction                                   **5 points**

**Recall**
  Ask for three objects used in the registration test, one point being awarded
  for each correct answer                                                        **3 points**

**Language**
  one point each for two objects correctly named (pencil and watch)              **2 points**
  one point for correct repetition of 'No, ifs, ands and buts'                   **1 point**
  three points if three-stage commands correctly obeyed                          **3 points**
      'Take this piece of paper in your right hand, fold it in half, and place it on the floor'
  one point for correct response to a written command such as 'close your eyes'  **1 point**
  Have the patient write a sentence. Award one point if the sentence is meaningful,
  has a verb and a subject                                                       **1 point**
  Test the patient's ability to copy a complex diagram of two intersected pentagons  **1 point**
                                                                    **Total Score  30**

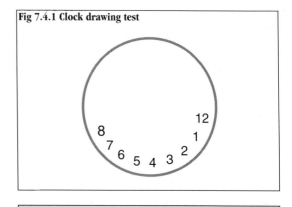

Fig 7.4.1 Clock drawing test

Table 7.4.3
**Examples of treatable causes of dementia-like syndrome**
Hypothyroidism
$B_{12}$ deficiency
Folate deficiency
Hypoglycaemia
Alcohol
Depression ("pseudo dementia")
Subdural haematoma
Normal pressure hydrocephalus

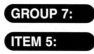 **GROUP 7:**

 **ITEM 5:**

# Geriatrics
# Depression

**Remember**
While the clinical features of depression in old age can be the same as in younger patients, somatic complaints, delusions, decline in cognition ("pseudo dementia") are more frequently noted in the elderly.

*(see also Group 16, Item 5)*

Depression as a condition is common in old age. Community studies have revealed a prevalence of 11.3% for depressive symptoms and three per cent for depression. Studies of elderly inpatients have shown that up to 33% have depression. It is common in the elderly with physical illness such as stroke, and may also be triggered by occult physical illness such as hypothyroidism, hypercalcaemia or carcinoma of lung.

## CASE HISTORY 1

A staff nurse noted that an 83-year-old man with a CVA is not eating well and losing weight. On direct questioning the patient admits to feeling depressed.

**Remember**
Ask patient about suicidal
thoughts/intent

## Assessment

• Geriatric depression scale (see box) as screening test
• Physical examination and investigations to detect/exclude physical causes of depression such as hypothyroidism, hypercalcaemia, malignancy etc. In a patient with a normal physical examination it is recommended that FBC, U&E, LFTs, $B_{12}$, Ca, $PO_4$, TFTs and chest X-ray are ordered

---

**Geriatric Depression Scale** – shorter version – is a reliable and valid screening instrument of depression in the elderly. A score greater than five indicates probable depression.
Choose the best answer for how you have felt over the past week:

| | |
|---|---|
| 1. Are you basically satisfied with your life? | YES/NO |
| 2. Have you dropped many of your activities and interests? | YES/NO |
| 3. Do you feel that your life is empty? | YES/NO |
| 4. Do you often get bored? | YES/NO |
| 5. Are you in good spirits most of the time? | YES/NO |
| 6. Are you afraid that something bad is going to happen to you? | YES/NO |
| 7. Do you feel happy most of the time? | YES/NO |
| 8. Do you often feel helpless? | YES/NO |
| 9. Do you prefer to stay at home, rather than going out and doing new things? | YES/NO |
| 10. Do you feel you have more problems with memory than most? | YES/NO |
| 11. Do you think it is wonderful to be alive now? | YES/NO |
| 12. Do you feel pretty worthless the way you are now? | YES/NO |
| 13. Do you feel full of energy? | YES/NO |
| 14. Do you feel that your situation is hopeless? | YES/NO |
| 15. Do you think that most people are better off than you are? | YES/NO |

The following answers **count one point**
Scores greater than five indicate probable depression

1. NO
2. YES
3. YES
4. YES
5. NO
6. YES
7. NO
8. YES
9. YES
10. YES
11. NO
12. YES
13. NO
14. YES
15. YES

Ref: Sheikh, J.I. and Yesavage, J.A. (1986) Geriatric Depression Scale (GDS); Recent evidence and development of a shorter version. Clinical Gerontologist 5: 165-173

## Management

Mild to moderately depressed patients can be treated successfully with selective serotonin reuptake inhibitors (SSRIs), tetracyclic or tricyclic antidepressants

Severely depressed patients with or without suicidal thoughts will require urgent referral to a psychiatrist for assessment

# Geriatrics

# Non-specific presentation of illness in the elderly

History should be obtained from patient, GP, district nurse, carers, relations and neighbours if necessary.

Many illnesses in the elderly population can present in a non-specific fashion. Taking a detailed and informative history can be very difficult. This could be the result of underlying memory loss that is exacerbated by an acute medical problem. Therefore, more information regarding the previous medical, mental, functional and social conditions should be obtained from the family doctor, district nurse, carers, relatives and neighbours, if necessary, to make an accurate assessment of the patient's current state.

These problems are highlighted in the following case.

## CASE HISTORY 1

Mr "S" is an 85-year-old who lived alone in a bungalow. It was noted by the neighbours that he failed to collect the milk from the front door for two days.

The family doctor was called in. He found the patient sitting in a chair with grossly swollen feet. In his letter referring the patient to hospital he confirmed that Mr "S" had been on salbutamol and ipratropium inhalers for a few years. He hadn't visited the surgery for sometime however.

On arrival in hospital he looked very confused and was unable to give a detailed history. His abbreviated mental test (AMT) score (table 7.4.1) was very low – three out of ten. He had a low grade temperature of 37.6°C, appeared breathless on minimal exertion, with a tinge of cyanosis and signs of gross heart failure; high JVP, an enlarged liver and leg swelling up to the groin. A chest X-ray showed signs of heart failure and there was right basal shadowing suggestive of chest infection.

It was not clear how long he had been confused for, nor the extent of his mobility before this problem.

His next of kin was a younger brother who lived far away. He was contacted by telephone and confirmed that the patient was not married and had been able to go out to the local shops a quarter of a mile away until three weeks ago. He also commented that the patient was mildly confused and needed some help in running his own affairs, but was self caring and didn't need much help at home.

Mr "S" was started on antibiotics and anti-heart failure measures. His general condition gradually improved and his AMT went up to seven out of ten.

With the help of the physiotherapist he was able to get back on his feet using a Zimmer frame. A home visit was successful and he went home with social support and follow up in the day hospital, to maintain his mobility.

**Remember**

It is important that an elderly person presenting to hospital with non-specific complaints has a full physical examination and investigations that include FBC, U&E, LFTs, Ca, phosphate, TFTs, ECG, MSU, chest X-ray and any other investigations as indicated by the findings on examination

## CASE HISTORY 2

An 89-year-old man was admitted after having had an unexplained fall. He was mildly confused but following direct questioning denied having any symptoms. On examination he had a tachycardia of 100/min, normal heart sounds and fine crackles at both bases. An ECG revealed raised ST segment in leads II, III and AVF, i.e. an inferior myocardial infarct.

- Illness in old age may present with any of the so-called 'giants' of geriatric medicine i.e. confusion, falls/instability and incontinence (see Group 7, Items 2, 3, 4 and 13)
- In addition, some illnesses present atypically. Examples of these include:
  – 'Silent' myocardial infarction (as illustrated by the case above)
  – Pneumonia without pyrexia
  – Pneumonia with no rise in white cell count
  – 'Silent' peptic ulcer perforation i.e. peptic ulcers may perforate with little or no pain

**GROUP 7:**

**ITEM 7:**

# Geriatrics
# Appropriate assessment scales

The Royal College of Physicians has already produced a list of useful assessment scales/tools for the day to day management of the elderly.

The following scales are recommended:

1. Barthel score for ADL (Activities of Daily Living Table 7.7.1).
2. Mini Mental State Examination – screening mental test for dementia and delirium (see Table 7.4.2).
3. Geriatric Depression Scale – screening test for depression (Group 7 item 5)
4. Waterlow Score – for risk quantification for pressure sores (Table 7.7.2)
5. Philadelphia Geriatric Morale Scale – for quality of life (Table 7.7.3)
6. Norton scale (Table 7.7.4)

---

**Table 7.7.1 – The Barthel Index**

| Item | Categories |
|------|-----------|
| **Bowels** | 0 = incontinent (or needs to be given an enema) |
| | 1 = occasional accident (once per week) |
| | 2 = continent |
| **Bladder** | 0 = incontinent/catheterized, unable to manage |
| | 1 = occasional accident (max once every 24 hr) |
| | 2 = continent (for over 7 days) |
| **Grooming** | 0 = needs help with personal care |
| | 1 = independent face/hair/teeth/shaving (implements provided) |
| **Toilet use** | 0 = dependent |
| | 1 = needs some help but can do something alone |
| | 2 = independent (on and off, dressing, wiping) |
| **Feeding** | 0 = unable |
| | 1 = needs help cutting, spreading butter etc |
| | 2 = independent (food provided in reach) |

| Item | Categories |
|------|-----------|
| **Transfer** | 0 = unable - no sitting balance |
| | 1 = major help (one or two people, physical), can sit |
| | 2 = minor help (verbal or physical) |
| | 3 = independent |
| **Mobility** | 0 = immobile |
| | 1 = wheelchair independent (includes corners) |
| | 2 = walks with help of one (verbal/physical) |
| | 3 = independent (may use any aid eg stick) |
| **Dressing** | 0 = dependent |
| | 1 = needs help, does about half unaided |
| | 2 = independent, includes buttons, zips, shoes |
| **Stairs** | 0 = unable |
| | 1 = needs help, (verbal, physical) carrying aid |
| | 2 = independent |
| **Bathing** | 0 = dependent |
| | 1 = independent (may use shower) |

The Barthel index should be used as a record of what a patient does, not as a record of what he could do. The main aim is to establish the degree of independence from any help, physical or verbal, however minor and for whatever reason. The need for supervision means the patient is not independent. Performance over the preceding 24 to 48 hours is important but longer periods are relevant. A patient's performance should be established using the best available evidence. Ask the patient or carer but also observe what the patient can do. Direct testing is not needed. Unconscious patients score '0' throughout. Middle categories imply that the patient supplies over 50% effort. Use of aids to be independent is allowed.

**Table 7.7.2 – Waterlow Pressure Sore Risk Assessment**

| Build/weight for height | | Visual skin type | | Continence | | Mobility | | Sex Age | | Appetite | |
|---|---|---|---|---|---|---|---|---|---|---|---|
| Average | 0 | Healthy | 0 | Complete | 0 | Fully mobile | 0 | Male | 1 | Average | 0 |
| Above average | 2 | Tissue paper | 1 | Occasionally | 1 | Restricted/ | 1 | Female | 2 | Poor | 1 |
| | | Dry | 1 | incontinent | | Difficult | | 14–18 | 1 | Anoretic | 2 |
| Below average | 3 | Oedematous | 1 | Catheter/ | 2 | Restless | 2 | 50–64 | 2 | | |
| | | Clammy | 1 | incontinent | | fidgety | | 65–75 | 3 | | |
| | | Discoloured | 2 | of faeces | | Apathetic | 3 | 75–80 | 4 | | |
| | | Broken/spot | 3 | Doubly incontinent | 3 | Inert/traction | 4 | 81+ | 5 | | |

| Special risk factors | | Assessment value | |
|---|---|---|---|
| 1. Poor nutrition eg terminal cachexia | 8 | At risk | 10 |
| 2. Sensory deprivation eg diabetes, paraplegia, cerebrovascular, accident | 6 | High risk | 15 |
| 3. High dose anti-inflammatory or steroids in use | 3 | Very high risk | 20 |
| 4. Smoking 10+ per day | 1 | | |
| 5. Orthopaedic surgery/fracture below waist | 3 | | |

**Table 7.7.3 The Philadelphia Geriatric Centre Morale Scale** – provides a multi-dimensional approach to assessing the psychological state of older people, ie well-being/life satisfaction/quality of life.

|  | High morale response | Low morale response |
|---|---|---|
| Do little things bother you more this year? | No | Yes |
| Do you sometimes worry so much that you canít sleep | No | Yes |
| Are you afraid of a lot of things? | No | Yes |
| Do you get mad more than you used to? | No | Yes |
| Do you take things hard? | No | Yes |
| Do you get upset easily? | No | Yes |
| Do things keep getting worse as you get older | No | Yes |
| Do you have as much pep as you had last year? | Yes | No |
| Do you feel that as you get older you are less useful? | No | Yes |
| As you get older, are things............than you thought? | Better | Worse or same |
| Are you as happy now as you were when you were younger? | Yes | No |
| How much do you feel lonely? | Not much | A lot |
| Do you see enough of your friends and relatives? | Yes | No |
| Do you sometimes feel that life isnít worth living? | No | Yes |
| Do you have a lot to be sad about? | No | Yes |
| Is life hard much of the time? | No | Yes |
| How satisfied are you with your life today? | Satisfied | Not satisfied |

Ref: Lawton, MP (1975) the Philadelphia Geriatric Centre Morale Scale: a revision. Journal of Gerontology, 30:85 -89

References
Report of a joint workshop with the Royal College of Physicians and the British Geriatrics Society. Standardised assessment scales for elderly people. Royal College of Physicians. London 1992

**Table 7.7.4 – Norton Scale for Pressure Sores**

| Physical | | Neural | | Activity | | Mobility | | Incontinence | |
|---|---|---|---|---|---|---|---|---|---|
| 4 | Good | 4 | Alert | 4 | Ambulant | 4 | Full | 4 | None |
| 3 | Fair | 3 | Apathetic | 3 | Walks with help | 3 | Slightly | 3 | Occasionally |
| 2 | Poor | 2 | Confused | 2 | Not bound | 2 | Limited | 2 | Usually |
| 1 | Very poor | 1 | Stupor | 1 | Bedfast | 1 | Very limited Immobile | 1 | Double |

Norton scale for pressure sores. Low scores carry a high risk.

**GROUP 7:**

**ITEM 8:**

# Geriatrics
# Stroke

**Information**

Each year in England about 100,000 (1.6-2 per 1000) people have a first stroke. Stroke is the commonest cause of severe disability in adult life. There are 64,000 deaths attributed to first or recurrent strokes which makes it the third commonest cause of death in the UK.

## CASE HISTORY

A 78-year-old man presents with reduced conscious level, weakness of the right arm and leg and unable to speak. His daughter thinks that he has had a stroke.

Definition of Stroke: Rapidly developing clinical signs of focal or global disturbance of cerebral function, with symptoms lasting 24 hours or longer, or leading to death, with no apparent cause other than of vascular origin.

### The questions you need to address are:

• Is it a stroke?
• What sort of a stroke?
• What part of the brain is affected?
• What is the prognosis?
• Are there complications to treat or prevent?

### Pathology

• 80 to 90% Ischaemic – due to thrombosis and embolism
• 10 to 20% Primary cerebral haemorrhage or aneurysm rupture

### Common sources of emboli

• Carotid artery and aortic arch atheroma
• Intracardiac sources, e.g. left atrium in AF, left ventricle mural thrombus
• Vertebral artery

### Uncommon causes of thrombosis

• Giant cell arteritis
• Vasculitides
• Haematological disorders, e.g. polycythaemia vera, hyperviscosity syndrome

## Typical signs of a stroke

| | |
|---|---|
| **Motor** | • Impaired sitting/balance |
| | • Hemiparesis |
| | • Monoparesis |
| | • Gait disturbance |
| | • Facial palsy |
| **Speech** | • Dysarthria |
| | • Dysphasia |
| |   - receptive |
| |   - expressive |
| **Swallow** | • Loss or impaired swallow |
| **Perceptual** | • Neglect |
| | • Sensory inattention |
| | • Visual field loss |
| | • Dyspraxia |

## Features of a stroke involving the brainstem

- Hemiplegia/Quadriplegia
- Ataxia/Vertigo/Tinnitus
- Dysphagia
- Dysarthria
- Gaze paresis
- Temperature control disturbance
- Altered respiratory pattern

## Is your diagnosis of a stroke correct?

Most strokes are easily diagnosed but errors do occur. Not all neurological impairments are due to stroke and other conditions may be misdiagnosed as stroke.

Unusual symptoms and signs should make you question the diagnosis, e.g.:

- Papilloedema
- Persisting headache
- Fluctuating signs
- Unexplained fever

## Examples of misdiagnosis

- Space occupying lesions:
  - primary tumours, metastases
  - subdural haematoma
- Infections – Acute confusional states due to:
  - systemic infections
  - meningitis
- Metabolic disturbance:
  - hypo/hyperglycaemia
  - hypo/hypernatraemia

– renal failure
• Intoxication/overdose:
  – alcohol
  – drugs – sedatives, tricyclics etc.
• Hypotension:
  – hypovolaemia
  – cardiac dysrhythmia
  – cardiogenic shock
• Old neurological deficits e.g. previous stroke:
  – Todd's paresis in epilepsy

**Remember**

The specific symptoms and signs detected will depend on site of lesion. Seventy-five per cent of strokes occur in middle cerebral artery territory. Fifteen per cent in the vertebro-basilar territory.

### How would you investigate?

CT scanning should be performed early in the course of a stroke so that appropriate treatment can be commenced i.e. aspirin. If CT scan is performed in first 24 hours it may appear normal, in cases with an infarct.

### Risk factors for stroke

• Smoking
• Hypertension
• IHD
• Peripheral Vasular disease
• Diabetes
• AF
• Hypercholesterolaemia

### Clinical problems and assessment

a) The neurological deficit:
  – motor deficit
  – conscious level
  – speech

**Investigations**

• FBCs, U&Es, BS, ESR
• ECG
• CXR
• CT or MRI Scan

b) Dysphagia and aspiration occur in up to 50% of patients at presentation. The ability to swallow should be tested by asking the patient to swallow a sip of water, not by putting a spatula in their throat.

If the patient's conscious level is impaired do not assess the swallow until it improves.

c) The condition of the skin:
  – are there any pressure sores?
  – are there any areas of skin at risk?

d) Bladder function:
  – incontinence can result from neurological problems or immobility
  – catheterisation is required if there is a risk of pressure sores

## How would you manage the patient?

The important aspects of management are:

- Hydration and/or feeding
- Prevention of complications
  - chest infection
  - DVT
  - pressure sores
  - contractures
- Rapid treatment of infection
- Aspirin/anticoagulation after CT scanning (to rule out haemorrhage)
- Hypertension – if persistent treat (Group 10 Item 20)
- Communicate with the patient and family: stroke is a major life event and both the patient and family need information

### Further management

- Physiotherapy
- Occupational therapy
- Speech and Language Therapist
- Continuing medical review

**Remember**

Poor prognostic signs in stroke are:

- Reduced conscious level
- Gaze paresis
- Early and persisting incontinence
- Sensory inattention
- Pre-existing disability
- Previous cognitive impairment

**GROUP 7:**

**ITEM 9:**

# Geriatrics

# Heart disease in the elderly

## CASE HISTORY

A 78-year-old man with long-standing atrial fibrillation was admitted with tiredness. Examination revealed a pulse of 96 (apical rate 110) in AF, a raised JVP, swollen ankles and crackles up to both mid zones. He suffered from dyspepsia and recent falls. He was taking digoxin 125μg daily and aspirin 75mg daily. ECG showed AF with poor R wave progression, CXR showed pulmonary oedema, and blood tests showed a microcytic anaemia, haemoglobin 9.8, MCV 70fl.

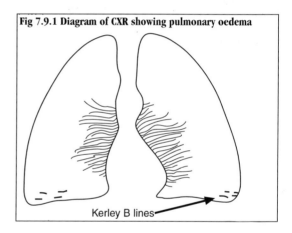

**Fig 7.9.1 Diagram of CXR showing pulmonary oedema**

Kerley B lines

- Cardiac failure in the elderly may present with non-specific symptoms such as tiredness and falls
- Benefits have been shown for anticoagulation of elderly patients in AF up to age 85, but care should be taken as the contraindications (such as falls or gastrointestinal haemorrhage) are more common in this population. In this case microcytic anaemia would need to be investigated before starting warfarin
- Risks of anticoagulation in the over 85s are high and no study has shown a benefit in this age group
- ACE inhibitors should be used with care in the elderly, and renal function closely observed due to increased risk of renal impairment. (Group 9, Item 4)

### Acute MI

The management principles of heart disease in the elderly are the same as those in young people with a few important exceptions:

Age alone is not a contraindication to thrombolysis in acute MI, in fact the greatest benefits are seen in older patients. However, other co-morbidities causing contraindications are more common in older people.

Acute MI may present silently (with no pain) more commonly in the elderly. (see Group 10, Item 6).

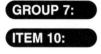

**GROUP 7:**

**ITEM 10:**

# Geriatrics
# Transient ischaemic attack

### CASE HISTORY

A 68-year-old man presents with weakness of the right arm and leg, expressive dysphasia and a facial palsy.

While being examined his symptoms and signs improve and have resolved when he returns from the X-Ray department. A diagnosis of a transient ischaemic attack (TIA) was made.

By definition this means the resolution of neurological symptoms within 24 hours.

### What are the important points to chart in the history?
• Previous similar episodes, especially recently
• Previous episodes of amaurosis fugax (sudden transient loss of vision in one eye)
• History of palpitations, hypertension, diabetes or high cholesterol
• Smoking
• Current and previous medication

### What are the important aspects of the examination?
• The neurological deficit
• BP
• Pulse rate and rhythm
• Presence of cardiac murmurs, carotid bruits
• Papilloedema, visual field deficit

**Investigations**
• FBC, ESR
• U&Es, BS, Cholesterol
• ECG / 24 hour tape
• CXR
• CT head
• Echo cardiogram in patients with suspected valvular disease or mural thrombus
• Carotid dopplers

Depending on the findings on examination and basic investigations, the CT, Echo and carotid dopplers could be performed as an outpatient.

### Should you admit this patient?

Reasons for admission:

- Doubt over diagnosis e.g. need to exclude space occupying lesion
- Multiple TIAs in short time – if appropriate these patients should be fast tracked to carotid endarterectomy
- Identification of pathology requiring intervention e.g. cardiac arrhythmia
- Background disability with poor social circumstances

### How would you manage a case of TIA?

Aspirin 75mg a day

- Anticoagulation with warfarin is used with atrial fibrillation.
- Treatment of risk factors e.g. hypertension, hypercholesterolaemia
- Advice to give up smoking
- Advice not to drive for one month following the event
- Follow up arrangements (Referral to appropriate consultant)
- Consider carotid endarterectomy

### Further Management – Carotid Endarterectomy (See also Group 15 Item 5)

Carotid endarterectomy is a treatment option for patients with TIAs and minor strokes who have 70% – 90% stenosis of the appropriate carotid artery and who are otherwise fit, with no major persisting disability.

Carotid artery angiography or MRI angiography is required prior to surgery. The former carries a small but distinct risk of inducing a stroke. Carotid endarterectomy has a 1 to 2% perioperative stroke risk in the most experienced hands but reduces the incidence of stroke by 75% over the next two to three years.

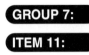

**GROUP 7:**

**ITEM 11:**

# Geriatrics
# Hypothermia

## CASE HISTORY

An 89-year-old female is found lying on the floor by her home help. On arrival at the A&E department she is noted to be confused and have a rectal temperature of 34°C.

### Information

Hypothermia is defined as core body temperature of <35°C. It is associated with some clinical conditions, but in most patients aetiology is multifactorial.

## Aetiological factors

- Exposure to cold
- Impaired thermoregulation
- Impaired shivering thermogenesis
- Low metabolic heat production
- Impaired temperature perception
- Drugs e.g. phenothiazines, hypnotics, alcohol
- Disease

## Clinical features

These vary with degree of hypothermia. While those with core temperature of 33° to 34°C may be confused and have slow cerebration, those with temperature of 30°C may be drowsy and have muscular stiffness.

Some patients with hypothermia may have features such as slow relaxing reflexes suggestive of hypothyroidism.

Electrocardiograph may show changes such as sinus bradycardia, slow AF, prolonged PR interval, 'J' waves (commonly seen in leads V3 – V4).

Complications of hypothermia include pancreatitis, oliguria, cardiac arrhythmias (particularly during re-warming) and aspiration pneumonia.

### Investigations

- Full blood count
- urea and electrolytes
- glucose
- amylase
- blood gases
- ECG
- chest x-ray
- thyroid function tests

(for measurement when the laboratory opens)

## How would you manage this patient?

- Nurse with space blanket in a warm room (allow temperature to rise by 0.5°C/hour)
- oxygen – remember that patients with COPD may require 24% oxygen.
- I.V. fluids (through blood warmer).
- Hypothyroidism, if present, should be treated with triiodothyronine 10µg IV 8 hourly.

A **severe hypothermic patient** will require admission to ITU and may require positive pressure ventilation, CVP line and ECG monitoring.

# Geriatrics
# Pressure sores

## CASE HISTORY

A 78-year-old lady with a residual right hemiplegia was brought to A&E having fallen at home. She had been on the floor for at least 24 hours as she was unable to get up. On examination a dusky area was apparent over the right hip overlying the greater trochanter which subsequently developed into a pressure sore.

Pressure sores are common. Ill elderly people are most at risk of developing pressure sores. The reported prevalence rates vary widely – on average five to 10% of this group.

### Other patients at special risk include those:

• Undergoing surgery particularly orthopaedic surgery
• With neurological disease
• With spinal cord injury including cord compression
• Having palliative care

### Why do pressure sores occur?

Pressure greater than the mean capillary pressure (25-32 mmHg) will occlude blood vessels and lead to anoxia of the skin. Hard surfaces can generate pressures greater than 100mmHg, therefore the damage to the skin results from the pressure applied and the length of time exposed to the pressure. In addition to pressure, shearing force is another significant factor.

Pressure sores can be graded into superficial (Grades 1-2) and deep (Grades 3-4).

### Risk factors for developing pressure sores

• Low body weight/excessive body weight
• Poor nutritional state
• Motor deficit/immobility
• Sensory deficit
• Presence of intercurrent illness
• Incontinence – bladder/bowel
• Use of some medication e.g. long term prednisolone

### Clinical Assessment

It is important to document pressure sores fully:
– the site, size and grade of pressure sore
– the condition of the surrounding skin
– the presence/absence of infection

**Remember**

Pressure sores are preventable. Litigation may arise following the development of pressure sores. "At risk" patients require immediate assessment of their pressure areas and appropriate management

### Investigations

- FBC – presence of anaemia will delay wound healing
- Albumin – marker of nutrition, low albumin will delay wound healing
- Blood sugar-diabetes delays healing
- Wound swabs for culture and sensitivity
- Blood cultures if appropriate
- If the wound is deep, overlies a bony prominence and has been present for sometime x-ray of the underlying bone should be performed to rule out osteomyelitis

### Remember

- Pressure sores can develop in one to two hours
- Beware leaving patients on hard A&E trolleys or X-ray tables for too long

General examination of the patient with special regard to:
- nutritional state including body weight
- full neurological examination
- abdominal examination, especially bladder and bowel

### How would you investigate?

Investigations will be directed by the physical examination, but special attention should be paid to those *in box*.

### How would you manage pressure sores?

Prevention is definitely better than cure.

- Relief of pressure with appropriate support mattress and/or cushion for chair:
- Low risk – a soft overlay to the mattress may be adequate
- High risk – an alternating pressure support system e.g. Pegasus air overlay/mattress, Nimbus mattress
- Appropriate dressings for wounds:
- Dry dressings should not be used on moist wounds. Examples of dressings include,
  - hydrocolloid for superficial granulating wounds
  - alginates for exuding or bleeding wounds
- Treatment of infection when present with appropriate systemic antibiotics

- General management of the patient
  a) Pain relief
  b) Treatment of medical conditions including anaemia
  c) Review of drug treatment, e.g. NSAIDs and steroids delay wound healing
  d) Review of nutrition – consider use of supplements including vitamin C and zinc
- Severe pressure sores may occasionally require debridement and skin grafting by plastic surgeons

Most hospitals now have tissue viability specialist nurses to advice on prevention and treatment of pressures sores. For quantification of risk, nurses may use the Waterlow score or Norton Scale (see Group 7, Item 7).

**GROUP 7:**

**ITEM 13:**

# Geriatrics
# Urinary tract infection and incontinence

### CASE HISTORY

An 80-year-old woman with mild dementia presented with increasing confusion and drowsiness. She had a three-day history of urinary incontinence and diarrhoea. She was taking Coproxamol for arthritis.

Examination revealed constipation with impaction and overflow, and a post void residual volume of 300mls. The urine was offensive smelling and positive to stix testing for nitrites, leucocytes, blood and protein.

### Particular points to note in the history

- Urinary tract infection in the elderly may present with non-specific symptoms such as confusion, drowsiness or falls
- Recurrent UTIs should be investigated (> 3 in a woman, > 1 in a man) with imaging of the kidneys and urinary tracts
- New urge incontinence may be precipitated by infection leading to unstable bladder
- Infection may be precipitated by obstruction – must commonly caused by constipation
- Drug history for precipitating causes – drugs causing constipation, diuretics, sedatives

### Examination of this patient should include:

- Physical examination for other coexisting causes of dementia, e.g. chest infection
- Rectal examination-important for constipation/overflow/prostate in men
- Neurological examination e.g. for old CVA

### What investigations would you perform?

- Stix testing positivity for both leucocytes and nitrites is highly specific and sensitive for infection-blood and protein stix are much less useful
- Bacteriuria without symptoms (urgency, frequency, dysuria or systemic symptoms) should not be treated
- In-Out catheterisation may be useful for obtaining specimens or assessing residual volumes but catheterisation should not be used as a treatment for incontinence
- FBC; blood cultures for evidence of infection
- U&Es, creatinine for evidence of renal impairment or dehydration
- AXR for evidence of constipation

• Consider further referral for incontinence if it doesn't settle on treatment of infection

### How would you treat?

• Treat infection with oral antibiotics
• Trimethoprim 200mg x2 daily is a good first line treatment. Only use parenteral antibiotics if very ill or vomiting
• Treat constipation – enemas and laxatives (see Group 4, Item 5). Repeat residual volumes as constipation is treated

This patient's constipation was due to the dextropropoxyphene in Coproxamol.

## Geriatrics
## Elements of provisional discharge plan

### CASE HISTORY

An 82-year-old widower was admitted with left sided temporal headache of three-days' duration. He is known to have IDDM, visual impairment, hypertension and a left hemiparesis. He lives alone in a house and has one son who lives far away.

### Medical Assessment

Detailed physical examination was performed. The left temporal and carotid arteries were pulsatile but tender. The investigations revealed a significantly elevated ESR. A clinical diagnosis of Temporal Arteritis (Group 8 item 7) was made. His response to steroids was very good.

### How would you organise his discharge?

The patient needs a multidisciplinary assessment before his discharge to ensure his safety. His son should also be contacted.

### General points for Discharge Planning

Discharge planning of an elderly person should start as early as possible after admission. Once the elderly person's medical problems have been accurately diagnosed and treated his potential for returning home should be assessed by a multidisciplinary team (MDT) of professionals taking into account the elderly person's views.

⚠️

**Remember**

A competent adult has a right to decide where he or she wishes to go home even if this decision is against the advice offered by some member/s of the MDT.

The assessment by MDT includes:

- Assessment by a physiotherapist to assess his/her mobility, transfers and ability to climb stairs
- Assessment by an occupational therapist to assess activities of daily living, kitchen assessment and/or a home visit
- Social work assessment that will take into account the assessments of other professionals to quantify his/her needs and care package to meet the identified needs of the individual
- Assessment by a speech and language therapist, dietician or a psychologist in some cases
- Referral to a district nurse for e.g. treatment of leg ulcers, monitoring of diabetic control
- Discussion with GP
- Following discharge it may be possible to continue further rehabilitation or monitoring of medical or nursing care in day hospital setting.

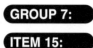

## Geriatrics

## Options for elderly patients who cannot return home

One of the aims of physicians looking after older people is to help them return to their own home after they have completed medical treatment including rehabilitation.

However, there are circumstances when it may be considered unsafe for an elderly person to return home from hospital (because he/she has made limited recovery) or after attendance at the accident and emergency department.

Under these circumstances it is important that the elderly person has full medical/functional and social assessment from all appropriate professionals that will allow the quantifying and meeting of his/her needs.

### An elderly person presenting A&E department who has:

- No clinical evidence of active medical problems and is able to walk and transfer independently, can be discharged home with same or increased support from community social services arranged via a social worker

- No clinical evidence of active medical problems but has functional problems – if these problems are known and supports are available in the community (this may require confirmation by contacting GP/carer or patient's social worker) he/she too can be returned home with same services. If these services are not in place, then duty social worker should be contacted and asked to assess the patient's needs and arrange services. If these cannot be arranged quickly it may be possible for the social worker to arrange temporary placement in a residential home. All this will require close liaison with social worker and carers/family if available.

### Elderly person in hospital who has not made a full recovery

This person's future placement will depend on findings of a multi-disciplinary team assessment. Most elderly can be cared for in their home and a care package arranged by social services with input from community health care workers such as district nurses. If it is not possible to provide the care at home then the options are:

- Residential home – suitable for someone who requires some help (usually from one person) with basic activities of daily living. They may be incontinent of urine but not incontinent of faeces

- Nursing home – suitable for someone who is more dependent, usually requiring help of two to transfer and may be doubly incontinent of urine and faeces
- Continuing care in hospital – this is suitable for minority of heavily dependent persons who have medical and/or nursing needs that require specialist care
- Home for elderly mentally ill – some private nursing homes may have some beds set aside for elderly who are very confused and have behavioural problems.
- In addition some districts may have beds within the department of mental health care of old people for severely impaired elderly. Need for such a facility will be determined by assessment by a psychiatrist in mental health care of older people

**Remember**

Admission criteria for residential home, nursing home or continuing care facility may vary from district to district.

---

**GROUP 7:**

**ITEM 16:**

# Geriatrics
# Acute hot joint

### CASE HISTORY

An 80-year-old man presents with a hot, painful, swollen knee joint.

### What are the possible causes?

- Acute gout (see Group 8, Item 6)
- Pseudo-gout (Pyrophosphate arthropathy) (see Group 8, Item 6)
- Septic arthritis (see Group 8, Item 11)
- Acute flare up of chronic arthritis e.g. rheumatoid arthritis (see Group 8, Item 2)
- Traumatic haemarthrosis with fracture of patella or tibial plateau
- Ruptured Baker's cyst in osteoarthritis (see Group 8, Item 1)

### Particular points you should elicit in the history?

- Trauma or injury – entry for infection
- Drug history – particularly diuretics
- Known arthritis or previous episodes e.g. of gout

### On examination you should look for:

- Temperature, pulse – systemic signs of infection
- Evidence of trauma

• Gouty tophi

• Other joint disease, including evidence of RA or OA (Heberdens/Bouchard's nodes)

### Investigations

• X-ray joint
• Tap joint under sterile conditions – fluid for culture, crystal detection and cell count
• Blood cultures
• FBC for WCC and ESR
• Serum uric acid
• Rheumatoid factor and auto antibody screen if appropriate

Joint fluid should be examined under polarised light. Urate crystals are distinguished by being negatively birefringent needles. Calcium pyrophosphate are weakly positively birefringent rhomboidal crystals.

### How would you manage this patient?

• Immobilise joint – plaster cast if appropriate for fracture
• Adequate analgesia
• Prophylaxis for DVT – low molecular weight heparin, e.g. enoxaparin 20mg a day if the patient is immobile.

• If *septic arthritis* is suspected, treatment should be started immediately as untreated septic arthritis has a high mortality in elderly people:
 – Benzyl penicillin 1.2g four times daily with flucloxacillin 500mg four times daily or Cefuroxime 750mg three times daily

• *Gout* – there are three acute options:
 – An NSAID – e.g. diclofenac with misoprostol one tablet three times daily
 – Colchicine – 1mg initially, 0.5mg every 2 hours until attack subsides or 0.5mg x 2 daily for 5 days if symptoms are not severe
 – Corticosteroids: intrarticular injection with methylprednislone 40mg
 Allopurinol should not be used acutely but only prophylactically to prevent further attacks of gout and started at least 6 weeks after the acute attack has settled.

• *Pseudogout*
 – Simple analgesics e.g. paracetamol 1g four times daily
 – NSAID e.g. diclofenac (50mg) with misoprostol one tablet three times daily
 – Joint injection – methyl prednisolone 40mg with 1ml 1% lignocaine

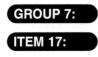

**GROUP 7:**

**ITEM 17:**

# Geriatrics
# Parkinson's Disease

## CASE HISTORY

An 80-year-old man with a history of hypertension presents with a fall. He has had numerous falls recently and on questioning said he had slowed down generally.

You noticed immediately a tremor in his left arm. The diagnosis is Parkinson's Disease.

### Features of Parkinson's Disease

• Akinesia/Bradykinesia
  – poor initiation of movement
  – poor repetitive movements
  – fatigue
• Rigidity
  – lead pipe
  – and/or cogwheel
• Tremor
  – rest tremor
  – 3.5Hz
  – absent in 30% at presentation
• Response to L-dopa
  – suggests true Parkinson's Disease

### What is the differential diagnosis?

• Essential tremor:
  – isolated tremor, may affect the head (Yes/Yes or No/No pattern)
  – becomes more prominent with increasing age
  – autosomal dominant inheritance
  – responds to alcohol, ß blockers, primidone
• Arteriosclerotic Parkinsonism:
  – history of cerebrovascular disease and hypertension common
  – wide based, short stepped gait 'Marche à petit pas'
  – upper part of body not affected
  – limited/transient response to L-dopa
• Drug induced Parkinsonism:
  – major tranquillisers especially depot preparations
  – metoclopramide
• Rarer causes of Parkinsonism
  – multiple system atrophy, Shy-Drager-Parkinsonism – autonomic failure and dementia

**Remember**
• You must question a diagnosis of Parkinson's Disease if:
• Poor response to L-dopa
• Early instability
• Pyramidal or cerebellar signs
• Early autonomic failure e.g. postural hypotension, incontinence
• Dementia early in course of disease
• Voluntary downward gaze palsy

– Steele Richardson Olszewski.-.Parkinsonism, with loss of voluntary conjugate deviation of gaze, and pseudobulbar dysarthria

### How would you manage this patient?

• Parkinson's Disease is a clinical diagnosis
• L-dopa is first line treatment e.g. Co-beneldopa 62.5mg twice daily. Dose requires titration depending on improvement and side effects of medication e.g. postural hypotension, nausea, hallucinations
• Other treatments are usually used as adjuncts. e.g. dopa agonists – bromocriptine, lisuride, pergolide, apomorphine
• Monoamine oxidase inhibitor (MAOI-B) – selegiline
• Catechol-O-Methyl transferase inhibitor (COMT) inhibitor eg tolcapone
• Pramipexole – a D3 agonist, has been introduced

---

**GROUP 7:**

**ITEM 18:**

# Geriatrics

# Drug treatment in older people/ drug treatment as a cause of illness and admission to hospital

Individuals over the age of 65 form approximately 18% of the population but represent 25 to 30% of drugs expenditure. Approximately 87% of the elderly take one prescribed medication and one third of this group take three or more drugs.

Age-associated increases in the incidence of adverse reactions have been well described for certain groups of drugs like benzodiazepines.

The most frequently used classes are cardiovascular drugs, analgesics, gastrointestinal preparations and sedatives.

### Drugs as a cause of illness and delayed discharge

### CASE HISTORY 1

A 75-year-old lady was admitted with infective exacerbation of COPD. She was started on amoxicillin 500mg three times a day, and erythromycin 500mg four times a day, in addition to nebulised salbutamol and ipratropium, with a good response. A few days later she developed watery diarrhoea which was bad enough to require I.V. fluids. Her stool analysis was positive for **clostridium**

| Some drugs that are more likely to produce adverse effects in the elderly | |
|---|---|
| *Drug* | *Adverse Effects* |
| Benzodiazepines | Sedation, drowsiness, confusion, ataxia |
| Non Steroidal Anti-Inflammatory drugs | Gastric erosions, fluid retention and drug interaction e.g. diuretics |
| Opiates | Sedation, confusion, constipation |
| Anticholinergic | Urinary retention, glaucoma |
| Antiarrhythmics | Confusion, urinary retention, thyroid problems |
| Major tranquillisers | Confusion, sedation, tardive dyskinesia, malignant hyperthermia |
| Diuretics | Dehydration, hyponatraemia, postural hypotension, gouty arthritis |
| Antibiotics | Renal and auditory injury, diarrhoea |

**difficile toxin**. She was prescribed a ten day course of metronidazole 400mg three times a day. Apart from transient nausea she made a good recovery and was able to go home.

## CASE HISTORY 2

A 71-year-old lady was admitted with malaise, fatigue, weight loss and generally feeling unwell. Clinically she looked anxious, underweight and tremulous with tachycardia. In the past she had suffered from atrial fibrillation and was taking amiodarone 200mg once daily. Detailed investigations revealed thyrotoxicosis (a side-effect of amiodarone) with undetectable TSH and very high free T3 and T4. The amiodarone was stopped and she was started on antithyroid therapy (propyl thiouracil 100mg three times a day) along with steroids (prednisolone 40mg once daily). Her response was slow and she remained an inpatient for a few weeks before her condition was brought under control

### Drug interaction

## CASE HISTORY 3

A 79-year-old lady with a background of NIDDM and ischaemic heart disease was admitted with uncontrolled diabetes and progressive shortness of breath. She was taking gliclazide 160mg twice a day and co-amilofruse (5mg amiloride, 40mg frusemide) one tablet daily. A few weeks prior to admission she complained of back pain and her GP prescribed diclofenac 50mg three times a day. Clinically, she was in acute left ventricular failure but there was no evidence of an acute ischaemic episode or chest infection. The NSAID was stopped and the dose of co-amilofruse was doubled. Her symptoms settled gradually over the next few days.

**Beware**

NSAIDS cause fluid retention.

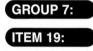

## Geriatrics
## Do not resuscitate (DNR) decision-making

### CASE HISTORY 1

A fit 80-year-old man presents with an acute myocardial infarct. If he has a cardiac arrest would you resuscitate him?

### CASE HISTORY 2

A 75-year-old lady presents with hypercalcaemia secondary to disseminated lung carcinoma. You treat her hypercalcaemia aggressively. A nurse asks whether the patient should be recorded for resuscitation or not.

### What would you say?

Cardiopulmonary resuscitation (CPR) is an everyday practice in UK hospitals. Despite the success in selected patients there is a consensus that CPR is inappropriate (e.g. in terminal illness) or ineffective (e.g. very severe pneumonia) in some patients.

All decisions should be discussed with senior medical colleagues.

### What are the principles which might guide you to decide to withhold CPR?

• Futility or ineffectiveness of CPR. Only six to 15% of CPR cases leave hospital alive. A number of factors have been identified which predict a poor outcome from CPR attempts. These include:
- pneumonia (0% survival)
- renal failure
- anaemia (<9g/dl)
- a high level of dependency including housebound lifestyle
- more than 2 acute medical conditions

**Remember**

- If no DNR decision is documented – the patient is for resuscitation.
- Any DNR decision made should be communicated to all members of the health care team involved with the patient.
- DNR decisions should be reviewed if appropriate (i.e. not necessarily in terminal illness).

- Patient autonomy, patient wishes, advance directives and living wills
  Mentally competent patients who express their wishes on treatment including CPR should have those wishes respected
- Justice. A decision to attempt CPR involves a commitment to continue the care of the patient whatever the outcome. This may entail the use of significant resources and may deprive other patients of their benefit
- Quality of life. This is the most difficult aspect to address. It includes the quality of life as it is now and also after a CPR attempt, which may be worse. Difficulties arise because it involves professionals making value judgements about other people's lives

References:

1. FLORIN D 'Do Not Resuscitate Orders: the need for a policy', 1993 Journal Royal College of Physicians of London 27, 2:135 – 138

2. WILLIAMS R. The 'do not resuscitate' decision: guidelines for policy in the adult 1993 Journal Royal College of Physicians of London 27, 2:139 – 140

# Notes

**GROUP 8:**

**ITEM 1:**

# Rheumatology
# Osteoarthritis (OA)

## CASE HISTORY

A 75-year- old woman attends the A & E Department with pain in the left groin. The pain has been present for several months and she has not sought medical advice until now. The pain is now severe, she is unable to walk more than a few yards and the pain is keeping her awake at night. She lives alone and is unable to manage either her pain or to cope alone at home. The casualty SHO has had a pelvis X-ray which shows OA of the hip. You are asked to see her for possible admission.

**Describe the main radiological features of OA of the hip.**

The radiograph may show joint space narrowing, periarticular sclerosis and cyst formation with osteophytes. These are the four classical features of osteoarthritis. (see Fig 8.1.1)

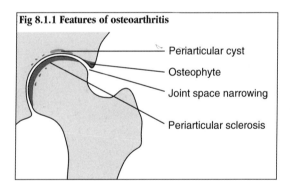

**Fig 8.1.1 Features of osteoarthritis**

- Periarticular cyst
- Osteophyte
- Joint space narrowing
- Periarticular sclerosis

**How would you assess her?**

The long standing history suggests a gradual onset of the pain and this should be clarified. A short history or systemic symptoms might indicate joint sepsis or a pathological fracture.

The main site of the pain – especially in the left groin radiating into the left thigh/knee indicates that the hip is the source of the pain. Beware referred pain either from the lumbar spine (common) or the knee (less common).

A full musculo-skeletal examination is needed. The GALS (Gait, Arms, Leg, Spine) is a useful screen (ref: Doherty M, Dacre J, Dieppe P, Snaith M: The GALS. Locomotor Screen. Ann Rheum Dis. 1992; 51: 1165). (see Figs 8.1.2a–d).

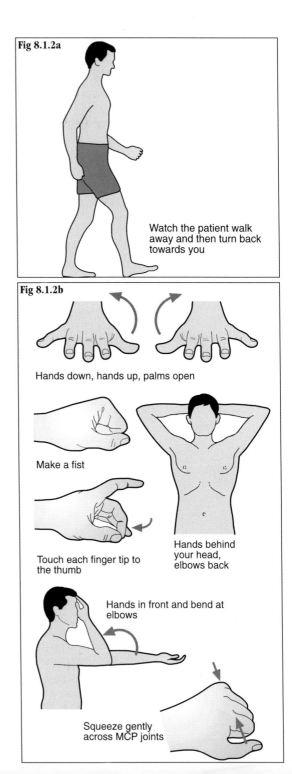

**Fig 8.1.2a**

Watch the patient walk away and then turn back towards you

**Fig 8.1.2b**

Hands down, hands up, palms open

Make a fist

Touch each finger tip to the thumb

Hands behind your head, elbows back

Hands in front and bend at elbows

Squeeze gently across MCP joints

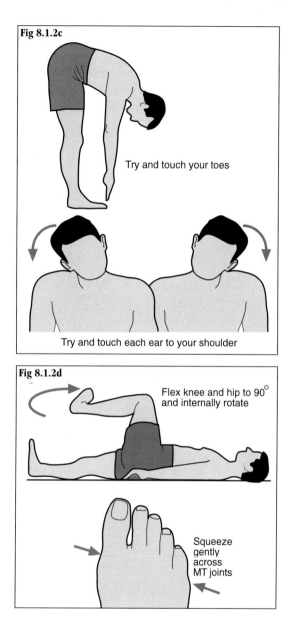

Fig 8.1.2c

Try and touch your toes

Try and touch each ear to your shoulder

Fig 8.1.2d

Flex knee and hip to 90°
and internally rotate

Squeeze
gently
across
MT joints

### Diagnostic clues

Look for: Heberden's/Bouchard's Nodes, 'square' hands, painful thumb, carpometacarpal joints that indicate 1° nodal Osteoarthritis. (Fig 8.1.3)

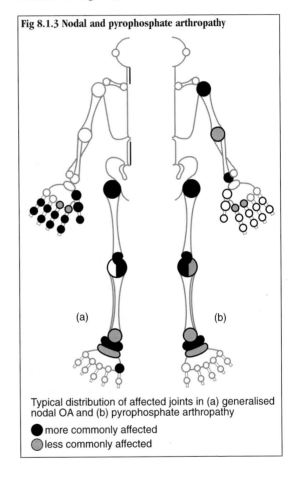

**Fig 8.1.3 Nodal and pyrophosphate arthropathy**

(a)

(b)

Typical distribution of affected joints in (a) generalised nodal OA and (b) pyrophosphate arthropathy

● more commonly affected
◐ less commonly affected

### Examine:

- other joints for evidence of inflammatory arthritis e g Psoriatic arthritis/RA
- Lumbar spine for referred pain
- Hips
  – ask patient to walk to assess gait
  – measure leg lengths
  – assess range of all movements fully and compare with right hip. Examine from behind to look for pelvic tilt and perform Trendelenburg's test.

## What points would you consider when deciding if admission is appropriate?

Full general medical examination is essential since comorbid conditions in this age group are common. For example in a patient with significant disabilities, consider the possibilities of pneumonia or urinary tract infections. Her nutrition may be poor raising the possibility of osteomalacia – a well described problem in the elderly..

A full assessment of her ability to cope is essential and you should ask her about her ability to wash, dress and feed herself. This disability assessment will weigh strongly when considering admission.

## How would you manage her initially?

Diagnosis is osteoarthritis or possibly avascular necrosis of the femoral head. A pathological fracture is less likely given the radiological appearances.

### Initial Treatment

- Admit because:
  - lives alone
  - no pain control
  - considerably disabled
- Analgesia: simple or compound analgesia as first line therapy e.g. paracetamol up to 4g/day

If this fails a short course of NSAID is reasonable. There is a high risk of G I toxicity with long term use in her age group and NSAIDs which only inhibit COX II can be used (eg rofecoxib). Opiates should be avoided unless essential because of sedation/confusion and constipation.

### Later Management

Refer to rheumatologist or medicine for the elderly consultant. In the meantime organise:

- Physiotherapy:
  - mobilise hip. Joint protection exercises
  - assess walking aids e.g. stick, Zimmer.
  - consider hydrotherapy
- Occupational Therapy and social work assessments
- Prior to discharge there should be careful planning including liaison with the GP and possibly a home visit

---

**Investigations**

If febrile:
- Blood cultures
- FBC
- CRP/ESR

---

### Indications for surgery

Referral to orthopaedics to consider surgery indicated for:

• Severe pain especially night pain
• Poor mobility

Consider general health of patient and history of surgery

# Rheumatology
# Rheumatoid arthritis (RA)

## CASE HISTORY

A 26-year-old woman presents at A&E with sudden onset of severe widespread joint pain and swelling affecting her hands, wrists and feet symmetrically. She has lost half a stone in weight and feels systemically unwell. Clinically you find symmetrical synovitis, joint restriction of the wrists, MCP and PIP joints and painful MTP joints. You suspect this is an acute onset of rheumatoid arthritis.

### What other conditions may give a similar clinical picture?

• Systemic lupus erythematosus
• Parvovirus B19 infection
• Post streptococcal arthritis
• Psoriatic arthritis
• Primary Sjogren's syndrome
• Some systemic vasculitides

In the first two differential diagnoses there are often other features. In systemic lupus erythematosus, there may be rashes that are photosensitive, hair fall, serositis and oral ulceration. Parvovirus B19 nearly always presents with flu-like symptoms and a widespread rash.

Post streptococcal arthritis may be preceded by a sore throat but is rare. Psoriatic arthritis is usually asymmetrical but may occasionally present with a symmetrical pattern. Psoriatic nail changes and other evidence of psoriasis are often also present but may develop after the onset of arthritis.

Sjogrens syndrome may be associated with intermittent parotid swelling and sicca symptoms: dry eyes (keratoconjuctivitis sicca) and dry mouth (xerostomia)

**Fig 8.2.1 Rheumatoid arthritis**

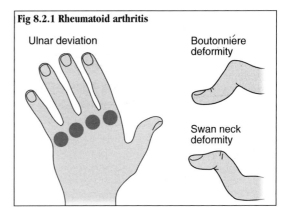

Ulnar deviation

Boutonniére deformity

Swan neck deformity

**Fig 8.2.2 Diagram of X-ray changes in rheumatoid arthritis**

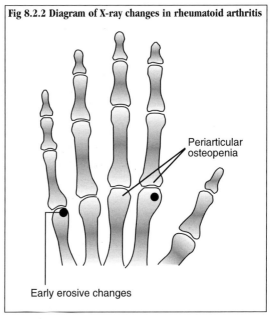

Periarticular osteopenia

Early erosive changes

## How would you manage her?

A careful history is required covering points that could assist the exclusion of the differential diagnosis. A full general medical examination is essential. Specific points:

**Remember**

Rheumatoid arthritis is a multisystem disease so look carefully for pulmonary, cardiac or neurological involvement though these are less common at presentation.

- Look for nodules or vasculitis – uncommon at first presentation
- A full musculoskeletal examination noting the symmetry of the joint involvement
- Look for PISA: Persistent Inflammatory Symmetrical Arthritis. The most common cause of this is rheumatoid arthritis

## Investigations

- FBC/ESR, chemistry including globulin level, CRP (the finding of a high ESR but normal CRP is characteristic of SLE)
- ANA/Rheumatoid factor
- X-Ray hands and feet for erosions, periarticular osteopenia (figure 8.2.2)
- ASO titre if sore throat
- Blood cultures if febrile
- Parvovirus B19 titres if the ANA/RhF are negative

The most commonly involved joints at onset in rheumatoid arthritis are: wrists, MCPs, PIPs and MTP joints (see Fig 8.2.1). Other joints such as knees and hips only become involved later in the disease course.

### How would you manage this patient?

Consider admission if the patient is very unwell systemically and to exclude other pathology –

- Initial management: A short period of bed rest, ice packs if only a few joints involved
- NSAIDS: Ibuprofen – safest. Other NSAIDs have a higher risk of GI toxicity though this patient is young. NSAIDs that inhibit COX II only are becoming available.
- Disease Modifying Agents. These should be considered at the earliest opportunity since rheumatoid arthritis is a systemic disease that leads rapidly to joint damage and disability. It is no longer acceptable to treat RA with NSAIDs alone. There is accumulating evidence to show that early DMARD use delays joint damage and functional disability.

Initial DMARDs commonly used include sulphasalazine, methotrexate or azathioprine. Others such as gold i.m. or D-penicillamine are less commonly used but still effective.

Hydroxychloroquine and auranofin are the least effective but may be used in combination regimens. Combination therapies are showing excellent short-term benefits.

All drugs need careful explanation to the patient and close monitoring for toxicity.

Prednisolone is not used in young patients but intramuscular methyl prednisolone 40-120mg stat gives excellent short-term benefit.

The addition of prednisolone 7.5mg to existing DMARD therapy may retard the progression of erosions, but studies in this area remain controversial and this is not recommended for general use at present.

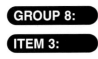

**GROUP 8:**

**ITEM 3:**

# Rheumatology
# SLE and vasculitis

## CASE HISTORY

A 28-year-old woman is referred to you by her general practitioner. Six weeks ago she delivered her first baby and the pregnancy and delivery were uneventful. Two weeks after delivery she developed a widespread polyarthritis affecting her hands, feet, and knees and a photosensitive rash on her face. In the last week or two she has become extremely unwell with weight loss and painful lesions on her hands and feet.

Clinically, she is clearly unwell with a facial rash and severe oral ulceration. Examination of her hands and feet shows extensive digital infarctions with necrotic ulceration on the palms, finger pulps and soles of the feet. There are splinter haemorrhages and nail-fold infarctions.

### Discuss the differential diagnosis, investigation and management of this lady.

The differential diagnosis clearly includes an inflammatory connective tissue disease such as systemic lupus erythematosus which has developed after delivery of her baby. The lesions on her hands (Fig 8.3.1) and feet are strongly suggestive of vasculitis which is a serious prognostic factor that requires immediate therapy.

**Remember**

The major risk of vasculitis is organ involvement including renal, cerebral and pulmonary involvement, which can be life-threatening.

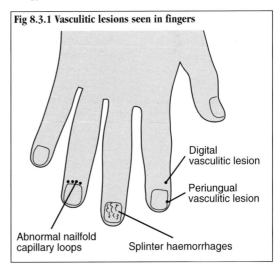

**Fig 8.3.1 Vasculitic lesions seen in fingers**

Digital vasculitic lesion

Periungual vasculitic lesion

Abnormal nailfold capillary loops

Splinter haemorrhages

Investigations are therefore directed at looking for the possibility of major organ involvement which may be vasculitic. Her urine must be dipped immediately for blood and protein and sent for urine cytology looking for fragmented red cells and/or casts. The presence of an "active" urine sediment with fragmented or dysmorphic red cells and granular casts has a >90% specificity for glomerulonephritis.

| | |
|---|---|
| FBC: | Immune cytopenias especially neutropenia and thrombocytopenia are common in SLE. There may be anaemia of chronic disease or haemolytic anaemia – check Coomb's test. |
| ESR: | the pattern of a high ESR but normal CRP is characteristic of SLE |
| Renal function: | U+E, 24 hour urine protein/creatinine clearance |
| Liver biochemistry | |
| Lupus serology | |
| ANA | present in 95% of SLE patients |
| ds DNA | specific marker for SLE |
| ENA | Ro/La  photosensitivity/Sjogrens |
| | RNP/Smoften seen in severe SLE |
| Complement | low values indicate activator or rarely congenital deficiency |
| ANCA | a marker of vasculitis – a systemic vasculitis is an alternative to SLE |

Once the diagnosis of lupus and vasculitis is established on clinical and serological grounds, therapy is with prednisolone and intravenous pulse methyl prednisolone 500-1000 mg intravenously on alternate days for three doses.

Consideration should be given to immunosuppressive therapy and one commonly used approach is to consider intravenous cyclophosphamide therapy given fortnightly or monthly, 500mg per pulse. The patient should be carefully counselled about the risks and benefits of cyclophosphamide and these include the adverse effects of cyclophosphamide such as cytopenias, haemorrhagic cystitis, infections including herpes zoster and infertility. If the patient is breast feeding, this should be discontinued as cyclophosphamide and other immunosuppressives such as azathioprine are excreted in breast milk. Plasma exchange is no longer routinely used.

⚠

**Remember**

Specialist advice from a rheumatologist or immunologist should be sought.

**GROUP 8:**

**ITEM 4:**

# Rheumatology
## Acute multi-system connective tissue disease

### CASE HISTORY

A 33-year-old Afro-Caribbean woman is admitted acutely through A&E complaining of breathlessness and swollen legs. Two years ago she was admitted acutely with a psychotic illness that had features of schizophrenia and improved with anti-psychotic medication.

In the last six months she has developed a symmetrical small joint inflammatory arthritis, mouth ulcers and photosensitive facial rashes. Over the last two weeks she has become breathless and her legs have become severely swollen.

Clinically, she is anaemic with a pulse of 120/min. with pulsus paradoxus. She has bilateral pleural effusions, a high jugular venous pressure and pitting oedema to her waist. There is synovitis of the small joints of her fingers and she has florid splinter haemorrhages. Her BP is 90/60. Her urine showed proteinuria.

### What is the likely diagnosis?

The diagnosis is likely to be systemic lupus erythematosus complicated by the nephrotic syndrome. In addition she may have cardiac tamponade from a pericardial effusion.

SLE is nine times commoner in females and is more common in Afro-Caribbean and Far Eastern patients. It may also be more severe in these ethnic groups. This patient has many characteristic features of SLE: inflammatory polyarthritis, mouth ulcers, photosensitive rashes, psychotic illness, serositis with pleural and probably pericardial effusions and renal disease with nephrotic syndrome. The high JVP might indicate early tamponade.

### How would you manage this patient?

The most urgent priority is to consider whether this patient has cardiac tamponade. The low BP and the presence of pulsus paradoxus, tachycardia and raised JVP with cardiomegaly on CXR are strong pointers to this. The overwhelming majority of patients with lupus who have cardiac tamponade associated with a pericardial effusion respond to high dose oral corticosteroids and do not need pericardiocentesis. This should, however, be considered if the patient deteriorates despite corticosteroid therapy or if sepsis is present. A normal CRP makes infection less likely.

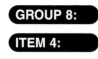

## Investigations

- FBC with reticulocyte count/ Coombs (Direct antiglobulin test): the anaemia might be haemolytic
- U + E – Renal impairment may be present
- LFTs – Serum albumin will be low
- Twenty-four hour urine protein and creatinine clearance should be commenced
- Urine cytology for fragmented red cells and granular casts: (a useful marker of glomerulonephritis)
- CXR —To document pleural effusions and cardiomegaly – fig 8.4.2
- Echocardiogram – To document pericardial effusion and possible valve lesions.
- ECG
- Blood gases
- Blood cultures/ urine cultures to exclude sepsis, especially endocarditis, prior to corticosteroid and immunosuppressive therapy
- Full auto-antibody screen: ANA, DNA, ENA, Rh factor Anticardiolipin antibodies Lupus Anticoagulant, ANCA
- Complement studies
- A diagnostic renal biopsy may be required later

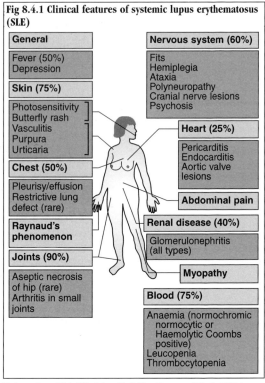

**Fig 8.4.1 Clinical features of systemic lupus erythematosus (SLE)**

| General |
|---|
| Fever (50%) |
| Depression |

| Skin (75%) |
|---|
| Photosensitivity |
| Butterfly rash |
| Vasculitis |
| Purpura |
| Urticaria |

| Chest (50%) |
|---|
| Pleurisy/effusion |
| Restrictive lung defect (rare) |

| Raynaud's phenomenon |
|---|

| Joints (90%) |
|---|
| Aseptic necrosis of hip (rare) |
| Arthritis in small joints |

| Nervous system (60%) |
|---|
| Fits |
| Hemiplegia |
| Ataxia |
| Polyneuropathy |
| Cranial nerve lesions |
| Psychosis |

| Heart (25%) |
|---|
| Pericarditis |
| Endocarditis |
| Aortic valve lesions |

| Abdominal pain |
|---|

| Renal disease (40%) |
|---|
| Glomerulonephritis (all types) |

| Myopathy |
|---|

| Blood (75%) |
|---|
| Anaemia (normochromic normocytic or Haemolytic Coombs positive) |
| Leucopenia |
| Thrombocytopenia |

Redrawn from *Clinical Medicine*, 4th Edition, Kumar and Clark, 1998, by permission of the publisher WB Saunders

The next priority is to determine the extent and severity of the renal disease. Serum creatinine, albumin, 24-hour urine protein and creatinine clearance will be useful. If there is an active urine sediment e.g. , fragmented red cells and granular casts, indicating glomerulonephritis, renal biopsy is indicated.

**Fig 8.4.2 Diagram of a CXR showing pleural effusions and cardiomegaly**

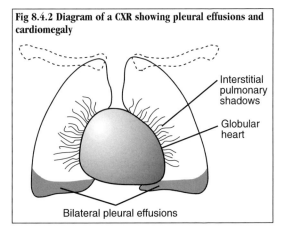

Interstitial pulmonary shadows

Globular heart

Bilateral pleural effusions

## Other points to consider

• Thrombosis prophylaxis. This patient is at high risk of DVT/PE. TED stockings and prophylactic low molecular weight heparin should be given.

• Is the anaemia haemolytic? If so, it should respond to corticosteroids.

• Once blood pressure has been corrected, consider an ACE inhibitor. This is especially useful in proteinuric patients.

• If renal biopsy confirms proliferative glomerulonephritis, the treatment of choice is corticosteroid therapy and intermittent intravenous cyclophosphamide followed by azathioprine.

• This patient's lipid profile may well be deranged, especially in the context of nephrotic syndrome. This will need to be assessed and managed actively.

• Prophylaxis against corticosteroid induced osteoporosis. A baseline DEXA scan should be performed and calcium supplementation should be considered.

## Long term prognosis

The majority of patients with SLE have a good prognosis though clearly this patient has serious disease with life threatening complications. Mortality in SLE occurs at two peak periods: those patients who die from overwhelming disease, thrombosis or sepsis and those who die prematurely from accelerated atherosclerosis. Prognosis has been considerably improved by earlier recognition and effective therapy.

**GROUP 8:**

**ITEM 5:**

# Rheumatology
## Thrombosis and the antiphospholipid syndrome

### CASE HISTORY

A-25-year old woman presents with a two-day history of left leg swelling and on the day of admission she notices breathlessness and chest pains which are worse on deep inspiration.

In the past medical history you find that she has had three miscarriages and one successful pregnancy. This pregnancy was complicated by hypertension and intra-uterine growth retardation with a premature delivery at 31 weeks. On further questioning you note that she has had oral ulceration, rashes that are worse in the sunlight and headaches.

### Drug history

She is on the oral contraceptive pill.

### On examination

You find she has extensive splinter haemorrhages on most fingers. Her pulse is 100 and BP 110/70 and she is not cyanosed. Her heart sounds are normal but there is a soft murmur of mitral regurgitation and also a soft left pleural rub. Abdominal examination and neurological examination are normal. The left calf is swollen and the calf circumference is 3 centimetres greater than on the right. You note extensive livedo reticularis on her arms, thighs and knees.

### What is the differential diagnosis and your management?

This young lady on the oral contraceptive pill clearly has a deep venous thrombosis and a pulmonary embolus until proved otherwise.

A full blood count may well reveal thrombocytopenia which is commonly seen in the antiphospholipid syndrome – see box.

An echocardiogram and blood cultures are essential as differential diagnosis includes Libman-Sacks endocarditis or bacterial endocarditis.

### The differential diagnosis

In this case includes the antiphospholipid syndrome with a DVT and pulmonary emboli, along with an increased risk of thrombosis from the oral contraceptive pill. The history is rather suggestive of systemic lupus erythematosus and this should be

---

### Investigations

- An ECG – looking for the classical (but seldom seen) S1 Q3 T3 pattern of PE Figure 8.5.1.
- A Chest X-ray – but is likely to be normal. It is important however, to exclude other causes of pleuritic chest pain including infective causes
- An ultrasound scan of the leg veins to document the extent of the left calf thrombosis or a venogram
- *A V/Q scan to show the extent of the pulmonary emboli
- *Plasma D-dimers – If undetectable the diagnosis of PE and DVT is excluded
- *Spiral CT with contrast` – good specificity and sensitivity for medium sized PEs
- *Choose the imaging techniques according to local availability.

### Information

- The Antiphospholipid Syndrome is due to the presence of antibodies which bind phospholipids leading to both venous and arterial occlusion.
- Most commonly seen in SLE, but may occur in isolation: Primary Antiphospholipid Syndrome.

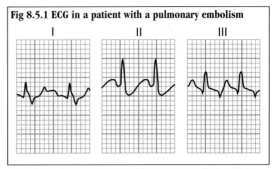

**Fig 8.5.1 ECG in a patient with a pulmonary embolism**

Redrawn from *Clinical Medicine*, 4th Edition, Kumar and Clark, 1998, by permission of the publisher WB Saunders

investigated further with auto-antibodies to ANA, DNA and ENA with complement studies. The features favouring a diagnosis of the antiphospholipid syndrome in this case would include the three previous miscarriages and one pregnancy complicated by intrauterine growth retardation and premature delivery. There is accumulating evidence in the literature to suggest that the intra-uterine growth retardation is due to recurrent placental thrombosis and this is often manifested by reduced umbilical artery flow patterns on doppler studies with an increased resistance index, notching or even reversed flow in the umbilical vessels.

## Information

Further reading
Hughes G R V: "Hughes' Syndrome – The Antiphospholipid Syndrome" Journal of the Royal College of Physicians of London June 1998 Vol 32 pp260-264
Khamashta MA et al: "The Management of Thrombosis in the Antiphospholipid Syndrome" New England Journal of Medicine 1995; 332: 993.

## The Antiphospholipid Syndrome

Anti cardiolipin antibodies and a full thrombophilia screen with the lupus anticoagulant should be performed. Both the anticardiolipin antibodies and the lupus anticoagulant are antiphospholipid antibodies and both should be requested since a small percentage of patients have either one or the other antibody but not both. The thrombophilia screen is important to look for other factors including the factor V Leiden mutation. Patients with the antiphospholipid syndrome also have reduced protein C and S levels which are associated with the lupus anticoagulant.

## Libman-Sacks Endocarditis

Splinter haemorrhages and a mitral murmur indicate Libman-Sacks endocarditis which is a feature of the antiphospholipid syndrome and SLE. These patients get a mucinous degeneration of the mitral valve leaflets and occasionally thrombus (which may embolise) is seen on the damaged valves. Similarly the damaged valves may become secondarily infected leading to infective endocarditis. The splinter haemorrhages may represent micro emboli and are a feature of both antiphospholipid syndrome and infective endocarditis.

### How would you manage this patient?

This lady should be admitted and commenced on heparin. The heparin may be given intravenously as a continuous infusion, but many hospitals are now switching to once-daily low molecular weight heparin, for example tinzparin. Warfarin should be commenced and the eventual target INR should be 3.5.

If the diagnosis of the antiphospholipid syndrome is confirmed then therapy with warfarin will be life-long at the target INR. These patients are often resistant to warfarin and occasionally require high doses – for example, of 15-20 mg daily of warfarin.

In terms of the mitral valve disease she will need counselling about antibiotic prophylaxis prior to any surgical procedure including dental work. Providing infective endocarditis has been excluded these patients will need to be monitored since a small percentage of patients require mitral valve replacement.

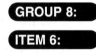

**GROUP 8:**

**ITEM 6:**

# Rheumatology
# Gout and pseudo-gout

## CASE HISTORY

A 73-year-old woman was admitted a week ago having had a right hemiparesis. You have been asked to see the patient who has developed a hot, swollen right knee, for your advice on whether this may be a septic arthritis.

**Investigations**

- Full blood count
- ESR
- Urea and electrolytes
- Bone and liver biochemistry
- Serum urate
- X-ray of the knee and blood cultures are required
- The joint should be aspirated with a sterile technique and fluid sent for cells, crystals and culture

On further questioning, this lady has attended the hypertension clinic for many years and has been taking bendrofluazide. She has also complained of knee pain intermittently over the last five years, but the joint has never previously swelled up. She is making a reasonable recovery from her stroke and there is no other relevant history.

Clinically there is no evidence of tophi. The knee is hot and movement is restricted due to a large tense effusion. She is afebrile.

### How would you manage this patient?

The X-ray may well show chondrocalcinosis (see Fig 8.6.1) and will probably show patello-femoral and tibio-femoral osteo-arthritis. The serum uric acid is likely to be elevated given that she is taking a thiazide diuretic. The differential diagnosis thus includes gout or pseudo-gout of which pseudo-gout is probably more likely in this clinical context.

**Fig 8.6.1 Chondrocalcinosis of the knee**

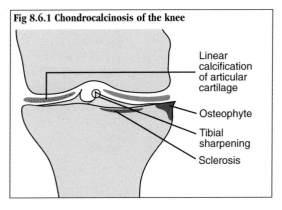

Linear calcification of articular cartilage

Osteophyte

Tibial sharpening

Sclerosis

## Pseudo-Gout

This patient has the typical presentation of pseudo-gout – an acute onset of a swollen joint in an elderly patient who has been admitted for other reasons – usually a stroke, MI or chest infection.

The commonest crystal associated with pseudo-gout is calcium pyrophosphate crystals – figure 8.6.2 which are diagnosed on synovial fluid analysis using polarised light microscopy. These crystals are rhomboidal and positively birefringent and may be idiopathic or associated with osteoarthritis. A number of metabolic conditions are also associated with calcium pyrophosphate deposition, these include hypo-thyroidism, hyperparathyroidism, acromegaly, Wilson's disease, haemo-chromatosis, hypophosphatasia and hypomagnesemia.

The differential diagnosis of gout is also made on crystal examination. These crystals are negatively birefringent needle-shaped crystals.

**Fig 8.6.2 Calcium pyrophosphate and urate crystals**

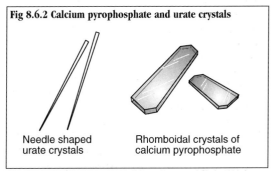

Needle shaped urate crystals

Rhomboidal crystals of calcium pyrophosphate

Redrawn from *Clinical Medicine*, 4th Edition, Kumar and Clark, 1998, by permission of the publisher WB Saunders

## Management

Septic arthritis, although unlikely should clearly be excluded, and providing joint aspiration and synovial fluid culture and blood cultures are all negative, the knee should be aspirated to dryness and injected with a steroid such as 40 mg of methylprednisolone . Risk factors should be minimised and in particular, the thiazide diuretic (which can precipitate gout) should be switched to an alternative antihypertensive medication. Intensive physiotherapy is important with particular attention to quadriceps exercises and maintaining mobility and hydration in the patient.

**GROUP 8:**

**ITEM 7:**

# Rheumatology
# Polymyalgia rheumatica/cranial arteritis

## Investigations

The following investigations are essential:
- Full blood count
- ESR or CRP
- Urea and electrolytes
- Liver biochemistry

## CASE HISTORY

A 73-year-old woman presents to A&E feeling non-specifically unwell. On further questioning she has a headache, and joint aches, particularly of her shoulders and hips in addition to widespread aches and pains. She has marked joint stiffness particularly of the shoulders and hips, lasting for several hours each morning, and may occasionally last all day. The headache is predominantly right-sided and the patient says that it is painful when she brushes her hair. In addition she has pains in the left jaw on talking or eating.

On examination the scalp is tender and it is difficult to palpate the temporal arteries. The rest of the examination is normal. Her shoulders and hips ache at the extremes of the range of movement but are otherwise normal.

### Differential diagnosis and management

The likeliest diagnosis is temporal arteritis with polymyalgia rheumatica and there is therefore a significant risk of blindness from arteritis of the opthalmic artery. A differential diagnosis includes malignancy of any cause and myeloma can also mimic polymyalgia rheumatica. This lady should be commenced on 40-60 mg of prednisolone immediately and a temporal artery biopsy should be arranged within the next 24 hours.

The response to steroids is usually dramatic in these patients and a response is often seen within 24 to 48 hours. The steroid therapy should be reduced reasonably quickly (over a few weeks to 15-20 mg daily) and if this is not possible then a steroid sparing agent such as azathioprine should be added to achieve this. She is also at high risk for osteoporosis and subsequent vertebral fractures and calcium and vitamin D supplementation should be co-prescribed routinely. A baseline DEXA (Dual Energy X-ray Absorptiometry) should be requested – if there is already osteoporosis, bisphosphonates should be considered.

**Patients who fail to respond to steroids**

Should be investigated in detail for an underlying malignancy. Occasionally other conditions such as severe hypothyroidism may also present with similar joint aches but the clinical picture of temporal arteritis is usually characteristic enough to establish the diagnosis.

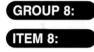

# Rheumatology
# Acute back pain

## CASE HISTORY

A 36-year-old drayman presents acutely to A&E. Having just lifted a barrel of beer he experienced severe buttock and back pain. The pain radiated down the left leg to the sole of the foot with associated parasthesiae. On further questioning he finds that it is extremely painful to move his back and the pain is worse on coughing or sneezing. The pain is worse in the leg than in the back. He says that he has not passed any urine for six hours .

### On examination

He is in severe pain and is lying flat on the examination couch. He finds it too painful to stand up but examination of the hips, knees and other joints are all normal. Straight leg raising on the right is 40° and on the left is only 10° with a strongly positive sciatic stretch test. The femoral nerve stretch test is strongly positive on the left and neurological examination reveals an absent left ankle jerk and sacral anaesthesia.

### Discuss your further investigations, diagnosis and management.

The history and clinical examination are almost diagnostic for a large L5/S1 disc protrusion with compromise of the cauda equina (Figure 8.8.1) which can lead to urinary retention. This is therefore a neurosurgical emergency.

The most urgent investigation is imaging of the lumbar spine and pelvis and the most rapid and easily accessible imaging is with a CT scan of the lumbo-sacral spine. If available, magnetic resonance imaging will give greater detail and definition of the soft tissues. The patient should be catheterised and analgesia given which may include intramuscular non-steroidals such as i.m.diclofenac or opiate analgesics including morphine or pethidine if needed. The patient should be referred immediately to

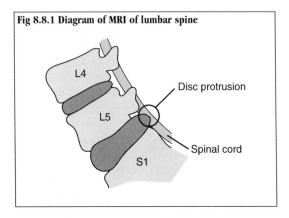

Fig 8.8.1 Diagram of MRI of lumbar spine

a neurosurgeon or orthopaedic surgeon with an interest in acute spinal problems to consider urgent decompressive surgery with a laminectomy and discectomy. Any delay in diagnosis or decompression may lead to a permanent neurological deficit .

In patients without sacral anaesthesia or neurological deficit, the evidence based advice is not to recommend bed rest but to mobilise the patient as soon as possible using adequate analgesia. Rapid access to physiotherapy may improve outcome and procedures such as sacral or lumbar epidurals may be considered to relieve pain while recovery occurs.

**GROUP 8:**

**ITEM 9:**

# Rheumatology
# Severe back pain/osteoporosis

## CASE HISTORY

A 71-year-old woman presents with severe thoracic spinal pain which came on suddenly six hours previously. The pain is severe and radiates around the thoracic spine and front of the chest and is worse on coughing or sneezing. In the past medical history she has had rheumatoid arthritis for the last 25 years and is currently taking 7.5mg of prednisolone. Her rheumatoid arthritis has been in remission for five years on this therapy and she is on no other medication; previous disease-modifying agents have either induced toxicity or have been ineffective.

Clinically there is evidence of quiescent rheumatoid arthritis with classical rheumatoid deformities, nodules and synovial thickening, but no active synovitis. On examination of the thoracic spine there is a marked kyphosis and she is exquisitely tender over T8. The thoracic spine is markedly restricted on rotation reproducing her pain radiating around the chest to the anterior aspect of the chest.

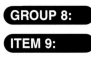

**Investigations**
- Full blood count
- ESR
- Renal function
- Bone and liver biochemistry
- C-reactive protein

**What investigations would you do? Discuss your differential diagnosis and management in this case.**

The likeliest diagnosis is a steroid-associated osteoporosis with an acute vertebral fracture. The differential diagnosis should include myeloma and other malignancies as they may also present with vertebral fractures.

Imaging should include a chest X-ray and specific views of the dorsal spine which is likely to show one or more vertebral crush fractures. Crush fractures have a fairly characteristic appearance and on the AP view of the thoracic spine all the pedicles should be visible. Should any pedicles be missing this should immediately raise the suspicion of metastatic malignancy as a cause of the vertebral fracture.

Later a myeloma screen including a protein electrophoresis strip and urine for Bence-Jones protein should be done.

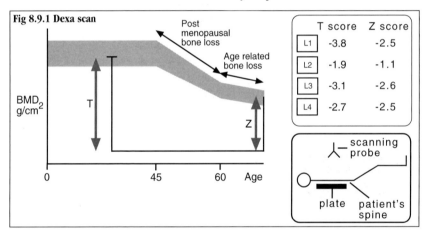

**Fig 8.9.1 Dexa scan**

| | T score | Z score |
|---|---|---|
| L1 | -3.8 | -2.5 |
| L2 | -1.9 | -1.1 |
| L3 | -3.1 | -2.6 |
| L4 | -2.7 | -2.5 |

A DEXA scan is performed to establish the degree of osteoporosis. The DEXA scan gives an accurate index of bone mineral density in relation to the normal range for an age, sex and race matched population. The World Health Organisation definition of osteopenia is a T score of between -1.5 and 2.5. The definition of osteoporosis is a T score of greater than -2.5 standard deviations below the mean and established or severe osteoporosis is a T score of greater than -2.5 with an established fracture. (Figure 8.9.1)

**Initial management**

In the acute setting of a recent vertebral fracture salmon calcitonin 50 units three times a week increasing to 100 units three times a week for six weeks has a very good analgesic effect and works rapidly. Its main adverse effects include hypotension and flushing with nausea although most patients are able to tolerate 50 units 3 times a week.

## Later management

Providing malignant causes have been excluded, this patient should commence specific therapy for osteoporosis. The most effective therapy is with hormone replacement therapy although most women of this age are unlikely to tolerate HRT as they are often unable to tolerate the adverse effects which include breast tenderness and a return of menses. A new alternative is raloxifene which is a tamoxifen derivative which has been shown to increase bone mineral density and may be a very suitable alternative.

Other alternative therapies include cyclical etidronate with calcium or alendronate. Both these therapies are well tolerated in this age group although alendronate is associated with a small but significant risk of oesophagitis. Both these bisphosphonate drugs are poorly absorbed and should be taken at least two hours before a meal with a full glass of water and in particular with alendronate the patient should not lie down for at least two hours after taking the medication to reduce the risk of oesophagitis.

There is good evidence that these medications increase bone mineral density over a three- to five-year period and also reduce fracture risk.

Other factors are also important in reducing the risk of further osteoporosis and include stopping smoking, keeping alcohol intake to a moderate level and encouraging active weight-bearing exercise. Attention to diet is crucially important particularly in this age group and a broad varied diet is important. Particular attention should be paid to calcium intake and if necessary a specific dietician referral would be helpful. These patients should be monitored with annual DEXA scan to check on progress.

### Remember

The main adverse effects of raloxifene include a risk of thrombosis and possible endometrial/uterine malignancy. There is some evidence that raloxifene may protect against the risk of breast cancer.

### Information

Other alternative medications not yet licensed include nasal calcitonin and newer generation bisphosphonates and tamoxifen derivatives are currently under development.

**GROUP 8:**

**ITEM 10:**

# Rheumatology
# Osteomyelitis

### CASE HISTORY

A 56-year-old Asian woman presents with a two-month history of upper back pain and weight loss. She has just arrived home after visiting relatives in Bangladesh for the last year.

There is no relevant history and she is taking no medication.

Clinically she is in pain and looks thin. Her pulse is 110 per minute and regular, her temperature is 38°C. Cardio vascular, respiratory and abdominal examinations are all normal and neurological examination including reflexes and plantars are within normal limits.

All her joints are normal but she is tender over the thoracic spine which is exquisitely painful on rotation of the thoracic spine.

A thoracic spine radiograph is required but may well be normal. A chest X-ray is also needed to look for evidence of tuberculosis. Later a bone scan may reveal other "hot spots"

### What is the differential diagnosis in this lady?

The differential diagnosis is spinal tuberculous osteomyelitis – Potts disease. A differential diagnosis may include staphylococcus aureus discitis although this tends to affect the lumbar spine whereas tuberculous spinal disease characteristically affects the thoracic spine, or the thoraco-lumbar junction.

The most useful investigation will be an MRI scan of the thoracic spine which will document the level of the tuberculous osteomyelitis and discitis and may well reveal a paravertebral abscess with bone destruction. Depending on the degree of bony destruction this lady may well need a neurosurgical opinion since there is a high risk of cord compression in the event of a vertebral collapse. Aspiration of the vertebral abscess is essential to culture the tubercle bacillus and to obtain the sensitivities. Therapy is with at least quadruple anti-tuberculous chemotherapy for a total of nine months. Other risk factors should always be considered, such as immunosuppression, and HIV disease.

Providing that vertebral collapse is avoided, prognosis is usually excellent in these patients if the organism is fully sensitive to therapy and compliance with therapy is maintained.

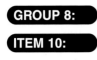

**Investigations**
- Full blood count
- ESR
- Urea and electrolytes
- Liver and bone biochemistry
- CRP

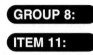

**GROUP 8:**

**ITEM 11:**

# Rheumatology
# Septic arthritis

---

**Investigations**

- Full blood count
- ESR
- Biochemistry including a serum urate

---

## CASE HISTORY

A 21-year-old man presents with pain and swelling of his right knee. On further questioning he is homosexual and there is no relevant past medical history. Specifically he has had no diarrhoea, urethritis, rashes or oral ulceration and has had no problems with inflammation of the eyes. (see Fig 8.11.1)

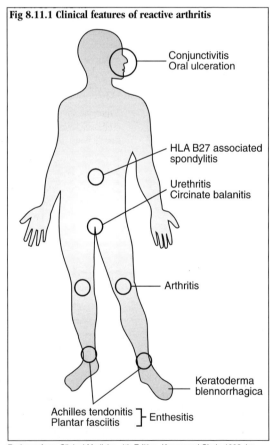

**Fig 8.11.1 Clinical features of reactive arthritis**

- Conjunctivitis
- Oral ulceration
- HLA B27 associated spondylitis
- Urethritis
- Circinate balanitis
- Arthritis
- Keratoderma blennorrhagica
- Achilles tendonitis
- Plantar fasciitis
- Enthesitis

Redrawn from *Clinical Medicine*, 4th Edition, Kumar and Clark, 1998, by permission of the publisher WB Saunders

### Discuss how you would investigate and manage this gentleman

The most common diagnosis in a young man with a monoarthritis is a reactive arthritis associated either with diarrhoea or with urethritis that may be gonococcal or chlamydial in origin. However, clinical questioning has excluded any associated features that may point to Reiter's disease (classical triad of urethritis, arthritis and conjunctivitis) and septic arthritis should be considered as the likeliest diagnosis raising the possibility of HIV disease.

The joint should be X-rayed and a series of blood cultures performed after the patient has been admitted.

Using sterile technique the joint should be aspirated and the fluid sent for microscopy, culture and crystals. The most common organism is staphylococcus aureus which is seen in between 40 and 70 per cent of patients. Gram negative organisms are the next most common but a careful search for gonorrhoea should be conducted and the patient should be referred to the genito-urinary medicine clinic for urethral swabs.

This gentleman is clearly at risk for HIV and should be counselled carefully before considering an HIV test. Should HIV be proven then microbiology assessment of the synovial fluid is crucial particularly for atypical organisms such as mycobacterium avium intracellulare and other forms of tuberculosis. Should HIV be established, then specialist referral would be helpful to consider anti-viral therapy.

In this man a septic arthritis was confirmed on blood and synovial fluid culture and requires six weeks of intravenous antibiotics, e.g. flucloxacillin and a cephalosporin such as Cefuroxime. Consideration should be given to arthroscopic drainage and washout of the joint to minimise joint damage.

---

**Examination of Synovial Fluid**

The fluid can be examined directly in a clear syringe or sterile pot. The characteristics of synovial fluid show a trend from clear to purulent which indicates roughly the type of arthritis.

| Colour | Diagnosis | WCC per mm$^3$ |
|---|---|---|
| Clear, yellow and viscous | OA | <3000 |
| Translucent and thin | RA | |
| Very cloudy | Seronegative arthritis | |
| | Reiter's disease | 3,000–40,000 |
| | Crystal arthritis | |
| | Sepsis | 750,000 |

**Polarized light microscopy** with a red filter needs to be undertaken by an expert:
• Gout – negatively birefringent, needle-shaped crystals of sodium urate
• Pyrophosphate arthropathy (pseudogout) – rhomboidal, weakly positively birefringent crystals of calcium pyrophosphate

**Gram staining** is essential if septic arthritis is suspected and may identify the organism immediately. Joint fluid should be cultured and antibiotic sensitivities requested.

RA = rheumatoid arthritis; OA = osteoarthritis

From *Clinical Medicine*, 4th Edition, Kumar and Clark, 1998, with permission

# Notes

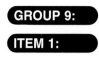

**GROUP 9:**

**ITEM 1:**

# Renal Disease

## Fluid balance and electrolytes: assessing fluid status

### How do you assess?

#### Clinical

Examine the patient. (see Fig 9.1.1)

| ✔ Useful | ✘ Not so useful |
|---|---|
| BP (especially postural drop) | Skin Turgor |
| Oedema | Eye Turgor |
| JVP | Mucous Membranes |
| Peripheral Perfusion | |
| Pulse | |
| Basal Crackles | |

#### Traps

- Mouth breathing can dry oral mucous membranes
- Autonomic neuropathy also causes POSTURAL DROP of blood pressure
- Ill patients often have basal crackles secondary to basal lung collapse
- Skin turgor depends on age
- Peripheral oedema does NOT always imply an adequate circulatory volume

#### Charts

| ✔ Useful | ✘ Not so useful |
|---|---|
| Serial weight (on same machine) | Fluid balance (input/output) |

#### Additional tools

| ✔ | ✘ |
|---|---|
| CVP line - use dynamically | CVP - absolute |
| CXR | Urine Na |
| Pulmonary artery flow catheter | Osmolality |

**Remember**

Examine the patient again!

(later today)

(tomorrow)

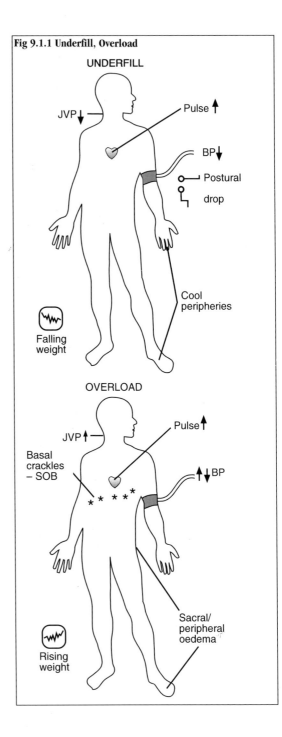

Fig 9.1.1 Underfill, Overload

**CVP GUIDE**
- Use dynamically

TAKE READING
↓
GIVE IV BOLUS (100mL N/saline) FLUID CHALLENGE
↓
REPEAT READING      ↑ FULL
                   → ↓ NOT FULL

- There is no ABSOLUTE value
- DO THIS YOURSELF!
  (If done correctly this gives accurate information)

**Fig 9.1.2 Fluid Challenge**

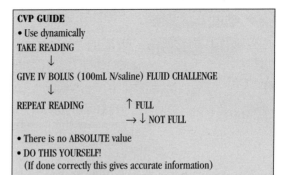

**Physiology Box**

Your patient is a "Box" with three compartments. The diagram shows these with the physical signs.

**Fig 9.1.3**

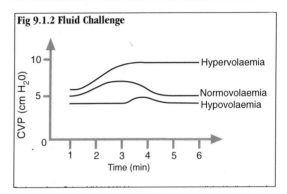

| INTRACELLULAR | INTERSTITIAL |
|---|---|
| Skin | Oedema |
| Mucous Membranes | |
| Cerebral Oedema | |
| | CIRCULATION |
| | BP, Pulse, JVP, Perfusion |

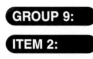

**Renal Disease**

**Fluid balance and electrolytes: sodium problems**

### What are you ACTUALLY measuring when you measure the serum sodium?

A ratio of:

EXTRACELLULAR $Na^+$      mmol
EXTRACELLULAR WATER      litres

Using this concept you can now describe how serum $Na^+$ becomes abnormally low (Hyponatraemia) or high (Hypernatraemia) (Table 9.2.1).

**Table 9.2.1 Hyponatraemia and hypernatraemia**

| | 'RATIO' ($Na^+$:water) | EXTRACELLULAR WATER |
|---|---|---|
| Hyponatraemia | WATER ↑ <br> WATER ↑>$Na^+$↑ <br> $Na^+$ ↓ | → or ↑ <br> ↑↑ <br> ↓ |
| Hypernatraemia | WATER ↓ <br> WATER ↓>$Na^+$ ↓ <br> $Na^+$ ↑ | → or ↓ <br> ↓↓ <br> ↑ |

### How do I work out why?

The key is to determine extracellular water. GO EXAMINE THE PATIENT (see Assessing Fluid Status Fig 9.1.1)

**Hyponatraemia**

### CASE HISTORY

The gynaecology SHO is worried about a 53-year-old lady who is three days post-op following a transabdominal hysterectomy. She has a serum $Na^+$ that has fallen to 119 mmol/l. "Shall I give some TWICE NORMAL SALINE?"

The polite answer is NO!

### Management

• Fluid assessment
• Examine fluid charts

In this case the patient showed no features of fluid depletion – this excludes true $Na^+$ depletion.

**Remember**

- "Wherever Na+ goes water is sure to follow," and vice versa
- However, you discover the patient has been receiving 5% dextrose IVI since surgery.

This is probably the most common cause of hyponatraemia in a hospital inpatient

## Action

- STOP I.V. fluids & WAIT i.e. RESTRICT FLUIDS

## Other causes of hyponatraemia (not in this case!)

- Diuretic therapy
- Syndrome of inappropriate ADH production
- Severe heart failure
- Advanced liver cirrhosis

## Hypernatraemia

Three main causes in practice:

- Impaired thirst – unconscious patient
- Osmotic diuresis e.g. diabetic ketoacidosis
- Water loss e.g. diabetes insipidus

These ALL equal WATER DEFICIENCY.

**Remember**

True Na+ overload is invariably IATROGENIC and gives a clinical picture of FLUID OVERLOAD

## Treatment

- Avoid rapid correction (see Fig 9.2.1).
- INITIALLY give I.V. N/Saline. This stays in extracellular compartment
  (see assessing fluid status Item 1)
- Ensure slow correction

## Key Points

- Examine the Patient – know where their water is
- Slow correction
- Hyponatraemia is more common
- Hypernatraemia is generally found in ITU

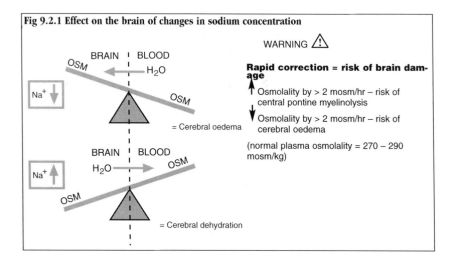

Fig 9.2.1 Effect on the brain of changes in sodium concentration

WARNING ⚠

**Rapid correction = risk of brain damage**

↑ Osmolality by > 2 mosm/hr – risk of central pontine myelinolysis

↓ Osmolality by > 2 mosm/hr – risk of cerebral oedema

(normal plasma osmolality = 270 – 290 mosm/kg)

---

**GROUP 9:**

# Renal Disease

**ITEM 3:**

# Patient stopped passing urine

### CASE HISTORY

The surgical House Officer calls you at 10pm. I have a 62-year-old man, two days post laparotomy, who isn't passing urine. Help!

DO: See the patient

DON'T: Simply give telephone advice

### Common causes

- Urine retention –(always catheterise)
- Dehydration – assess fluid status. See Fig 9.1.1
- Shock – see table 9.3.1.
- Drugs – look at medicines chart

**Table 9.3.1 SHOCK – failure of organ perfusion**

|  | BP | Peripheral Perfusion | CVP | Brief Action |
|---|---|---|---|---|
| Hypovolaemia | ↓ | ↓ | ↓ | Look for overt/covert loss & replace with appropriate fluid e.g. saline or blood |
| Cardiogenic | ↓ | ↓ | → ↑ | MI may need inotropes |
| Septic | ↓ | → ↑ | → ↓ | Look for source, give antimicrobials ±inotropes |

## Initial Management

Most cases are fluid depleted and therefore need careful FLUID REPLACEMENT:

- Normal Saline (0.9%) I.V.
- Write up initial regimen – modulate according to patient age, size and severity
- Reassess fluid status REGULARLY
- When in doubt use a CVP LINE

## Aim

To establish a DIURESIS of at least 100ml per hour. In most cases a failure to achieve this is because of inadequate fluid replacement.

## Other actions

- Us and Es
- Stop potentially nephrotoxic drugs
- Stop antihypertensive drugs
- Ask nurses to record daily weights

## Still no urine?

- Are you certain the patient is adequately fluid replete?
- Check that the urine catheter is NOT blocked or misplaced
- GIVE A LOOP DIURETIC
- Investigate further
- Take steps to PREVENT FLUID OVERLOAD
- Patient may now have established renal failure. REFER TO NEPHROLOGIST

## Key Points

- Don't miss urine retention
- Recognise shock
- Assess fluid status regularly
- Most cases will need fluid replacement, and failure to achieve this will result in established renal failure

**Remember**

Shock is a life threatening condition that often requires a critical care environment. CALL FOR HELP

**Remember**

HYPERKALAEMIA NEEDS URGENT MANAGEMENT see Group 9 item 5

**Table 9.3.2 Intravenous fluids in general use for fluid and electrolyte disturbances**

| | $Na^+$ (mmol/l) | $K^+$ (mmol/l) | $HCO_3^-$ or equivalent (mmol/l | $Cl^-$ (mmol/l) | $Ca^{2+}$ (mmol/l) | Indication (see footnote) |
|---|---|---|---|---|---|---|
| Normal plasma values | 142 | 4.5 | 26 | 103 | 2.5 | |
| Sodium chloride 0.9% | 150 | - | 150 | - | 1 | |
| Sodium chloride 0.18% + glucose 4% | 30 | - | - | 30 | - | 2 |
| Glucose 5% + potassium chloride 0.3% | - | 40 | - | 40 | - | 3 |
| Sodium bicarbonate 1.26% | 150 | - | 150 | - | - | 4 |
| Compound sodium lactate (Hartmann's) | 131 | 5 | 29 | 111 | 2 | 5 |

1. Volume expansion in hypovolaemic patients. Rarely to maintain fluid balance when there are large losses of sodium. The sodium (150 mmol/l) is greater than plasma and hypernatraemia can result. It is often necessary to add KCl 20-40 mmol/l.
2. Maintenance of fluid balance in normovolaemic, normonatraemic patients.
3. To replace water. Can be given with or without potassium chloride. May be alternated with normal saline as an alternative to (2).
4. For volume expansion in hypovolaemic, acidotic patients alternating with (1). Occasionally for maintenance of fluid balance combined with (2) in salt-wasting, acidotic patients. To induce forced alkaline diuresis, e.g. in severe salicylate poisoning.
5. Used for maintenance of fluid balance after surgery. The potassium content may be dangerous in renal failure but occasionally useful in the diuretic phase of acute tubular necrosis where hypokalaemia occurs.

Redrawn from *Clinical Medicine*, 4th Edition, Kumar and Clark, 1998, by permission of the publisher WB Saunders

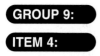

# Renal Disease
## Left ventricular failure

### CASE HISTORY

A 65-year-old 50kg woman who smokes 20 cigarettes per day, with a past history of intermittent claudication, presented to A&E with acute shortness of breath. She is on no medication. On examination she was centrally and peripherally cyanosed, and peripherally cold and clammy, with a raised JVP, gallop rhythm and bilateral coarse crackles to both mid-zones. She had absent foot pulses and bilateral femoral bruits. Her BP at presentation was 195/98. Her ECG showed only hypertensive changes, and CXR showed bilateral perihilar shadowing.

### Initially her biochemistry was:

Na      142mmol/l
K̇       3.1mmol/l
Urea    12mmol/l
Creatinine 115μmol/l

She responded well to oxygen, I.V. opiate, I.V. loop diuretic and a vasodilator (Captopril 12.5mg)

### But four days later her biochemistry was:

Na      142mmol/l
K       6.0mmol/l
Urea    54mmol/l
Creatinine 500μmol/l, (see Fig 9.4.1)

### What has gone wrong?

It is very likely that she has underlying renovascular disease.

### Clinical suspicion of renovascular disease

- Most patients will have disseminated atheroma and will have missing pulses and/or bruits.
- Abdominal/renal bruits (although they have a very strong association with Renal artery stenosis (RAS) are rare.
- 'Flash pulmonary oedema' (without an obvious precipitant is a good predictor of renovascular disease.
- Brittle response to volume loading or off-loading (see Fig 9.4.3)

**Her renal function was abnormal at presentation**

### Fig 9.4.1 INTERPRETING SERUM CREATININE

The serum creatinine in the healthy population is normally distributed according to muscle bulk. Only large, well muscled men will usually have a creatinine >110 if their renal function is normal.

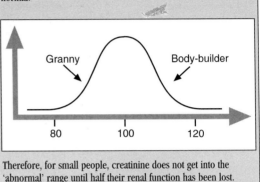

Therefore, for small people, creatinine does not get into the 'abnormal' range until half their renal function has been lost.

---

## *i*

**Information**

'THE FIRST REFLEX OF THE ISCHAEMIC KIDNEY IS TO RETAIN SALT AND WATER'

(Dr C Ogg, Guy's Hospital)

---

**ACE inhibitors can cause acute renal failure in patients with renovascular disease**

Fig 9.4.2a – d Effect of ACE inhibitors

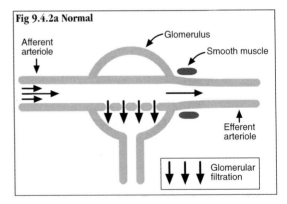

Fig 9.4.2a Normal

## Fig 9.4.2b

STIMULUS

Reduced renal perfusion ⟶ reduced trans-glomerular pressure ⟶ reduced GFR

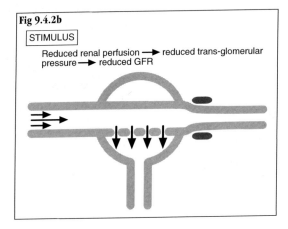

## Fig 9.4.2c

RESPONSE

Intra-renal activation of Renin/Angiotensin system leads to preferential efferent arteriolar vasoconstriction ⟶ restores trans-glomerular pressure ⟶ restores GFR

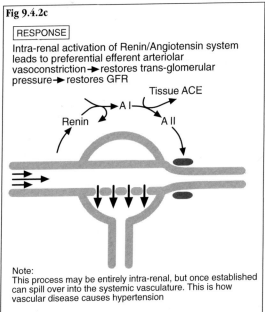

Note:
This process may be entirely intra-renal, but once established can spill over into the systemic vasculature. This is how vascular disease causes hypertension

Group 9 • Renal Disease

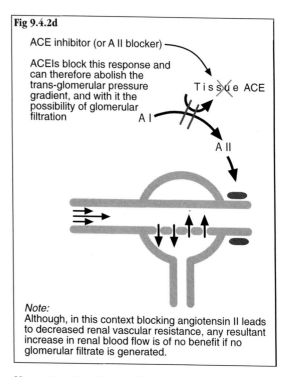

**Fig 9.4.2d**

ACE inhibitor (or A II blocker)

ACEIs block this response and can therefore abolish the trans-glomerular pressure gradient, and with it the possibility of glomerular filtration

Tissue ACE

A I

A II

*Note:*
Although, in this context blocking angiotensin II leads to decreased renal vascular resistance, any resultant increase in renal blood flow is of no benefit if no glomerular filtrate is generated.

**How should patients like this to be managed?**

The key to successful management is very careful fluid control.

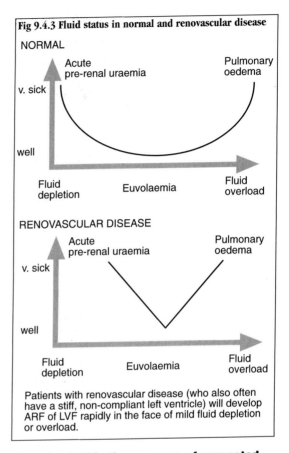

**Fig 9.4.3 Fluid status in normal and renovascular disease**

NORMAL

Patients with renovascular disease (who also often have a stiff, non-compliant left ventricle) will develop ARF of LVF rapidly in the face of mild fluid depletion or overload.

### Managing LVF in the presence of suspected renovascular disease

- Do treat the pulmonary oedema – it is a dangerous and very distressing condition
- Avoid ACEIs/AII blockers – use other vasodilators
- Avoid rapid volume off-loading – titrate diuretic dose against renal function
- Insert a CVP line and use it properly (see Fig 9.1.1)
- Examine (and weigh) patient regularly. Consider using low-dose dopamine (can be given via peripheral line at 2.5mg/kg/min) for its natiuretic effect

### Fig 9.4.4 ON THE NATURAL HISTORY OF ATHEROMATOUS RENOVASCULAR DISEASE

1. ACEI/AII blockers will only cause ARF if both kidneys are affected by RAS, or only one functioning kidney is present. BUT atheroma is diffuse and progressive. Complete renal artery occlusion with total loss of renal function on one side is usually clinically SILENT.

2. Anatomical renovascular disease is very common, and much of

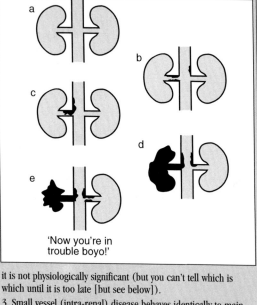

'Now you're in trouble boyo!'

it is not physiologically significant (but you can't tell which is which until it is too late [but see below]).

3. Small vessel (intra-renal) disease behaves identically to main renal artery disease (but you can't treat it).

### Further renal imaging investigations

- Ultrasound – Unequal renal size ( > 2cm difference) is a good predictor of renovascular disease, but its absence does not exclude RAS

- Isotope renography – Unequal function, slow transit, altered dynamics with captopril are all suggestive. Can be used as a screening test to save those with low probability of having RAS from having to undergo angiography.

- Intra-arterial angiography – Gold Standard should be done by experienced radiologist with care and minimal contrast load (risk of precipitating LVF).

- Other modalities – e.g. Doppler U/S/Magnetic resonance angiography/Spiral CT: techniques being evaluated.

**GROUP 9:**

**ITEM 5:**

# Renal Disease
# Hyperkalaemia

*"Don't let your patient die tonight . . ."*

**Remember**
This is a life-threatening condition

## CASE HISTORY

A 70-year-old woman has been admitted by the vascular surgeons with an acutely ischaemic limb. She is on an ACE inhibitor and diuretic for hypertension and also on an NSAID

It is 2am.

The surgical SHO calls you because her $K^+$ has come back at 7.2 mmol/l

The surgical SHO is panicking

### What do you do next?

If $K^+ > 6.5$ mmol/l DO THIS:

**Remember**
There are no usual symptoms of life-threatening hyperkalaemia

- Immediate cardio protection – 10ml of 10% Ca Gluconate over 10 min
- Get $K^+$ inside cells – 50ml of 50% glucose with (or followed by) 20 U insulin. 5mg of nebulised salbutamol can be tried.

See Fig 9.5.1

NOW YOU HAVE TIME TO STOP AND THINK: $K^+$ is usually telling you that something has gone badly wrong. Find it and treat it!

### Common reversible causes of $K^+$

- Tissue hypoxia/damage
- Acidosis
- $K^+$ sparing diuretics
- ACEI
- Blood transfusion
- Acute renal failure

**Remember**
If $K^+$ is not responding your patient may need dialysis – refer to nephrologist.

### Quick and simple ways to stop or reverse underlying causes of raised $K^+$.

- Establish a diuresis
- Stop $K^+$ sparing diuretics/ACEI/NSAID/slow $K^+$
- Stop blood transfusion
- Successfully treat systemic sepsis

### While you are thinking

- Assess volume status
- Look for ischaemic/damaged tissue – have you considered bowel ischaemia?

• Get an ECG
• Check ABGs
• Check Drug Chart

### If you can't promptly reverse the cause

• Give a loop diuretic
• Consider giving $NaHCO_3$ – small aliquots – see controversy box 9.6.2, e.g. 25-50ml 8.4%
• Consider getting a surgeon to remove any ischaemic tissue (or revascularise it)
• Treat tomorrow's $K^+$ with $Ca^{++}$ resonium
  (15gm orally with 10ml lactulose or 30gm PR)

### Now go back and re-examine the patient

• Fluid status
• Peripheral perfusion
• Acid/base status
• Re-check U&E

**Remember**

1ml of 8.4% NaHCO3= 1mmol $Na^+$. Don't kill your patient with sodium overload – see fluid status assessment fig 9.1.1}

**Remember**

Myths that are NOT true
• A normal ECG implies your patient is not in danger
• $Ca^{++}$ resonium will alter tonight's $K^+$

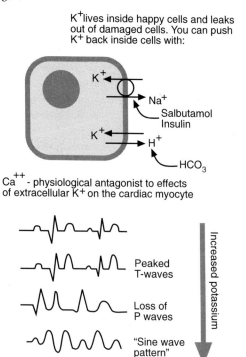

**Fig 9.5.1**

$K^+$ lives inside happy cells and leaks out of damaged cells. You can push $K^+$ back inside cells with:

$K^+$
$Na^+$
Salbutamol
Insulin
$K^+$
$H^+$
$HCO_3$

$Ca^{++}$ - physiological antagonist to effects of extracellular $K^+$ on the cardiac myocyte

Increased potassium

Peaked T-waves

Loss of P waves

"Sine wave pattern"

### Less common causes of hyperkalaemia

- *Endocrine:*
  Addisons
  Isolated hypoaldosteronism
  C-21 hydoxylase deficiency
  Congenital adrenal syndromes e.g. 3 β hydroxydehydrogenase deficiency
- *Additional drugs:*
  Cyclosporin
  Succinylcholine
  NSAIDs
- *Others:*
  Tumour lysis syndrome
  Periodic hyperkalaemia paralysis
  Malignant hyperthermia
  Familial hyperkalaemia acidosis

**GROUP 9:**

**ITEM 6:**

# Renal Disease
# The acidotic patient

## CASE HISTORY

A 50-year-old woman with chronic renal impairment developed laryngeal oedema as an idiosyncratic reaction to a phenothiazine. She became hypotensive and oliguric.

On admission her blood gases showed:

- pH 6.9
- $pO_2$ 6.0
- $pCO_2$ 8.2
- $HCO_3$ 15

On intubation, ventilation and fluid resuscitation, her B.P. rose to 145/70. Her blood gases returned to normal over the next 12 hours.

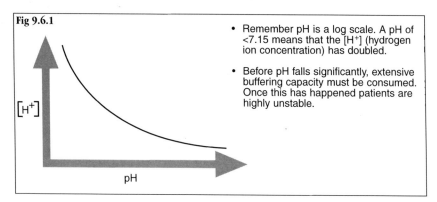

**Fig 9.6.1**

- Remember pH is a log scale. A pH of <7.15 means that the $[H^+]$ (hydrogen ion concentration) has doubled.

- Before pH falls significantly, extensive buffering capacity must be consumed. Once this has happened patients are highly unstable.

## How to manage severe acidosis

- Airway
- Breathing
- circulation

} Problems with any of these will contribute to acidosis and must be corrected

## Identify and treat underlying problem

Tissue damage/hypoxia is by far the commonest cause of metabolic acidosis. Examples include:

- Sepsis
  – Hypotensive patient with warm peripheries
  – Often apyrexial and/or normal WBC on presentation, especially if very sick or elderly
  – Sometimes develop $PO_4\downarrow$

**Remember**

Less than 5% of patients admitted with pH, 7.0 survive to discharge from hospital. This is because severe acidosis is a reflection of serious underlying problems.

- Rhabdomyolysis
  - Areas of muscle necrosis not always clinically evident
  - $PO_4\uparrow$, $K^+\uparrow$
  - May have biphasic $Ca^{++}$ pattern (initially $\downarrow$ due to binding to damaged muscle, then $\uparrow$)
- Bowel ischaemia
  - Severe acidosis
  - $PO_4\uparrow$, $K^+\uparrow$
  - Often have evidence of peripheral vascular disease
- Heart failure
  - Pump failure leading to tissue hypoperfusion
  - Often accompanied by renal hypoperfusion and impaired renal function

**Remember**

Find and treat the underlying cause

**Fig 9.6.2**

The role of I.V. $HCO_3$ is not clear

Remember, 8.4 % $HCO_3$ = 1mmol/ml $Na^+$. It is very easy to precipitate volume overload

May be indicated if pH < 7.25 in an attempt to reduce the depression of myocardial function produced by severe acidosis
BICARBONATE WILL NOT SAVE YOUR PATIENT IF YOU DON'T CORRECT THE UNDERLYING CAUSE OF ACIDOSIS (but it might help keep them alive until you do).

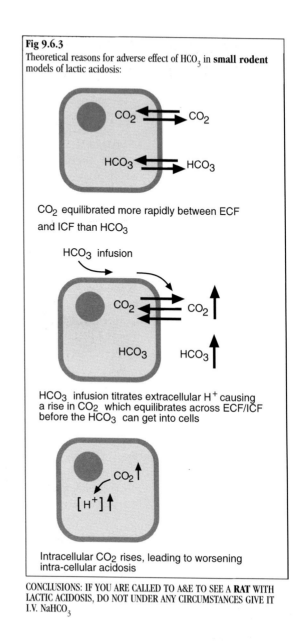

**Fig 9.6.3**

Theoretical reasons for adverse effect of $HCO_3$ in **small rodent** models of lactic acidosis:

$CO_2$ equilibrated more rapidly between ECF and ICF than $HCO_3$

$HCO_3$ infusion

$HCO_3$ infusion titrates extracellular $H^+$ causing a rise in $CO_2$ which equilibrates across ECF/ICF before the $HCO_3$ can get into cells

Intracellular $CO_2$ rises, leading to worsening intra-cellular acidosis

CONCLUSIONS: IF YOU ARE CALLED TO A&E TO SEE A **RAT** WITH LACTIC ACIDOSIS, DO NOT UNDER ANY CIRCUMSTANCES GIVE IT I.V. $NaHCO_3$

**GROUP 9:**

**ITEM 7:**

# Renal Disease
# Acute renal failure

## CASE HISTORY

Consider a 75-year-old man with a five-day history of anorexia, nausea, vomiting and lethargy. The GP has made the following findings:

- Hb          10.0 g/dl
- Urea        48 mmol/l
- creatinine  820 µmol/l

The previous history includes mild hypertension and osteoarthritis

### What are your priorities?

### a) SAFETY

- Treat life-threatening HYPERKALAEMIA (see Group 9, Item 5)
- Fluid assessment (see Fig 9.1.1)
  - DRY    Treat with fluids
  - WET    Treat with fluid restriction
  - OKAY

In this case the patient has a $K^+$ of 5.6mmol/l and his fluid status is okay. At this stage review /stop any drug therapy

Now, you have to consider:

- Why does this man have renal failure?
- Is it potentially reversible?
- Do you need to refer to a renal unit?

### b) TEST THE URINE (& send MSU)

Blood + Protein = 'Active' Urine and suggests active glomerular disease in the absence of infection.

### c) RENAL TRACT IMAGING

**Investigations**
- Immunological markers
- Serum protein electrophoresis
- Twenty-four hour urinary protein loss

### What investigation would you arrange?

- Ultrasound (see below)

In this case the renal ultrasound is NORMAL, and this tells you:

- There is a low probability of obstruction
- There is the potential that there is a reversible component

### d) REFER TO A RENAL UNIT

- DON'T DELAY! The commonest concern expressed by Renal Units is that the referring teams wait too long and end up transferring the case in a critical condition
- BE PREPARED – See 'Questions you will be asked' (below).

## Guide to indications for dialysis

There is no MAGIC level of urea or creatinine.

Dialysis is indicated in:

- Uncontrolled hyperkalaemia
- Unresponsive pulmonary oedema
- Patient symptoms

## Outcome

In this case the patient turned out to be taking an NSAID. He required haemodialysis for uncontrolled vomiting and subsequently had a renal biopsy. This showed INTERSTITIAL NEPHRITIS secondary to NSAID and responded well to a short course of steroids.

## Questions you will be asked when referring to a Renal Unit

- Is the patient passing urine?
- What is the fluid status of the patient?
- Have you done a Renal Ultrasound?
- Is the Urine 'active'?
- Any Nephrotoxic drugs?
- Hepatitis Status?

## Renal tract imaging

### Ultrasound

- Non-invasive
- Independent of renal function
- Can measure size (renal length and cortical thickening)
- Limited or NO view of ureters
- Low detection rate of renal calculi
- Operator dependent

### Intravenous urogram (IVU)

- Good visualisation of pelvico-calyceal system and ureters
- Gives some functional information
- Demonstrates parenchymal scarring
- No value when creat. > 250 µmol/l
- Exposure to ionising radiation
- Risk of contrast toxicity

### Summary of renal tract imaging
KEY POINTS

- In renal failure ultrasound is first choice investigation
- A normal renal ultrasound does NOT always exclude obstruction
- When investigating haematuria BOTH ultrasound and IVU are indicated

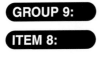

## Renal Disease
## Chronic renal failure

### CASE HISTORY

A 35-year-old lady registers with a new GP and is found to be hypertensive (180/105), with blood and protein in her urine. Blood tests reveal:

- Hb          8.5 g/dl
- Urea        18.0 mmol/l
- Creatinine  310 µmol/l

| HISTORY | Asymptomatic | Comment<br>CRF is an insidious disease with no specific symptoms |
|---|---|---|
| EXAMINATION | Pallor<br>BP<br>Grade II hypertensive retinopathy | Apart from hypertension, these cases have few specific physical signs<br>EXCEPT    * Polycystic kidneys<br>              • Renal bruits |
| INVESTIGATION | Renal ultrasound | Small, non-obstructed kidneys |

This lady has irreversible renal failure and subsequent follow-up showed a progressive rise in creatinine.

### How do you manage this case?
A multi-disciplinary approach (Fig 9.8.1)

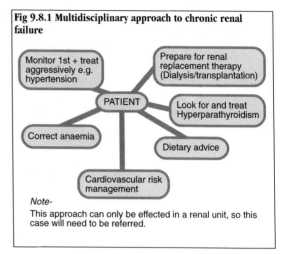

**Fig 9.8.1 Multidisciplinary approach to chronic renal failure**

Monitor 1st + treat aggressively e.g. hypertension

Prepare for renal replacement therapy (Dialysis/transplantation)

PATIENT

Look for and treat Hyperparathyroidism

Correct anaemia

Dietary advice

Cardiovascular risk management

Note-
This approach can only be effected in a renal unit, so this case will need to be referred.

**Remember**

- CRF is an insidious condition with no specific symptoms. In some cases the patient does not present until they have reached the stage when dialysis is required
- Preparing the patient for dialysis is a specialist task – REFER PLEASE!
- CRF is a major cardiovascular risk factor – the average dialysis patient is approximately 15 times at risk

**Remember**

CONTROL OF HYPERTENSION IS THE SINGLE MOST IMPORTANT FACTOR

## Preparing the patient

- Educate – need for specialist counsellor
- Decide on mode of therapy (haemodialysis vs peritoneal dialysis)
- Plan access surgery – an AV-fistula requires at least six weeks before it can be used

## Hyperparathyroidism

- Measure PTH – radiographs only become diagnostic in advanced cases
- Control phosphate
  - dietician
  - phosphate binding drugs (e.g. calcium carbonate)
- Vitamin D analogues (e.g. alfa calcidol)
- Monitor $Ca^{2+}$ and phosphate

## Anaemia

- Correct iron deficiency (if present)
- Erythropoietin – can only be given by sub-cutaneous injection x3 weekly
- Target Hb 12.0 g/dl
- Monitor BP

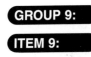

# Renal Disease

# Multi-system vasculitis/acute glomerular nephritis

## CASE HISTORY

A 54-year-old man with a month's history of cough and SOB which has not responded to two courses of antibiotics from his GP (Amoxicillin, then Clarithromycin and Co-Amoxiclav), re-presented to his GP complaining of fatigue, muscle aches and pains. He requested a 'tonic'.

A week later he came to A&E complaining of acute SOB. His CXR showed fluffy bilateral patchy alveolar shadowing, and his creatinine was 350. On further investigation, he was c-ANCA positive. Renal biopsy showed focal necrotising glomerulonephritis. He responded well to immunosuppression.

## Inflammatory auto-immune vasculitis: microscopic polyangiitis/Wegeners granulomatosis

Very non-specific presentation – typically vague arthralgia and myalgia with fatigue, anorexia and malaise

At a later stage they may develop:

• Vasculitic rash
• Mono-neuritis multiplex
• Arthritis

At which point the diagnosis is more obvious, BUT

THESE DISEASES RESPOND WELL TO TREATMENT IF DIAGNOSED EARLY.

## Pulmonary haemorrhage

• Commonest disease related cause of death in ANCA +ve vasculitis and anti-GBM (glomerular basement membrane) disease (Goodpasture's syndrome)
• CXR appearances very variable but usually patchy alveolar shadowing (can mimic, or be accompanied by pulmonary oedema or chest infection)
• Often precipitated by pulmonary oedema/infection/smoking
• Can be diagnosed non-invasively by finding Kco↓

### Information

Most GPs will see many patients with vague muscle aches and pains in a day They will see few, if any, patients with multi-system vasculitis in their working lifetimes.

To identify patients with multi-system vasculitis, dipstick the urine and don't ignore microscopic haematuria.

### Remember

If diagnosed late, these diseases have difficult and life-threatening complications.

## What to do

- Requires urgent nephrology and ITU referral: these patients can become very sick very quickly, and may need ventilation and plasma exchange

### How to diagnose multi-system vasculitis?

If you find microscopic haematuria in a patient with non-specific malaise/myalgia

- Enquire specifically for suggestive symptoms:
  - nasal congestion/nose bleeds (in Wegeners granulomatosis)
  - rash
  - neurological symptoms
- Examine carefully for:
  - splinter haemorrhages
  - nail fold infarcts
  - mouth ulcers
  - rash
  - neuropathy
- Don't assume that microscopic haematuria is due to UTI – send an MSU.
- If there are suggestive symptoms or signs:
  Discuss with a nephrologist.
- If there are no suggestive symptoms or signs but MSU is -ve:
  Check renal function, if it is abnormal, discuss with a nephrologist.

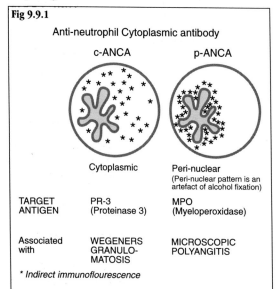

**Fig 9.9.1**

Anti-neutrophil Cytoplasmic antibody

c-ANCA          p-ANCA

Cytoplasmic          Peri-nuclear
                     (Peri-nuclear pattern is an
                     artefact of alcohol fixation)

| TARGET ANTIGEN | PR-3 (Proteinase 3) | MPO (Myeloperoxidase) |
| --- | --- | --- |
| Associated with | WEGENERS GRANULO-MATOSIS | MICROSCOPIC POLYANGITIS |

* Indirect immunoflourescence

> ⚠️
>
> **Remember**
>
> These diseases will irretrievably damage your patient's kidneys in a matter of weeks. Prompt diagnoses and treatment can make the long-term difference between life on dialysis and life on a small dose of steroids.

**ANCA points** (see Fig 9.9.1)

- False +ves occur in situations of polyclonal B-cell activation (usually on immunohistology but not against specific target antigens)
- ANCA -ve small vessel vasculitis can be clinically and pathologically identical to ANCA +ve vasculitis
- Changes in antibody titre may be unrelated to, lag behind, or precede changes in disease activity in different patients
- ANCA subtypes are being recognised, e.g. x ANCA

**Other markers of disease activity**

ESR↑ CRP↑ Thrombocytosis

**Other rapidly progressive glomerulonephritides (GN)**

- Goodpasture's disease is rare. It is classically described as a "one hit" disease, and is less likely to be preceded by a non-specific pro-drome than ANCA +ve vasculitis
- IgA nephropathy, mesangiocapillary GN, and diffuse proliferative GN in SLE can all present with a rapidly progressive, crescentric nephritis

**GROUP 9:**

**ITEM 10:**

# Renal Disease

# Intercurrent illness in dialysis and transplant patients

*(Or - How to kill a patient so fast you won't know what hit you...)*

## CASE HISTORY 1

A 72-year-old type II diabetic haemodialysis patient was brought in by urgent ambulance to his local DGH complaining of chest pain and SOB. He was due to be dialysed later that day at the nearest renal unit (five miles away). On admission he had signs of mild biventricular heart failure. His ECG showed lateral ischaemia and his Hb was 8.2 gm/dl.

He was given I.V. nitrates and two units blood under cover of 40mg frusemide.

As the second unit of blood ran through, he complained of acute shortness of breath, then suffered a cardio-respiratory arrest, from which he could not be resuscitated.

**Other things NOT TO DO in dialysis patients**

**a) ACCESS PRESERVATION**

**Remember**

- DON'T give blood transfusion in dialysis patient unless a nephrologist tells you to
- You may precipitate lethal hyperkalaemia and volume overload (and the normal methods of treating these complaints will be ineffective).
- ALSO: Even if your patient survives, you may sensitise them to HLA antigens in the blood, thereby denying them the chance of a renal transplant.
- AS A GENERAL RULE. Dialysis patients should be transfused while on dialysis

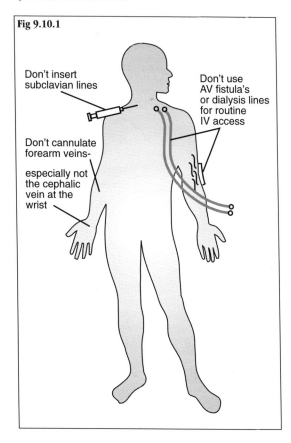

Fig 9.10.1

Don't insert subclavian lines

Don't use AV fistula's or dialysis lines for routine IV access

Don't cannulate forearm veins-

especially not the cephalic vein at the wrist

Dialysis access is essential for life-preserving treatment and potential sites for it are limited and easily damaged irretrievably.

Use veins in hands or feet or the antecubital fossa. For central access use the internal jugular

**b) FLUIDS**

Dialysis patients DO NOT need 2l/day of I.V. fluid post operatively.

**Things to watch out for in dialysis patients:**

- **Vascular disease**
  Ischaemic heart disease is very common in dialysis patients – even young ones.
  It is often unmasked by anaemia.

• **Infection**

Dialysis patients are significantly functionally immunosuppressed.

They cope poorly with sepsis and rapidly become systemically unwell.

Infections in access sites (lines, fistulas, PD catheters) are common and may not be clinically evident e.g. subacute infective endocarditis and osteomyelitis – always think of these complications.

• **Electrolytes**

• Haemodialysis patients are often chronically hyperkalaemic pre-dialysis (and invariably hypokalaemic immediately post-dialysis).

• They will often present with hypercalcaemia (too much vit-D or $Ca^{++}$ based $PO_4$-binders) or hypocalcaemia (too little).

• Poorly compliant patients are routinely hyperphosphataemic, if they then start taking their "prescribed" doses of vit-D (1–$\alpha$ calcidol) and $Ca^{++}$ based phosphate binders, their $Ca^{++}$ x $PO_4$ product may exceed 7mmol/l, precipitating ectopic calcification.

## CASE HISTORY 2

A 23-year-old renal transplant recipient (primary renal disease – vesico-ureteric reflux), on standard triple-therapy immuno-suppression (Prednisolone, Azathioprine, Cyclosporin), presented with a hot, swollen, exquisitely painful ankle.

The joint was aspirated and moderate pus cells, with birefringent crystals were seen on microscopy.

The symptoms responded to colchicine after which allopurinol was started (300mg OD).

Three weeks later, the patient presented, shocked with pancyto-penia, developed multi-organ failure, and died.

### Beware

• DRUG INTERACTIONS THAT MATTER IN TRANSPLANTATION
• Allopurinol and Azathioprine
• Azathioprine is metabolised to 6-mercaptopurine, which is metabolised by xanthine oxidase. Allopurinol inhibits xanthine oxidase and effectively trebles or quadruples the functional dose of azathioprine leading to significant bone-marrow depression
• Cyclosporin

| Increase CyA levels e.g. | Reduce CyA levels e.g. |
| --- | --- |
| • Macrolides e.g. Erythromycin | • Rifampicin |
| • Calcium channel blockers | • antiepileptics |
| • Triazoles | |

### Things to watch out for in renal transplant patients

• Infections

The level of immunosuppression is high initially, and then reduced.

A wide range of opportunistic infections can occur:

| Viral | Bacterial | Protozoal | Fungal |
|-------|-----------|-----------|--------|
| CMV | TB | Pneumocystis | Candida |
| EBV | Listeria | Toxoplasma | Aspergillus |
| HSV | Nocardia | | |
| VZV | Salmonella | | |

• Vascular disease

Remains very common after transplantation. Death (with a functioning graft) from IHD is the biggest cause of graft loss.

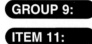

**GROUP 9:**

**ITEM 11:**

# Renal Disease
# Nephrotic syndrome

Nephrotic Syndrome is not a diagnosis but a set of signs and symptoms.

• Oedema
• Proteinuria – usually > 3g per day
• Hypoalbuminaemia
• Hypercholesterolaemia. This is a secondary phenomena due to increased liver synthesis associated with increased protein synthesis
  – it can be very resistant to lipid lowering drugs
  – treat the primary condition
• Thrombophilia. Nephrotic syndrome is associated with an increased clotting tendency and risk of thromboembolic disease. It is also a secondary condition. However, while the patient is nephrotic, anticoagulation is indicated especially in membranous nephropathy.

## CASE HISTORY

An 18-year-old girl presents with a two-week history of swollen ankles and mild dyspnoea on exertion.

Nephrotic syndrome is confirmed by:

• Serum albumin 19g/l
• Twenty-four hour urine protein 5.6g per day

**Remember**

In Nephrotic Syndrome there is a reduction in circulating volume in the presence of oedema – look for a POSTURAL BP DROP (See Assessing Fluid Status figure 9.1.1).

• Fasting cholesterol 8.7 mmol/l

## Management

The aim in ALL cases is to make a diagnosis.

## How?

Although various non-invasive tests may hint at the diagnosis, in most adult cases a RENAL BIOPSY is required.

## Renal biopsy findings

Don't panic – you do not need to know about renal histo-pathology!

However, here is a list of some common diagnoses and therapeutic strategies.

This case turns out to have minimal change disease and responds promptly to oral steroids.

| DIAGNOSIS | TREATMENT |
|---|---|
| Minimal change disease | steroids (1st line) |
| | CyA |
| Membranous Nephropathy | None |
| | or ACE-Inhibitors |
| | or steroids |
| | or steroids + azathioprine |
| Lupus Nephritis | Immunosuppression |
| Diabetic Nephropathy | ACE-Inhibitors for hypertension |
| | Improve glycaemic control |
| Vasculitis | Immunosuppression |
| Amyloid | 1° – consider myeloma chemotherapy |
| | 2° – treat underlying condition |

**Remember**

The use of IV albumin is controversial, but its use is declining. However, where severe reduction in circulating volume threatens renal function, its use may help prevent acute renal failure.

# Notes

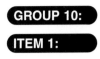

## Cardiology

## Syncope

*(see also Group 15, Item 13)*

Simple faints are a common and benign condition, but anyone witnessing a faint will know that patients can look awful, and it is not surprising that many are brought to hospital for assessment. Unfortunately, too, a lack of first aid knowledge in the general public means that patients who faint are often sat in a chair or even stood up – either causing a recurrence or delaying recovery.

### CASE HISTORY 1

A 25-year-old man is brought to hospital having fainted at work. He still appears pale but clinical examination is normal. He had a similar episode two years earlier.

### What are the key questions in establishing the diagnosis?

- Reliable witness account – if not available, make a phone call to work!
- Prodromal symptoms – non-specific but almost always present for some minutes before
- Precipitating cause – anything from the sight of blood to a hangover
- Circumstance of event: frequently in:
  - pub (even without alcohol)
  - restaurant – before or after food
  - church, synagogue or mosque
  - warm environment

There are also some specific forms of vasovagal syndrome:

- Cough syncope
  - after a paroxysm of coughing, usually in a patient with obstructive airways disease
- Micturation syncope
  - usually occurs in the night when going to pass urine, or during micturation itself. As the patient may get wedged in the toilet the ambulance may well be called!

### What is the differential diagnosis?:

There are many other causes of blackouts and all may need to be excluded:

- Cardiac Arrhythmia

– associated with both profound bradycardia and tachycardia. Symptomatic palpitations may be a pointer but often not present. Outflow obstruction eg Aortic stenosis or HOCM cause syncope.

Note: A cardiac cause should be sought in all patients with known structural heart disease.

• Neurological
  – epilepsy and cerebrovascular disease are the most common causes. A good witness account is key to the diagnosis.

Note: Some jerky movements of the limbs and even incontinence can occur in a prolonged vasovagal attack, especially if the patient remains upright.

• Hypoglycaemia
  – well known in diabetics. In non-diabetic, circumstances usually the clue. Spontaneous hypoglycaemia (from insulinoma) is rare.

**Hyperventilation**

• light headedness, a feeling of being distanced from their surroundings, chest pain, paraesthesiae, numbness in arms occur. Pallor and peripheral cyanosis can be striking in a full blown attack. Circumstances provoking an attack can often be the same as for a faint (e.g. warm room, stressful situation).

Note: If hyperventilation suspected, symptoms can usually be readily reproduced by voluntary hyperventilation.

## CASE HISTORY 2

A 68-year-old man passed out suddenly at the wheel of his car and ran into the car in front. His wife reports that he was pale and sweaty, but loss of consciousness was brief and he recovered quickly. His ECG showed LBBB. ambulatory monitoring subsequently showed periods of asymptomatic second degree heart block. A pacemaker was implanted without any recurrence.

### Information
"Medical Aspects of Fitness to Drive" HMSO Publication)

### Practice points
• Sudden loss of consciousness without warning must be assumed to be a cardiac arrhythmia until proved otherwise
• Altered consciousness whilst driving has important legal implications and the patient must be warned not to drive again until the diagnosis is established

### Investigation

The history of the event is the key to further investigation and blanket investigations are unrewarding without some clinical pointers as to the cause. A single faint requires no further investigation, but if there is some diagnostic doubt the symptoms can usually be reproduced by a Tilt Test.

This is usually carried out with a mechanised tilt table giving a head up tilt of 60° for 45 minutes, with continuous ECG and BP monitoring. Although false positive results can occur, if the prodrome before the faint reproduces the symptoms, it provides strong support for the diagnosis.

## Treatment

Most vasovagal attacks require no treatment except for some general advice to the patient and family. In recurrent attacks betablockers are often valuable.

## CASE HISTORY 3

JR is a 26-year-old physiotherapist. Her first episode of unconsciousness occurred on a ward outing. A nursing colleague thought that she was pulseless at the time of the collapse. The possibility of excess alchohol was considered, but on arrival in A&E at a nearby hospital she was intubated and ventilated overnight.

She was quite well the next day. A second collapse occurred under rather similar circumstances when she was in the pub with medical and nursing colleagues. On this occasion she was found to be hypotensive on arrival at A&E (at a second different hospital) and again required ventilation but was fine the following day.

A third episode occurred when she had had nothing to drink; she was taken to a third hospital but did not require ventilation. She was investigated with 24 and 48-hour ECG, echocardiography and CT scanning of the head but no abnormality was found. Since all of these investigations were unhelpful an electrophysiological study was performed to exclude the possibility of tachyarrhythmias. During this study she spontaneously became bradycardic and hypotensive.

A tilt table test was performed the following day. 60° head-up tilting produced bradycardia, hypotension and syncope. A DDD pacing system has been implanted which is programmed to produce a tachycardiac response to bradycardia of sudden onset and so far she has had no more attacks.

---

⚠

**Remember**

TILT TEST

Not for the faint-hearted – Syncope is often accompanied by 10 to 20 seconds of ASYSTOLE, which recovers as soon as the patient is tilted flat. A doctor should always be in the vicinity while tilt is being carried out.

---

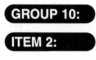

**GROUP 10:**

**ITEM 2:**

# Cardiology

# A clinical approach to patients with tachycardia

The main reason people have difficulty assessing tachyarrhythmias is they get entangled in the ECG changes without thinking about the patient to whom the ECG belongs. This section offers a simple approach to looking at both at the same time.

Imagine you are in A&E and you are asked to see a 54-year-old man who has a tachycardia. His heart rate is 165 beats/min.

There are three simple questions you need to ask yourself as you approach a patient with an acute tachyarrhythmia.The first is:

### What is the heart rate?

What are the other two simple questions that you need to ask yourself as you approach the bedside?

### Has the patient hit the deck?

In other words, is the patient compromised by the tachycardia or not?

In assessing the degree of cardiovascular collapse take the heart rate into account. Remember that the maximal heart rate which you would expect a patient to achieve on the treadmill is 220 minus age.

Someone with a heart rate at this level is going at the same rate you would expect if they had just hurried up several flights of stairs. If they are profoundly compromised by this rate it is likely that they have a seriously impaired ventricle; what is more, it is likely that the arrhythmia is secondary to their LV problem.

In contrast, if the man in our example is not very worried by the tachycardia then it is a good bet that he has a good ventricle. People with heart rates substantially above their predicted maximum who tolerate the situation well are likely to be suffering from a primary electrophysiological problem rather than an arrhythmia secondary to LV disease.

### Broad or narrow ECG complexes?

Divide tachycardias into broad or narrow complexes rather than try to split them into SVT and VT at the first glance. If you follow this approach you will not treat VT as SVT which is the important error to avoid.

Having answered these questions (and taking account of the heart rate) you can construct a simple matrix

**Remember**

The default position is to diagnose VT so:

Always regard a broad complex tachycardia as being VT unless it is PROVEN to be an SVT

| | Broad Complex | Narrow Complex |
|---|---|---|
| **Hit the deck** | A patient with a broad complex tachy who is compromised is likely to have a VT. If the collapse occurred at relatively low rates it is likely that there is some primary LV problem such as ischaemia or cardiomyopathy. | Many of these patient's are in AF secondary to LV disease. Otherwise it is relatively rare for people to be compromised with narrow complex tachycardia. |
| **Did not hit the deck** | The faster the heart rate the better view you can take of their LV. These patients have to be considered very carefully. In many patients SVT and conduction aberration present like this but so do patients with primary VF. Young people in this group may have the Wolff Parkinson White (WPW) syndrome. | This is a common category and will contain many of the younger patients who have primary arrhythmias such as re-entrant tachycardia and AV nodal tachycardia. |

All this can be done in seconds and the matrix makes the first important decision for you.

### When should you admit the patient to hospital?

| | Broad Complex | Narrow Complex |
|---|---|---|
| **Hit the Deck** | Needs to be admitted from A&E*. Do not give Verapamil or other negatively inotropic drugs. (Case 2) *Usually need immediate cardioversion. | Will probably need to come into hospital. Is the patient in Heart Failure? |
| **Did not hit the Deck** | The most difficult category to sort out. Will probably need admission to sort out diagnosis. Irregular tachycardia in this group may be due to WPW with AF – do not give verapamil. | Can probably go home if tachycardia stops on treatment (case 1). Needs outpatient assessment. Is this a recurrent problem? Would they benefit from radiofrequency ablation of their pathway or their atrial focus? |

Having made this rapid assessment there are two important things to do in every case.

- Measure the electrolytes
  – many arrhythmias are secondary to hypokalaemia.
- Take a 12 lead ECG of the arrhythmia
  – this is essential to sort VT from the SVT.
  It is also valuable in sorting out the mechanisms in narrow complex tachycardias; the retrograde P waves can be seen in the ST -T segments in re-entrant tachycardias but they may only be seen in some leads.
- Treatment – this is discussed later on.

### Summary

The two by two matrix approach helps you to think about the ECG and the clinical context at the same time. It focuses you on the underlying state of the ventricle. To be safe:

• Always assume a broad complex tachycardia is VT
• If in doubt use DC cardioversion rather than drugs
• Seek advice if your first drug does not work
• Beware of Verapamil and other negatively inotropic drugs
• Check the electrolytes before using drugs

### Some definitions

• Broad Complexes
  – QRS complex of > 120 ms. (3 small squares on the standard ECG). May have a typical Bundle Branch Block pattern.
• Re-entrant tachycardia
  – the WPW (Wolff Parkinson White) syndrome is the classic example of a re-entrant tachycardia. The depolarisation wavefront "re-enters" the atrium through the bundle of abnormal conducting tissue between ventricle and atrium. In some cases a bundle is present but is not visible on the resting ECG so that it is a "concealed pathway". This is a common cause of SVT. Similar mechanisms are involved with re-entry within the AV node.
• Atrial tachycardia
  – an SVT from a focus in the atrium rather than due to re-entry.

### The ECG In Tachycardia

In discussing the ECG in tachycardia we have assumed that a 12 lead ECG of the tachycardia is available

### Narrow complexes (Fig 10.2.1)

In narrow complex tachycardias it is clear that the arrhythmia is arising above the level of the bundle of His.

### Fig 10.2.1 Narrow complex tachycardia

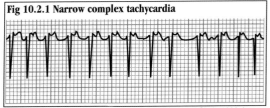

Redrawn from *Clinical Medicine*, 4th Edition, Kumar and Clark, 1998, by permission of the publisher WB Saunders

## Look for

- Irregularity in rhythm and irregularity of the baseline. This suggests atrial fibrillation.This can be easier to see after giving adenosine.
- Flutter waves. A regular tachycardia at a rate of around 150 is highly likely to be flutter. Again adenosine may help in revealing the flutter waves.
- Retrograde P waves hidden in the ST segments and the T waves. These represent retrograde depolarisation of the atria and are found in re-entrant tachycardias.

### Broad complexes (Fig 10.2.2)

- **Conduction aberration**
  – the ECG may show perfectly normal conduction at normal heart rates. However in patients who have a diffuse abnormality of the conducting system an arrhythmia arising above the AV node will produce a broad complex tachycardia. This is because one of the bundle branches may be capable of conducting normally at slow rates but may show delayed conduction (bundle branch block) at higher rates.

### Fig 10.2.2 Broad complex tachycardia

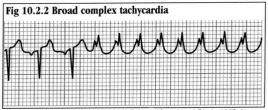

Redrawn from *Clinical Medicine*, 4th Edition, Kumar and Clark, 1998, by permission of the publisher WB Saunders

## Features suggestive of a ventricular arrhythmia

- A QRS duration of >140 ms. strongly suggests a ventricular origin
- The frontal and horizontal axes are grossly discordant with that in sinus rhythm. Most people are used to looking at frontal QRS axis in the limb leads. The horizontal axis is estimated by seeing where the predominantly negative QRS complexes become equiphasic as you look across from V1 towards V6. This equiphasic point is called the zone of transition and is usually at V3 or V4. In VT there may be no transition zone or it may be far to the right, or left of V4
- QRS Morphology: The pattern is not typical of LBBB or RBBB. These are specific appearances which strongly suggest VT eg concordance; seek help if unsure
- Fusion beats. These are beats where there is simultaneous activation of the ventricles from a focus of arrhythmia and from the atria via the AV node at the same time. These beats will look like a cross between the standard VT complex and the patient's normal complexes in sinus rhythm.
- Capture beats. Occasionally the atria may 'capture' a normal complex in the midst of a tachycardia
- You may be able to see evidence of both atrial and ventricular activity. If there is no constant relationship between the P waves and the QRS complexes it suggests a ventricular origin and this is called atrioventricular dissociation

### Remember
Differentiating VT from SVT in broad complex tachycardia can be very difficult and you should always regard the tachycardia as being VT.

### Features suggesting that a tachycardia may be an SVT

- Normal LBBB or RBBB morphology; but be careful VT from RV outflow tract with LBBB morphology can look like SVT. A small stubby R wave in V1-2 is characteristic of VT
- You may be able to see evidence of both atrial and ventricular activity. If there is a constant relationship between the P waves and the QRS complexes it suggests a supraventricular origin
- The frontal and horizontal QRS axes are in the same general direction as that in sinus rhythm
- It slows with manoeuvres designed to increase vagal tone such as carotid sinus massage
- If the onset is witnessed you may see a P wave which is premature

### Torsade de Pointes

Torsade de Pointes is an uncommon form of VT with a characteristic ECG pattern. The complexes appear to twist around the baseline by virtue of their changes in amplitude. It is particularly associated with syndromes involving a long QT interval. CORRECT diagnosis of torsade de pointes is important as the treatment is very different from VT.

### The acute treatment of arrhythmias

⚠️

**Remember**

It is always important to think about the underlying state of the ventricle when treating an acute arrhythmia.

- The use of drugs in patients with acute arrhythmias can be dangerous. The dangers flow from two problems:
- Many arrhythmias arise as a result of pre-existing disease of the LV so that any drug which further suppresses LV function can be dangerous
- A drug which is ineffective for the rhythm in question may also depress ventricular function without alleviating the rate related stress on the ventricle

Because of these problems it is often safer to use DC cardioversion than drugs.

The final catch when you are treating arrhythmias with drugs (see fig 10.2.3) is that ischaemia may alter the electrophysiogical activity of drugs. This means that drugs which are anti-arrhythmic under normal circumstances may become pro-arrhythmic in ischaemic myocardium. This limits the use of drugs in many patients since it is often difficult to exclude the possibility of ischaemia, – particularly chronic management of arrhythmias.

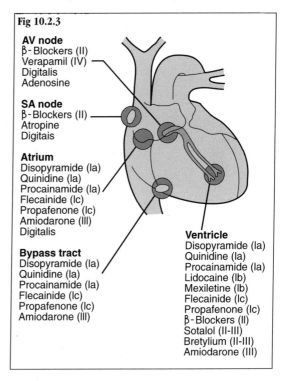

**Fig 10.2.3**

**AV node**
β-Blockers (II)
Verapamil (IV)
Digitalis
Adenosine

**SA node**
β-Blockers (II)
Atropine
Digitais

**Atrium**
Disopyramide (Ia)
Quinidine (Ia)
Procainamide (Ia)
Flecainide (Ic)
Propafenone (Ic)
Amiodarone (III)
Digitalis

**Bypass tract**
Disopyramide (Ia)
Quinidine (Ia)
Procainamide (Ia)
Flecainide (Ic)
Propafenone (Ic)
Amiodarone (III)

**Ventricle**
Disopyramide (Ia)
Quinidine (Ia)
Procainamide (Ia)
Lidocaine (Ib)
Mexiletine (Ib)
Flecainide (Ic)
Propafenone (Ic)
β-Blockers (II)
Sotalol (II-III)
Bretylium (II-III)
Amiodarone (III)

Numbers in brackets refer to the Vaughan-Williams classification (see Kumar and Clark 4th Edition p673 1998

## CASE HISTORY 1

A 35-year-old man presents with a narrow complex tachycardia at a rate of 180 per minute. He is not seriously compromised by his tachyarrhythmia and the BP is 128/64.

The ECG shows an SVT (narrow complex tachycardia).

### Management

This rhythm is likely to respond to adenosine (see below). If it fails, consider intravenous beta blockade. If either the beta blocker or verapamil fails it is best to go straight to DC cardioversion (start with 50J).

⚠️

**Remember**

Verapamil can be dangerous in WPW; if uncertain it is safer to cardiovert

### Adenosine

Adenosine has revolutionised the diagnosis and management of acute tachycardias. The major limitation is that is should not be used in asthmatics. Otherwise the drug will cardiovert many SVTs. It does not usually cardiovert AF or flutter but will slow the rate transiently (often for only one or two complexes – have the ECG running) and enable you to see the baseline. It is safe to give adenosine to patients in VT, however it will not usually cardiovert the problem although it may slow the rate.

## CASE HISTORY 2

A 57-year-old woman presents with a tachycardia at a rate of 132 per minute. She is hypotensive (106/58) and looks pale and shocked. The 12 lead ECG shows an axis of $-120°$ and the complexes are predominantly positive across the chest leads (broad complex tachycardia).

### Management

This is a ventricular tachycardia. Set up lignocaine infusion following a bolus and measure the electrolytes whilst preparing for DC cardioversion. If the arrhythmia recurs then intravenous amiodarone with a repeat DC cardioversion is the best strategy. This patient has clinical evidence of poor LV function BUT in a patient who has a good LV sotalol might be preferred. Finally, in patients refractory to treatment, remember the possibility of Torsade de Pointes with low magnesium and potassium levels.

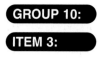

**GROUP 10:**

**ITEM 3:**

# Cardiology
# Atrial fibrillation

### Prevalence and mechanisms

Atrial fibrillation (AF) remains one of the most common and challenging of arrhythmias. It is estimated that 10% of the population may suffer from AF at some stage of their lives. Patients who remain in AF after their hospital admission face a long-term risk of embolism and stroke. This is reduced by the use of anticoagulation but long-term anticoagulation also carries a risk. In an ideal world all patients would be cardioverted to sinus rhythm but this is often not possible when there is underlying heart disease.

### Clinical strategies

The treatment of patients who have chronic atrial fibrillation remains controversial. The difficulty lies in deciding whether cardioversion should be used on an elective basis or whether it is better to leave the patient in AF and promote good rate control.

**Remember**

The problem with this strategy is that AF becomes more stable over time, and may be less easy to cardiovert the longer you wait.

When patients present with acute AF the first question is whether they should be cardioverted. The reason for this lies in the need for anticoagulation on the one hand and the electrophysiogical characteristics of AF on the other.

In those who are in obvious heart failure (Such as Case 1) acute cardioversion will almost certainly be unsuccessful in reverting to AF. Where AF is primarily electrophysiogical in origin, acute cardioversion is much more likely to be effective.

Cardioversion can be undertaken in acute AF without risk of embolus in the first 24 hours (some authorities say within the first 48 hours ). If this opportunity is missed then the patient must wait until they have been on anticoagulation for at least four weeks.

The final point to make is that AF is unlikely to be converted to persistent sinus rhythm in the presence of an enlarged left atrium. The doctrine of perfection is to obtain an echocardiogram before embarking upon acute DC cardioversion. In fact the chest X-ray is very helpful in this situation; a patient in acute AF with a large heart on PA chest X-ray is unlikely to be cardioverted into persistent sinus rhythm.

### Mechanisms of AF

Atrial fibrillation is a very stable arrhythmia. The stability of the rhythm and the difficulty in maintaining sinus rhythm is easy to understand once the mechanism of AF is understood (Fig 10.3).

AF results from wavelets of depolarisation which move around the atria. The mechanism is explained in the following diagrams.

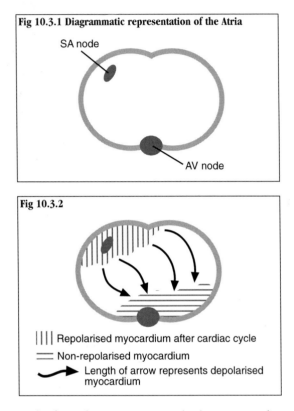

**Fig 10.3.1 Diagrammatic representation of the Atria**

SA node

AV node

**Fig 10.3.2**

|||| Repolarised myocardium after cardiac cycle

≡ Non-repolarised myocardium

Length of arrow represents depolarised myocardium

In this figure the arrows represent depolarisation spreading through the atria.

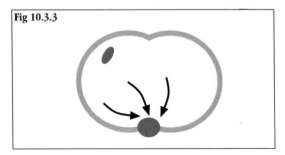

**Fig 10.3.3**

In this figure the atrium is enlarged. The electrophysiological characteristics are unchanged so that the arrows are the same length

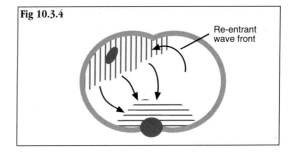

Fig 10.3.4

Re-entrant wave front

This enables a re-entrant wave front to depolarise myocardium which has already repolarised.

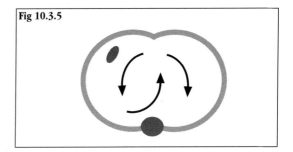

Fig 10.3.5

Leading to four or five wave fronts "chasing" depolarised myocardium around the atria – in other words atrial fibrillation.

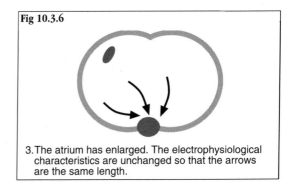

Fig 10.3.6

3. The atrium has enlarged. The electrophysiological characteristics are unchanged so that the arrows are the same length.

The same effect may take place in a normal sized atrium that has delayed conduction velocity. The area of myocardium which is depolarised during a single cycle is less (represented by shorter arrows) so that re-entry may occur.

## CASE HISTORY 1

A 68-year-old woman with a history of hypertension presents with a rapid heart rate of 160 accompanied by breathlessness. The ECG is compatible with atrial fibrillation (AF). The BP is 116/70.

### Management

This lady is likely to have AF in association with CCF. This must be the assumption on which you move forward. The CXR may show evidence of pulmonary oedema. The first priority is to treat the CCF (diuretics, etc.) Rate control of the AF with digoxin is important but remember that a tachycardia may simply be an indication of poorly controlled failure even in AF. There are some patients in whom the poor LV function is secondary to poor rate control but this is much less common than poor rate control being secondary to poor control of CCF. In such cases where digoxin fails to control the rate it may be reasonable to use amiodarone.

## CASE HISTORY 2

A 70-year-old woman with a history of hypertension presented to the hospital with a history of six hours of palpitations. She had been taking 75mg of aspirin prescribed by her GP for two years. The ECG shows atrial fibrillation at a rate of 132 beats per minute. The patient looked well and had a BP of 142/78 and there was no cardiomegaly on X-ray. She was clear that the symptoms started acutely six hours previously. She reverted to sinus rhythm in response to a 50 Joule shock and was started on sotalol. She remained in sinus rhythm at follow up six months later.

The choices facing clinicians with a patient in AF are:

• Should I attempt to cardiovert?
• What precautions should I take against embolisation at the time of cardioversion?

• What should I do to promote good rate control in the long term if cardioversion fails?
• Should I give prophylactic medication to prevent AF if sinus rhythm is achieved?

### Should I cardiovert?

Yes. Cardioversion can be achieved with drugs or with DC cardioversion.

Amiodarone and class 1c drugs such as flecainide both promote cardioversion. Fig 10.2.3 shows the sites of action of drugs on the heart.

DC Conversion with 50–100 joules may revert AF to sinus rhythm in 80% of patients. This is the best treatment for AF less than 24 hour duration (Case History 2).

### What precautions should I take to prevent embolism at the time of cardioversion?

Cerebral embolism can be prevented by anticoagulation and patients who have been in AF for more than 24 hours should be anticoagulated for a minimum of three weeks before and four weeks after cardioversion.

The use of ultrasound techniques to assess the risk of embolism is currently under investigation. Transoesophageal Echo may detect those patients who can safely be cardioverted without anticoagulation, although this is not yet standard practice.

### What should be done to promote good rate control in the long term if cardioversion fails?

Digoxin is effective in rate control (although there is a clinical impression that good rate control is only achieved in relatively inactive people). There is no evidence that digoxin promotes conversion to sinus rhythm and can worsen symptoms in paroxysmal atrial fibrillation.

Where digoxin fails to control rate, beta blockers and verapamil are usually effective. Amiodarone is also effective and can be used in poor LV function, but does have long term side effects. However AF can often be controlled with a dose of only 100mg of amiodarone daily, with a lower risk of side effects.

### Should I give prophylactic medication to prevent AF if sinus rhythm is achieved?

Quinidine or disopyramide should be used with caution, because of the risks of proarrythmia. Discuss the pros and cons with your cardiologist.

**GROUP 10:**

**ITEM 4:**

# Cardiology
# Bradycardia and pacing

Bradycardia is a common finding in health due to increased vagal tone, and is seen in an extreme form in vasovagal attacks when periods of asystole can occur. A similar vagal reaction can be seen with severe pain or after vomiting in some patients, and responds promptly to atropine.

Bradycardia is an increasing problem in the elderly and very elderly, and reflects degenerative disease of the conducting system at all levels:

• Sinus node     – sick sinus syndrome
• AV node         – complete heart block
                        – slow atrial fibrillation
• HIS-Purkinje system – bifascicular block (left axis deviation and right bundle branch block)

## CASE HISTORY 1

A 78-year-old man without any prior cardiac disease was brought to hospital after collapsing at home with brief loss of consciousness. On arrival he had fully recovered and the ECG showed bifascicular block. During monitoring overnight he was shown to have periods of complete heart block. He subsequently had a dual chamber pacemaker (DDD) implanted without any recurrence.

## Diagnosis

• Difficulties arise in establishing arrhythmia as a cause of dizzy spells when the condition is intermittent as it often is in the early stages
• Twenty-four hour ECG is the most important investigation, but repeat tapes may be needed to demonstrate an abnormality when the history is very suggestive

### Remember
Bradycardia and even transient conduction disturbance can occur in healthy people during sleep, and great caution is needed in interpreting rhythm disturbances at night.

---

**Classification of pacemakers**

Notation is by a 3/5 letter abbreviation

Chamber sensed (A = atria, V = ventricular, D = both or dual)

Chamber paced (A = atria, V = ventricular, D = both or dual)

Response to sensing (I = inhibited, T = triggered, D = both T+I, O = none)

Programmability (R = rate modulation)

Anti-tachycardia function

Examples:

VVI = ventricular sensing, ventricular pacing, inhibition of pacing when beat is sensed

DDDR = dual sensing, dual pacing, inhibition and triggered as appropriate when beat is sensed, rate response mode available

## Pacemakers in common use
- VVI – for slow AF
- DDD – for complete heart block
- AAI – for sick sinus syndrome

DDDR/VVIR/AAIR used where patient has lost chronotropic response i.e. cannot increase heart rate with exercise/stress.

## Pacemaker problems
- Infection
  - Potentially very serious. Even slight redness around the scar should be treated promptly with antibiotics e.g. flucloxacillin 500mg x3 daily. Usually occurs early after implantation.
- Technical problems
  - With time pacemaker thresholds can change as fibrosis occurs around the pacemaker tip, but not usually enough to affect function.

### Remember
Failure to capture can be due to lead failure which in a 'pacing-dependent' patient can be life-threatening.
ALWAYS seek specialist cardiology advice if this is seen on any ECG tracing in a patient with a pacemaker.

## CASE HISTORY 2

A 78-year-old man is admitted for a routine hip replacement and the pre-operative ECG shows pacing spikes with intermittent failure to capture (Fig 10.4.1).

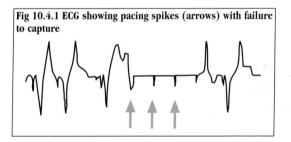

**Fig 10.4.1 ECG showing pacing spikes (arrows) with failure to capture**

On checking the pacemaker it was found that the pacing threshold was 1.5mv but the sensing threshold had risen. On re-adjusting the sensing threshold, pacing returned to normal.

### 'Pacemaker Syndrome'

Often rather vague feelings of weakness or dizziness in patients with VVI pacemakers and complete heart block. Not seen with dual chamber pacing.

### Mechanisms

Loss of synchrony between atrial and ventricular contraction leading to episodic falls in BP

Retrograde conduction of pacing impulse from ventricle to atria leading to simultaneous atrial and ventricular contraction

### Remember
Always take dizzy spells in a patient with a pacemaker seriously. Formal evaluation is usually required.

### Thrombo-embolism

Systemic emboli are relatively common in patients with pacemakers especially in:

• slow AF
• sick sinus syndrome/complete heart block with VVI pacemaker

Prophylactic anticoagulants may be needed in many of these patients.

## Cardiology
## Basic life support

You are walking alone along an isolated corridor of your hospital. Just ahead, you observe a man collapse to the ground. As you approach you notice he is one of the hospital porters. He is lying motionless.

### What are you going to do?
• Check for danger
• Shake and shout to check responsiveness
There is no response

• Shout for help
No one immediately appears in response to your shout for assistance

• Open the airway

### What two methods could you use to open the airway?
Head tilt, chin lift or a jaw thrust

### What are the indications for using a jaw thrust?
Suspected cervical spine injury

### Assess for breathing
Look, listen and feel for breathing for 10 seconds
There are no signs of breathing

**Information**

The chance of survival from ventricular fibrillation is generally agreed to deteriorate by five to 10 per cent per minute (Cummins [1989]). It is therefore imperative that a defibrillator is brought from A&E as soon as possible. Alerting the team is a priority. Give a prerecordial thump if appropriate.

**You are still on your own at this point.
What must you do now?**

You must leave the porter and go to the nearest telephone to initiate the cardiac arrest call

You have initiated the emergency call from a telephone further along the corridor. On your return there is a visitor leaning over the porter wondering what to do.

**What should be your next action?**

Commence basic life support by delivering two effective breaths

The bystander asks if she can help. She tells you she has never performed basic life support before, but seems very keen to assist you.

**Should you allow her to help?**

No. You have alerted the arrest team and should continue the assessment and basic life support yourself without wasting any time explaining the procedure to the bystander

**What do you need to assess for at this stage?**

Circulation. Carotid pulse check, also looking for other signs of circulation, including colour and movement for ten seconds

There are no signs of circulation after your assessment. The porter is cyanosed and motionless.

**What do you need to commence at this stage?**

Chest compressions. Carefully observing the following:

• Hand position. Place the heel of the hand on the sternum, two fingers breadth above where the rib margins meet.
• Arm position. Lock the elbows and lean directly over the porter.
• Rate. Aim to maintain a rate of 100 per minute.
• Depth. Compress the chest one third of the resting diameter of the chest.
• Ratio. Single rescuer CPR at a ratio of 15:2 (15 compressions to 2 breaths).

**How long would you continue this for?**

Until the defibrillator arrives

• Another person now arrives before the arrest team and knows how to perform basic life support.
• Two person CPR.

## How would this alter the ratio of chest compression and ventilations?

• You would commence five chest compressions followed by one ventilation

## Summary

**Check responsiveness**
Shake and shout
**Unresponsive**
Shout for help
**Open the airway**
Head tilt, chin lift or jaw thrust
**Check for breathing**
Look listen and feel for 10 seconds
**Breathing present**
Recovery position
**No breathing**
Give two effective breaths
**Assess for circulation**
Look for movement and check carotid pulse for 10 seconds
**Circulation present**
Continue breathing, check circulation every minute
**No circulation**
Commence chest compressions, 100 per minute, 15:2 ratio

## Information

Cummins R.O., Annals Emergency Med. 1989 18 : 1269 -1275

Recommended reading

A J Handley et al, the 1998 Resuscitation Council guidelines for adult single rescuer basic life support. Resuscitation 37 (1998) 67 – 80.

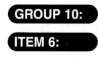

**GROUP 10:**

**ITEM 6:**

# Cardiology
# Chest pain

**Remember**

• The management depends on a FAST TRACK approach with an initial assessment of whether the patient is having a heart attack as 'TIME IS MUSCLE'.

**Remember**

• If the initial ECG is normal – DO NOT DISCHARGE THE PATIENT

• Repeat the ECG every 20 minutes for at least an hour

• Consider other causes of chest pain

**Remember**

DON'T MISS AN AORTIC DISSECTION!

## CASE HISTORY 1

You are called to assess a 68-year-old woman who gives a 90-minute history of central chest pain radiating down her left arm and through to her back. She has a history of treated hypertension but has not smoked for 15 years. How are you going to manage her?

### Initial Assessment

Within 10 minutes of arrival:

• Brief history
• Risk factor profile
• Brief examination (BP, pulse, murmurs, chest)
• ECG
• Give aspirin 300mg orally
• Relieve pain eg if ischaemic ECG give diamorphine 5-10 mg IV and anti-emetic
• Take blood for markers of cardiac damage

### Learning point

Every year patients are inappropriately discharged from A&E departments with a myocardial infarction because their initial ECG is normal. If in doubt admit the patient.

### Non-cardiac causes of chest pain

• Aortic dissection – see later
• Pericarditis – sharp central pain, related to posture and respiration
• Pleurisy – sharp, usually lateral, related to respiration
• Muscular – related to posture, localised tenderness
• Herpes zoster – nerve root distribution, rash may appear later
• Gastro-oesophageal reflux disease – retrosternal burning pain but can be very similar to angina

Note: Many episodes of chest pain do not easily fit into any category and patients are often admitted with a diagnosis of "ischaemic heart disease; unstable angina"

The patient's symptoms should be assessed in conjunction with their risk factor profile (smoking, hypertension, lipids, family history, age, gender)

## What features would make you suspect a dissecting aneurysm?

- Pain tends to radiate to back
- The pain starts abruptly
- The pain is often intense and described as tearing
- Additional problems may appear e.g. absent arm or leg pulses, murmur of aortic regurgitation, different BP in arms
- ECG may be normal or show an inferior MI
- A stroke may be a complication

### Remember

- Aortic dissection is a rare but important differential diagnosis of chest pain.
- With the necessity to give rapid thrombolytic treatment for acute myocardial infaction (MI) there is a risk that inappropriate and potentially dangerous treatment could be given to a patient with a dissection.

## If you clinically suspect a dissecting aneurysm

- Get a chest X-ray to look for mediastinal widening
- Get a senior opinion
- Do not give thrombolytic therapy or aspirin
- Carefully reduce BP
- Refer to cardiac centre
- Consider CT/MR/trans-oesophageal Echo (TOE) dependent on facilities

**Fig 10.6.1 Types of aortic aneurysm**

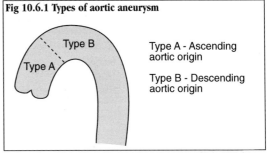

Type A - Ascending aortic origin

Type B - Descending aortic origin

Redrawn from *Clinical Medicine*, 4th Edition, Kumar and Clark, 1998, by permission of the publisher WB Saunders

## CASE 1 (CONTINUED)

### INITIAL ECG now changes at approximately 20 minutes

There could be three types:
- S-T elevation of 2mm in 2 contiguous chest leads
- S-T/T wave changes
- Left Bundle Branch Block

If the initial or this later ECG show significant S-T elevation (i.e. myocardial infarction), give thrombolytic therapy unless there is a contraindication:

### Thrombolytic therapy

Drug of first choice:

- Streptokinase 1.5 million units (in 100mls of 5% dextrose or 0.9% saline) over 60 minutes

or consider

- Alteplase (tPA, tissue-type plasminogen activator) 1mg/kg over 60 mins if:
  - allergy to streptokinase (Sk)
  - Sk within previous five days
  - ant. MI within four hours

### Contraindications to thrombolytic therapy

- Active bleeding
- Persistent BP > 180/110
- Prior stroke
- Major surgery < two weeks
- Other major illness

### Don't forget pericarditis!

\* S-T changes in pericarditis are often widespread involving inferior as well as anterior leads (Fig 10.6.2)

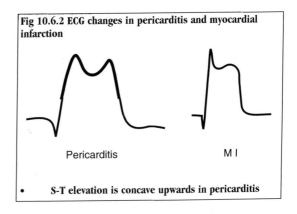

**Fig 10.6.2 ECG changes in pericarditis and myocardial infarction**

Pericarditis                    M I

• **S-T elevation is concave upwards in pericarditis**

### Other ECG "catches"

- LBBB
  If this is known to be old the diagnosis will rest on the history and cardiac enzymes as it is difficult to distinguish acute changes on a background of LBBB
  If it is known to be new it can be used to support the diagnosis
- Normal variants
  High S-T take off is seen more commonly in certain racial groups e.g. Afro-Caribbean

### Cardiac enzymes in the early assessment of a patient with chest pain (Fig 10.6.3)

Most cardiac enzymes take several hours to rise and may be misleading

Apart from the patient with known LBBB they should play a minor role in the evaluation of a patient with a suspected AMI

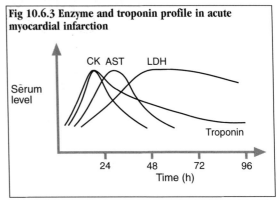

**Fig 10.6.3 Enzyme and troponin profile in acute myocardial infarction**

Redrawn from *Clinical Medicine*, 4th Edition, Kumar and Clark, p695, 1998

### How to differentiate unstable angina (UA) from an acute myocardial infarction (AMI)

#### UA

- Angina appearing for the first time
- A change in pattern of stable angina
- Angina occurring at rest, at night or on minimal effort
- Chest pain which resolves spontaneously or with GTN within 10 minutes

#### MI

- Persistent pain which is usually severe
- Lasts more than 20 minutes
- It is often associated with sweating, nausea and breathlessness
- Not relieved by GTN

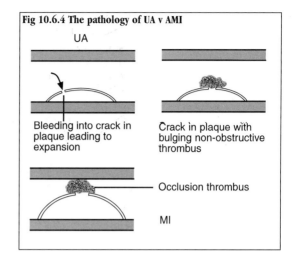

**Fig 10.6.4 The pathology of UA v AMI**

UA

Bleeding into crack in plaque leading to expansion

Crack in plaque with bulging non-obstructive thrombus

Occlusion thrombus

MI

| Investigations to differentiate UA from AMI | | |
|---|---|---|
| | UA | AMI |
| Cardiac enzymes (AST, CPK) | Normal | Usually raised |
| Troponin-I or T | Useful to assess prognosis Raised in high risk patients | Usually raised |
| ECG | Subtle S-T/T changes or normal | Usually abnormal |

## CASE HISTORY 2

A 60-year-old woman presents to a chest pain clinic with a one week history of a sudden worsening of her angina.

### How do you manage her?

• Admit
– to stabilise symptoms
– to assess severity of underlying disease
– to consider further investigation

• Therapy
– aspirin 300mg daily in hospital
– ß blocker (unless contraindicated)
– I.V. or buccal nitrates if chest pain at rest
– assess and correct risk factors (smoking, lipids, hypertension)

Glycoprotein (Gp), IIb, IIIa inhibitors (platelet receptor antagonists) have shown a modest benefit in clinical trials but are not yet in routine clinical practice.

- If symptoms settle:
  Perform exercise ECG on therapy
  If exercise test is strongly positive consider referral for further investigations e.g. angiography
- If symptoms continue:
  Refer for further investigation: angiography.

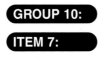

## Cardiology

## Myocardial infarction – educating the patient

### CASE HISTORY 1

A 50-year-old woman presents with a three-hour history of chest pain which she thought was indigestion. An ECG reveals an acute inferior myocardial infarction and she is admitted to the coronary care unit for monitoring.

Heart attacks are different from many other illnesses as there is an awareness that they can be fatal, creating a sense of anxiety and fear that may be absent in other diseases. These concerns are also felt by the wider circle around the patient and may lead to overprotection.

### Common reactions to initial phase

- Am I going to survive?
- Why me?
- What is a heart attack?

### Initial advice should be:

- Realistic
- Honest
- Consistent – ensure that all members of the team are giving roughly the same message
- Reassuring – most patients who survive to reach hospital after a heart attack will be discharged alive

### Information

- In-hospital mortality following an acute myocardial infarction is between 10 to 20%
- One-year mortality following discharge is approximately 10%

### CASE 1 CONTINUED

The patient is given thrombolytic therapy and aspirin together with a ß blocker. She mobilises without symptoms after two days.

### Questions and reactions during middle phase and discharge

*What can I do to prevent a further attack?*

– see Group 10 Item 11. Must stop smoking!

*Will this affect my work?*

– the majority of patients can return to work six to 12 weeks after a heart attack
– some may wish to ease back on a part-time basis
– keeping patients off work longer delays return to normality

*When can I drive?*

– after a month – the DVLA need not be informed but insurance companies should be informed
– HGV/PSV drivers must inform the licensing authorities as they will need a formal reassessment

*What can I do when I get home?*

– try not to be too proscriptive
– encourage a gentle increase in activity with the aim that the patient will be performing a full exercise test one month following discharge

*When can I resume sex?*

– patients who have returned to normal everyday activities can resume sex, usually at about a month

**Remember**

Some patients (often younger men) will minimise and attempt to deny their heart attack. The threat to life and livelihood in a previously apparently fit person may be difficult to come to terms with

*Why am I taking these drugs and how long do I need to stay on them? (see Group 10, Item 11)*

### Practice points

• Doctors have traditionally been poor at listening to and responding to the concerns of patients after a heart attack, as they have tended to concentrate on the physical aspects of the attack
• Listen to the patient and check that the advice you give is consistent with other members of the team
• Use the expertise of a cardiac rehabilitation counsellor
• Provide written information
• Reassure and be optimistic when you can be. Patients and their relatives are scared by heart attacks and need support

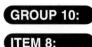

**GROUP 10:**

**ITEM 8:**

# Cardiology
## Myocardial infarction – heart failure and shock

Heart failure and cardiogenic shock usually reflect extensive cardiac damage, but cardiac 'stunning' may be present, and active treatment can save lives.

### Myocardial Stunning and Hibernating Myocardium

When heart muscle is subjected to acute ischaemia it may cease to contract but it may remain viable. This is a potentially reversible cause of haemodynamic problems in acute myocardial infarction.

If the blood supply to the relevant area is restored as a result of natural recanalisation of occluded arteries, pharmacological thrombolysis or angioplasty the functional capacity may return relatively quickly – that is over a matter of a few hours. Such myocardium is called stunned myocardium.

A similar state of affairs may occur on a more chronic basis, usually in severe three vessel disease. In this case the cellular ultrastructure may become seriously derranged even though the ischaemic myocytes are still potentially viable. This is known as hibernating myocardium and such myocardium can be restored by revascularisation.

However the major changes that have occurred at cellular level mean that the period of recovery may be over weeks or even months. PET scanning and radionuclide myocardial perfusion scanning are used to identify hibernating myocardium.

### Early Hypotension

Many patients with MI have a low BP at presentation, the causes being:

• Reflex response to pain
• Parasympathetic overactivity – especially in inferior MI
• Right ventricular infarction in inferior/posterior MI
• Extensive LV infarction or stunning, especially anterior MI

### Immediate treatment should be:

• Relief of pain: diamorphine intravenously (with antiemetic) in sufficient doses to give good pain relief (5-10mg usually a minimum)
• Atropine 600mcg intravenously if bradycardia/hypotension persist

**If hypotension persists after these measures the likely cause is:**
• Inferior MI – right ventricular infarction
• Anterior MI – extensive damage/stunning

## CASE HISTORY 1

A 58-year-old man is admitted with an inferior MI (Fig 10.8.1a) and successfully thrombolysed within six hours of the onset of pain. Although ST elevation largely resolves within one hour, he remains hypotensive with a systolic BP of 70-80mmHg associated with a low urine output.

A further ECG with right sided chest electrodes (Fig 10.8.1b) suggests right ventricular infarction with ST elevation in V3R – V4R. A fluid challenge of one litre of 5% dextrose given over half an hour intravenously, restores the BP to 110 systolic with a good urine output.

In the context of an acute MI, a fluid challenge is best given using intravenous dextrose; saline may precipitate left ventricular failure if there is significant LV damage.

Right ventricular infarction is:

• Diagnosed readily by elevation in ST in V3R – V4R on right sided ECG
• Associated with volume dependent hypotension
• Often associated with elevation of JVP without other evidence of heart failure

Note the raised ST segment and Q waves in the inferior leads (II, III and AVF)

**Fig 10.8.1a: An acute inferior wall myocardial infarction**

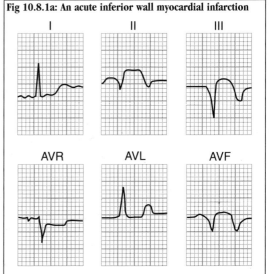

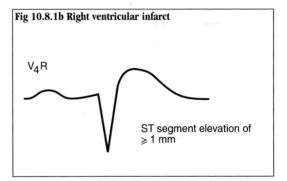

**Fig 10.8.1b Right ventricular infarct**

V$_4$R

ST segment elevation of
$\geqslant 1$ mm

• Also associated with a higher incidence of all post MI
  complications e.g. arrhythmias, rupture

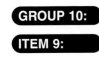

**GROUP 10:**

**ITEM 9:**

# Cardiology
## Cardiogenic shock

**Remember**

- An urgent echocardiogram is probably justified in every patient with cardiogenic shock. It is the only way to diagnose "silent" mitral regurgitation.

### Definition

Persistent hypotension (< 90mmHg systolic) associated with poor peripheral perfusion and urine output, usually the result of acute myocardial infarction, and associated with clinical/radiological evidence of LVF. Predisposing factors:

- Age
- Previous MI
- Anterior MI
- Prior hypertension/diabetes
- Inadequate (late) thrombolysis

### CASE HISTORY 1

A 68-year-old diabetic lady with a previous inferior myocardial infarct was admitted with a 12-hour history of chest pain and ECG changes of an extensive anterior MI. She was treated with streptokinase but remained hypotensive with a poor urine output. Her CXR showed early pulmonary oedema and echocardiography severe global left ventricular impairment.

**Remember**

- In patients on prior beta blockers, competitive blockade may persist for 24 hours or more and will require much higher doses of dobutamine/dopamine.
- It is probably simpler in this situation to use milrinone/enoximone which bypasses the β adrenoceptor.

### Management

- Check that patient is not fluid responsive (not in this case because there is evidence of LVF on chest X-Ray)
- Check that there is no structural cause
  – ventricular septal rupture (loud murmurs at left sternal edge)
  – papillary muscle damage/rupture giving severe mitral regurgitation (usually murmur but may be silent)
- Give inotropes intravenously

- digoxin
- catecholamines – dobutamine, dopamine
- phosphodiesterase inhibitors – enoxcimone, milrinone.
- Consider Intra-aortic Balloon Counterpulsation
  - this is a highly effective way of improving both peripheral and cardiac perfusion, and should be considered in any patient in whom there is a reasonable prospect of further definitive treatment (e.g. revascularisation/repair VSD). Cannot be used in the presence of significant aortic regurgititation.
- Consider immediate angiography if angioplasty available on site
  - this is particularly appropriate in the patient with an anterior MI and no previous history of IHD where cardiac stunning may be important

This lady was treated with intravenous dobutamine with some improvement in BP and peripheral perfusion, but 24 hours later developed acute pulmonary oedema and shock unresponsive to increasing inotropic support and died.

**GROUP 10:**

**ITEM 10:**

# Cardiology

# Heart failure following a myocardial infarction

The presence of heart failure, even if transient or only evident on CXR or ECHO, places the patient with a myocardial infarct in a bad prognostic group. All should be monitored closely and given secondary prevention with an ACEI e.g. Ramipril 2.5-5mg x2 daily or an angiotensin II receptor antagonist e.g. Losartan 50mg daily.

Acute pulmonary oedema: in the context of acute MI carries a very high in-hospital mortality (> 50%)

### Treatment
- I.V. diamorphine 2.5-10mg
- I.V. nitrates 12.5-100mcg/min intravenously – give as high a dose as the BP will allow
- I.V. frusemide 40-80mg
- consider I.V. digoxin
- consider I.V. inotropes (especially if hypotensive)

ACEI have been shown to reduce the mortality of this high risk group by 20-30%. Initiate once the patient is stable (day two to seven). Evidence for benefit exists for: captopril, lisinopril, ramipril, trandolapril.

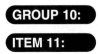

**GROUP 10:**

**ITEM 11:**

# Cardiology
# Myocardial infarction – secondary prevention

Once a patient has recovered from a heart attack, their most important concern is whether they will have another. As well as lifestyle changes there are now a wide range of drugs available for secondary prevention with strong evidence to support their use. The following should be undertaken:

- Stop smoking
- Control of blood pressure
- Diet modification
- Drug therapy

**Aspirin** – widely accepted with few contraindications

Dose: no clear agreement in the literature. Current practice 75-150mg daily.

Contraindications – clear history of Type I allergic reaction (angio-oedema, anaphylaxis).

If there is a history suggestive of active peptic ulcer disease consider co-prescription of H2 receptor antagonist. (NB. Check for helicobacter pylori and eradicate.)

**Beta blockers** – should be considered in all patients

Evidence: 20 to 25% mortality reduction; greatest benefit in the high risk group (prior MI, diabetes, transient heart failure). Probably a class effect but documentary evidence for: propranolol, timolol, metoprolol, acebutolol (not atenolol, though this is the most widely used drug in British practice). Contraindications: chronic obstructive pulmonary disease.

**Calcium channel blockers**

**Non-dihydropyridines** should be considered in patients with chronic obstructive pulmonary disease

Evidence: the mortality data is not as strong as for beta blockers, but the magnitude of the effect (20-30% reduction in events) is similar.

Verapamil: daily dose 240mg. Contraindicated in transient heart failure. Main side-effect is constipation.

Diltiazem: daily dose 180mg. Evidence for benefit in non-Q infarction, but remains controversial. Should not be used where transient heart failure is present.

**Dihydropyridines** – e.g. nifedipine, have NO place in secondary prevention and may be harmful.

**Angiotensin – converting enzyme inhibitors (ACEI):** should be considered in all patients with overt or transient heart failure

Evidence: strong evidence for mortality benefit in patients with heart failure or LV dysfunction, but some controversy about cost/benefit when used in all myocardial infarcts. May be a class effect, but evidence exists for: captopril, Ramipril, Lisinopril and trandolapril.

Contraindications: previous adverse reaction to ACEI, otherwise well tolerated but require monitoring of BP and renal function. Note: benefit appears to be additive with beta blockers.

**Remember**
Cough can be a problem with ACEI – if so use angiotensin II receptor antagonists e.g. losartan

**Lipid lowering drugs** – should be considered in all patients

Evidence: strong for mortality (20-30%) and morbidity benefit for 'statins' independent of:

• Age – evidence for up to 75 years at onset
• Sex – evidence from CARE/SSSS study
• Initial cholesterol – benefit seen at high (SSSS) and "normal" (CARE, LIPID) levels
• Other complications (e.g. heart failure, HT, diabetes)

Evidence from many dietary and fibrate studies show same trend but without mortality benefit

**Statins:**
• Evidence base for: simvastatin, pravastatin, but could be a class effect
• Use when the total cholesterol > 5.6mmol/l or the LDL cholesterol is>3.3mmol/l and TG < 4mmol/l (SMAC guidelines). This will account for about 80% of patients with acute MI. Aim to get the cholesterol below 4.
• Few contraindications – myalgia/myositis in first few weeks in some patients

**Remember**
After MI, the lipid levels may fall for up to two months. Ideally check lipid profile at this stage, though there is a trend to initiate statin therapy on the basis of a random cholesterol at presentation.

**Fibrates:**
• Evidence for gemfibrozil, bezafibrate
• Use where TG > 4mmol/l but care to exclude secondary causes (alcohol excess, hypothyroidism and poorly controlled diabetes)
• Few contraindications – myalgia/myositis in first few weeks in some patients

**Anticoagulation** – may be valuable in some patients

Evidence: evidence for benefit largely indirect but of significant magnitude to justify use.

Indications:

absolute -arterial embolus post MI. Should be continued for at least 6 months

relative – persistent atrial fibrillation
– markedly impaired LV function (Ejection fraction < 30%)

## Summary of drugs

- Aspirin for all
- Statins for majority
- Beta blockers for majority
- ACEI for patients with heart failure
- Verapamil/diltiazem for selected patients
- Anticoagulation for arterial embolisation + selected patients

**Remember**
High risk patients benefit most!

## Identifying 'high risk' survivors of MI

- Prior IHD, HT, Diabetes mellitus
- Heart failure (even transient)
- Late arrhythmias (> 24 hours after MI)
- Age >60 years
- Impaired ventricular function
- Unable to perform exercise tolerance tests (ETT) because of cardiac symptoms

## 'Low risk'

- Age <55 years
- No previous MI
- Event free course
- No angina on ETT

## Cardiology
## Post infarction arrhythmias

Arrhythmias – atrial and ventricular – are common in the first 24 hours after a myocardial infarction and may be life-threatening. Late arrhythmias (after first 24 hours) are of more prognostic significance and require specialist evaluation.

### Early Arrhythmias

• Ventricular
  – ectopics and non-sustained VT very common particularly in the one to two hours after thrombolysis ("re-perfusion arrhythmias") and usually require no treatment. Check K+, and correct if needed.
  – sustained VT or after VF: standard practice is lignocaine infusion (following 100mg IV bolus) for 24 hours after cardioversion
  – early use of I.V. beta blockers often reduces incidence of ventricular arrhythmias

### CASE HISTORY 1

A 56-year-old man without previous heart disease is admitted with an inferior myocardial infarct and successfully thrombolysed. He developed a nodal bradycardia 50 to 54/min with frequent ventricular ectopics and short runs of VT. Potassium was 4.1 mmol/l. He was given lignocaine but became hypotensive and it was discontinued after five minutes. Atropine 600mcg restored sinus rhythm (70-80/min) and the ventricular activity settled.

**Remember**
Ventricular 'escape' rhythms are common in bradycardia due to increased vagal tone, and usually respond to atropine.

### Heart block

Management is very different for inferior and anterior MI.

• Inferior MI:
  Conduction disturbance is common, but heart block is usually self limiting (up to two weeks) and very rarely requires permanent pacing.
• Anterior MI: Heart block is uncommon but always associated with extensive infarction. Immediate pacing mandatory; most require permanent pacing.

### CASE HISTORY 2

A 72-year-old woman with diabetes is admitted with an anterior MI and received thrombolysis eight hours after the onset of pain. The CXR showed pulmonary venous congestion. The ECG after thrombolysis:

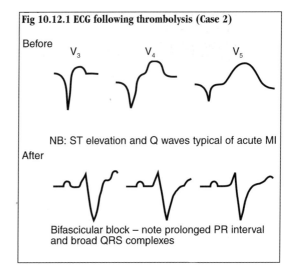

**Fig 10.12.1 ECG following thrombolysis (Case 2)**

Before $V_3$ $V_4$ $V_5$

NB: ST elevation and Q waves typical of acute MI

After

Bifascicular block – note prolonged PR interval and broad QRS complexes

---

**Information**

Anterior MI and complete heart block carries a very high in-hospital and one-year mortality

---

During the night, nurses observed some isolated non-conducted P waves but no action was taken. The next morning the patient collapsed with a heart rate of 28/min and complete heart block. A wire was passed via the internal jugular route and she was successfully paced. Despite this she developed increasing heart failure and died two days later.

## Practice points

- In an anterior MI bifascicular block is an indication for a prophylactic pacing wire, as the development of complete heart block (CHB) is common and unpredictable
- After thrombolysis temporary pacing should be via internal jugular or femoral routes and NOT by subclavian due to the risk of internal haemorrhage

## Late Arrhythmias

- Atrial Fibrillation/SVT – commonly associated with pericarditis or heart failure. Usually self-limiting or respond to digoxin. Treat pericarditis (indomethacin 50mg X3 daily for 2 days) or cardiac failure (diuretics + ACE1) actively
- Ventricular Tachycardia – As a late event carries a bad prognosis, consider:
- beta blockers
- amiodarone
- early angiography

Other anti-arrhythmics e.g. flecainide should be avoided because of the risks of producing an arrhythmia.

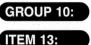

**GROUP 10:**

**ITEM 13:**

# Cardiology

# Acute myocardial ischaemia – who needs intervention?

Patients present to hospital with newly-diagnosed ischaemic heart disease with:

- Acute full thickness myocardial infarction
- Subendocardial (non Q) infarction
- Unstable angina

These latter two diseases are increasingly regarded as forming a continuous spectrum of disease.

As soon as the diagnosis of ischaemic heart disease has been made in a patient the question of revascularisation inevitably arises. The value of revascularisation – whether by surgery or by angioplasty in relieving persistent symptoms is beyond doubt.

However the value of revascularisation in extending life has only been established in prospective trials for the use of surgery in:

- Left main stem disease
- Three vessel disease and
- Two vessel disease where one of the two vessels is the proximal left anterior
- Descending coronary artery

The value of angioplasty in extending life has yet to be firmly established, although there is good evidence that it is similar to coronary artery bypass surgery in the trials which have compared the two techniques. However, the technology of angioplasty and stenting has been moving forward so quickly that the trials have not been able to keep up.

## CASE HISTORY 1

A 62-year-old man was admitted to hospital with a six-hour history of central chest pain radiating to both shoulders and to his jaw. The ECG in casualty showed 2mm of ST segment depression in the inferior leads and in lead V6. There was no acute rise in CPK. The pain settled with buccal nitrates, aspirin, intravenous heparin and oral atenolol.

He undertook an exercise test four days after admission where he reached the beginning of the second stage of the protocol (three minutes and 20 seconds) before developing pain. The test shows 1mm of ST depression developing in the inferior leads within the first four minutes of the test with subsequent ST depression developing in leads V3 to V6. Urgent outpatient angiography was arranged which showed an 85% occlusion in the mid portion of a dominant right coronary artery, a totally occluded circumflex and a 70% proximal occlusion in the anterior descending coronary artery. Coronary artery surgery was recommended and successfully undertaken.

## Acute angioplasty versus thrombolysis

The thesis is that the benefits of thrombolysis could be exceeded if acute angioplasty rather than acute thrombolysis were used. At the moment the evidence is mixed and suggests that acute angioplasty has short term benefits but the evidence of long term benefit is less clear. This strategy is in any case only available in a few centres.

### In-hospital angioplasty after Q wave infarction

Patients who develop new ischaemic pain more than 48 hours after a Q wave infarction should be considered for urgent investigation with a view to acute angioplasty.

### In-hospital angioplasty in non Q infarction

The place of angiography after non Q infarction has become a little clearer after the results of the VANQISH study. This study from the US used non-invasive exercise testing to assess the risk status in non Q infarct patients, only proceeding to angiography and intervention in the patients with evidence of ischaemia. The outcomes in this group were compared to the rapid angiography group who went straight to angiography and angioplasty as dictated by the angiogram appearances. The results suggested that the group who were treated more conservatively fared better.

It has been suggested that those patients who have ST segment depression rather than T inversion in association with an enzyme rise may have a worse prognosis and it may be reasonable to go straight to angiography in these patients. A pre-discharge exercise ECG test can be used to identify patients at high risk from ischaemia (those with marked ST depression at low work loads for example). Such patients should have angiography but others without evidence of ischaemia can be managed symptomatically.

### In-hospital angioplasty for unstable angina

Using such a conservative strategy, patients with acute unstable angina are given medical treatment and those whose symptoms fail to settle are offered acute angiography. It is also reasonable to suggest that patients whose symptoms do settle should be offered reasonably early non-invasive testing for ischaemia using exercise testing and those who have high risk positive test results should be offered angiography.

**Remember**

He is left on his atenolol for this exercise since the objective is to identify patients at high risk. The fact that the sensitivity of the test for ischaemia will be reduced by doing this is not of importance.

**Information**

There is no compelling evidence that acute angiography and subsequent angioplasty (and stenting) is superior to a conservative strategy.

## Uncertainty

The place of acute intervention during the hospital admission for an acute ischaemic syndrome remains controversial and there are many areas of uncertainty. Early coronary artery intervention may be thought to save myocardium and there is compelling evidence that the size of a myocardial infarction and the subsequent degree of left ventricular dysfunction are excellent predictors of a poor prognosis. This is the argument which drives practice towards early intervention that is being undertaken in many parts of the developed world at the moment.

The main areas of uncertainty

- Angioplasty in acute myocardial infarction has not been shown to be superior to acute thrombolysis in the longer term although there is evidence of short term benefit.

- Angioplasty and acute intervention is often recommended in patients whose pain fails to settle on the sound ground that intervention has been shown to be successful for symptom relief where medical management has failed. However it is important to remember that patients and their doctors vary in their assessment of pain. Even though angioplasty (and surgery if necessary) will relieve symptoms we will not be able to conclude that myocardium has necessarily been saved and that life has necessarily been prolonged. It is doubtful whether we will ever obtain controlled evidence in this area.

- The practice of intervening in patients with known high risk situations, such as the development of recurrent pain after the acute phase of a myocardial infarction has developed. The evidence that these patients are at high risk of losing further myocardium is good, and the evidence that the extent of myocardial loss determines prognosis is also good, although that is not the same as having controlled evidence that life will be prolonged by intervention.

- The need to stratify risk in those patients presenting to hospital for acute ischaemic syndromes is fairly well established. However, how risk should be assessed and when patients should be tested is not firmly established. Routine ECG based exercise testing is definitely less sensitive than radionucleide techniques or stress echocardiography. This lack of sensitivity may be an advantage rather than a disadvantage since the objective is to identify those at high risk. The diagnosis of ischaemic heart disease has already been established in the patients who have had an enzyme rise (or a raised troponin) and in the anginal patients who have definite ST segment changes which resolve with the resolution of their symptoms.

- If a patient presents within 12 hours to a hospital that has angiographic facilities, the case for angioplasty in high risk patients is more compelling. In the UK most patients are admitted to hospitals without these facilities and transfer adds to the overall risk.

**GROUP 10:**

**ITEM 14:**

# Cardiology
# Heart failure recognition and acute management

Differentiating heart failure from lung disease as a cause of breathlessness can be difficult as there is often a mixture of problems in patients. There is thus a tendency to give a concoction of therapy including diuretics, digoxin, ACE inhibitors and bronchodilators. This section will attempt to provide a diagnostic route to clarify the problem and seek therapeutic solutions.

## CASE HISTORY 1

An 80-year-old man is admitted at 3am with a four-day history of increasing breathlessness and cough. He lives alone in a first floor flat and smokes ten cigarettes a day.

### Is it heart failure?

| Differentiating symptoms | Heart failure | Lung disease |
|---|---|---|
| Breathlessness | Tends to be sudden | Often more gradual |
| Cough | Uncommon | Common |
| Orthopnoea | Usual | Possible |
| **Differentiating signs** | **Heart failure** | **Lung disease** |
| Raised JVP | Probable | Common in RV failure |
| Oedema | Common | Common in RV failure |
| Crackles at bases | Fine crackles | Coarse crackles |
| Wheeze | Uncommon | Common |
| Gallop | Moderately common | Rare |

### Practice point

As the clinical features can be confusing, reliance may have to be made on investigations in trying to identify whether the patient has cardiac failure:

| | Heart failure | Lung disease |
|---|---|---|
| ECG | Almost always abnormal | May be normal |
| CXR | Heart size often large | Heart size often normal |
| | Pulmonary oedema | Lungs clear or segmental defect |
| Echo | Abnormal ventricular function | LV function usually normal |
| | | Images may be poor |

## Information

- Systolic heart failure is associated with a decreased left ventricular ejection fraction. The heart is enlarged and there is frequently accompanying diastolic heart failure. The cause is often IHD.

- In Diastolic heart failure there is normal left ventricular systolic function with a small heart and delayed left ventricular filling. It often occurs in the elderly associated with hypertension.

## CASE 1 CONTINUED

The patient had a sudden onset of breathlessness, crackles at his lung bases and a BP of 190/110. His ECG showed an old anterior myocardial infarction.

In this patient the aetiology of the left ventricular failure appears to be a mixture of ischaemic heart disease and hypertension. The common causes of cardiac failure in this country include:

- Ischaemic heart disease
- Valvular heart disease
- Hypertension

Diabetes mellitus is an important risk factor

### Practice Point

If you can't identify an aetiology for the cardiac failure, and the ECG is normal, reconsider your diagnosis, but don't forget the possibilities of constrictive pericarditis or diastolic ventricular dysfunction. This latter diagnosis is difficult to make and confirm.

When cardiac failure appears, consider what has precipitated it and treat appropriately.

Could any of the following factors have been involved?

- Arrhythmia (e.g. atrial fibrillation)
- Myocardial infarction
- Excess fluid intake (e.g. post op I.V. fluids)
- Excess fluid retention (e.g. NSAIDs, renal failure)
- Anaemia, thyrotoxicosis
- Drug compliance

Correct the above if possible.

## Investigations

- Blood count – anaemia can precipitate failure
- Renal function – potassium, renal impairment
- ECG – ischaemia, LV+, arrhythmia
- CXR – large heart, pulmonary oedema
- Echo – valvular heart disease, LV dysfunction
- Atrial and brain natriuretic peptides are increased early in the presence of left ventricular dysfunction

## CASE 1 CONTINUED

Investigations in this man showed the old anterior MI on his ECG and pulmonary oedema on CXR.

### Management

This man needed rapid therapy to improve his clinical condition, with acute treatment to correct his breathlessness, followed by further therapy to maintain and improve left ventricular function.

The acute phase of therapy consists of:

- I.V. diuretics
- I.V. nitrates
  - these provide more rapid symptomatic relief than diuretics and should be given for the first 24 hours
- I.V. diamorphine
  - to relieve symptoms

- ACE Inhibitor
  - usually started after acute symptoms have settled
  - remember to watch renal function
  - recent evidence suggests that the use of higher doses of ACEIs is more effective
- Digoxin
  - valuable in atrial fibrillation
  - shown to reduce rate of hospitalisation in patients with sinus rhythm in the USA
- IPPV
  - patients who do not respond adequately to the previous measures may need short-term ventilation with PEEP

### Other lifestyle changes
- Reduce alcohol intake
- Reduce weight
- Reduce salt intake
- Take moderate regular exercise

His breathlessness and pulmonary oedema resolved after two days, and plans were made to discharge him when his condition was stable.

### Practice point

Patients are often left on excessively high doses of diuretics and may easily become dehydrated on discharge unless their therapy is reduced. However, patients developing heart failure whilst on diuretics usually require to be discharged on a higher dose than on admission. Aldosterone antagonists (spironolactone) have been shown to be beneficial.

The trend would be to increase the dose of the ACEI whilst reducing the diuretic dose, assessing the response by monitoring symptoms, signs and weight.

Further adjustments can be made in outpatients with reductions of frusemide (or equivalent) of 20mg.

### Selected Points
- Heart failure may be difficult to diagnose – especially with diastolic dysfunction
- A proportion of elderly patients are on diuretics but have no objective evidence of heart failure
- Echocardiography should be performed in most patients to identify an aetiology where this is in doubt, especially if a cardiac murmur is present
- ACEIs should be given to all patients unless contraindicated (i.e. renal impairment, aortic stenosis, renal artery stenosis)
- Look for precipitating causes (e.g. anaemia, NSAIDs) Adjust diuretic dose to minimum required
- Correct underlying causes (e.g. valvular heart disease)

*i*

**Information**

Increasing evidence shows that ß blockers improve prognosis in selected patients with heart failure, and are being increasingly used. A recent trial of bisoprolol was stopped early because of the significant survival benefit over placebo (CIBIS -II Trial). Carvedilol was also shown in a trial to be beneficial in these patients.

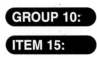

**GROUP 10:**

**ITEM 15:**

# Cardiology

## Aortic stenosis and other valvular heart disease

In the UK, valvular heart disease is now mainly degenerative rather than due to rheumatic fever. It is increasingly common over the age of 60, and needs careful assessment to select those who will benefit from surgery.

### Aortic Stenosis

Calcific, often on basis of a congenital bicuspid valve.

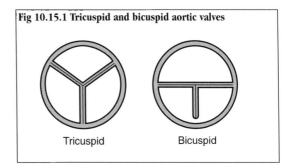

**Fig 10.15.1 Tricuspid and bicuspid aortic valves**

Tricuspid                    Bicuspid

### CASE HISTORY 1

A 75-year-old man is brought to hospital after he had blacked out running for a bus. He had fully recovered when he reached hospital. Cardiac examination revealed normal pulse, sinus rhythm, BP 180/90. The heart sounds were soft with a moderate systolic murmur heard all over the precordium. The CXR was normal and the ECG showed LBBB. A diagnosis of aortic sclerosis was made and he was sent home with an appointment to see a cardiologist. He was shown to have significant aortic stenosis with a gradient of 60mm Hg on echocardiography. He had a successful aortic valve replacement and has been symptom free since.

### Practice points

In degenerative aortic stenosis the physical signs can be misleading:

• Post exercise syncope in someone with a systolic murmur suggests significant aortic stenosis

• Aortic sclerosis is a dangerous diagnosis to make without full echo assessment

**Remember**

IF IN DOUBT REFER FOR ECHO
+ CARDIAC ASSESSMENT

- Soft heart sounds in the context of an aortic murmur suggest significant stenosis
- In older patients the pulse may not be anacrotic because of rigidity of the arterial tree and wide pulse pressure
- LVH in aortic stenosis is concentric and rarely produces cardiomegaly on CXR
- LBBB usually indicates significant LVH

**Fig 10.15.2 Pulse patterns in aortic valve disease**

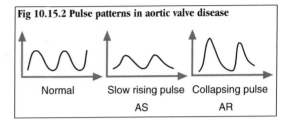

### Aortic regurgitation (AR)

- Aortic root dilatation (including Marfan's)
- Infective endocarditis (Group 10, Item 16)
- Rheumatic/degenerative/congenital valvular disease
- Hypertension

### Assessment of severity

- Clinical
  – wide pulse pressure, low diastolic BP, LVH
- ECHO
  – left ventricular dilatation – limits are now defined for surgical intervention

### Mitral valve disease

Mitral Stenosis/(MS) is increasingly uncommon and mainly seen in the immigrant population or in older age where often associated with mitral regurgitation and non-pliant valve.

Mitral Regurgitation (MR) has multiple causes:

- Functional in cardiac failure due to mitral ring dilatation
- Papillary muscle dysfunction/rupture
- Rheumatic
- Mitral valve prolapse
- Hypertrophic cardiomyopathy (Group 10, Item 18)

### Assessment of severity of MS and MR

- Clinical
  – RVH + evidence of pulmonary hypertension (MS)
  – LVH and 3rd heart sound (MR)
- Echo
  – mitral valve area (MS)
  – left ventricular dimensions (MR)

**Remember**

In acute AR (e.g. endocarditis) the murmur may become inaudible and replaced by a third heart sound. If this happens the patient needs URGENT surgical referral.

### CASE HISTORY 2

A 64-year-old man was admitted in heart failure with signs of mitral regurgitation. He had been in hospital six months earlier with heart failure and had been well since on maintenance treatment with digoxin, diuretics and an ACEI. He had gross cardiomegaly on chest X-ray and the ECG showed LVH and ST change. He responded to an increased dose of diuretics. Echo assessment confirmed severe MR due to papillary muscle dysfunction; the left ventricle was dilated and had some impairment of function (EF 45%). Cardiac catheterisation showed normal coronary arteries and confirmed the Echo findings. He had a mitral valve replacement and made a good recovery. He remains however on maintenance treatment with digoxin and diuretics and still has cardiomegaly on CXR one year later.

### Practice points

• Mitral valve replacement should be considered once a patient with MR has developed heart failure

• Outcome of mitral value replacement is largely determined by LV function

• Where there is impairment of LV function the decision to undertake surgery for MR can be very difficult (see below).

### Summary

### When should you consider surgery?

• *Aortic stenosis*
Usually well compensated for by LVH for many years but deterioration rapid once symptoms have developed. Operate when: dyspnoea, chest pain, syncope.

• *Aortic regurgitation*
Not very well compensated for by LV dilatation.
Symptoms poor guide for intervention.
Operate when: Echo evidence of progressive LV dilatation.
(End systolic dimension > 5.5cm).

• *Mitral stenosis*
Slowly progressive symptoms over decades; some compensatory RV hypertrophy.
Operate when: Mitral valve area < 1cm² and symptoms uncontrolled on medical treatment.
Any evidence of pulmonary HT.
(Note: threshold for intervention lower if suitable for valvotomy/valvoplasty).

• *Mitral regurgitation*
Slowly progressive symptoms as with MS; compensatory LV dilatation and hypertrophy with variable RVH/pulmonary HT.
Operate when: symptoms not controlled on medical treatment and any evidence of pulmonary HT. [Recent evidence suggests

**Remember**
Age is not a barrier to valvular surgery if LV function good and no major coronary disease is present.

that progressive LV dilatation on Echo also important – see AR above]. Functional mitral regurgitation can act as a 'safety valve' for a failing left ventricle; operation in these circumstances can be fatal.

(Note: needs careful assessment of LV function before operation considered).

### Prosthetic valves – common problems

- Heart failure – must be assumed to be due to valve malfunction until proved otherwise. NEEDS URGENT CARDIAC ASSESSMENT.
- Murmurs – paraprosthetic leaks common, but should be formally assessed by Echo.
- Infection – blood cultures must be taken for any febrile illness before giving antibiotics. Endocarditis of prosthetic valve should be referred to cardio thoracic centre.
- Anticoagulants – control is very important (INR 3.5). Take specialist advice before any surgical intervention.

## GROUP 10:
## ITEM 16:

# Cardiology
# Infective endocarditis

Untreated infective endocarditis is invariably fatal. Delay in the diagnosis of infective endocarditis may:

- Make medical treatment more prolonged
- Increase the risk of death
- Promote the need for surgery which might have been avoided had treatment been started earlier

It follows that endocarditis is a diagnosis which needs to be kept in mind when dealing with any pyrexial or constitutional illness in patients with valvular or congenital heart disease.

### CASE HISTORY 1

A 28-year-old man presents with a pyrexia. His doctor had prescribed amoxicillin for a flu like illness three weeks previously. He had a pyrexia of 38.5°. There was a mid systolic murmur radiating to the neck and the apex. Careful inspection of the nail beds and of the conjunctivae failed to reveal any splinter haemorrhages. However blood cultures taken in A&E on arrival in the hospital showed a growth of gram positive cocci in both bottles. These cocci were later identified as Strep. viridans. He was started on Amoxicillin and gentamycin to which the organism was sensitive. A transthoracic echocardiogram suggested that there was a vegetation on the aortic valve.

Blood cultures were negative from the onset of treatment and intravenous antibiotics were continued for two weeks. Oral antibiotics were prescribed for a further three weeks. The CRP levels were monitored and fell steadily through the course of the illness.

There are a number of difficulties which can occur in the management of the condition.

It is best to wait for the result of the blood cultures before starting treatment (three sets are appropriate). However it is sometimes necessary to start treatment particularly if staph. aureus is suspected.

- Prosthetic valve endocarditis is very difficult to manage and should be transferred to a cardiothoracic surgical centre.
- Haemodynamic deterioration may precipitate the need for surgery in endocarditis. The difficulty is that operative results are clearly better if the surgeons are able to operate in a field which is no longer infected. However, fatal haemodynamic deterioration can only be prevented by surgery in some patients.

**Remember**
The main problem with endocarditis is delay in the diagnosis.

• Aortic valve endocarditis often needs surgical intervention. It is wise to regard aortic valve endocarditis as being "a surgical condition which occasionally responds to medical treatment".

• Transthoracic echocardiography does not exclude a diagnosis of endocarditis. (Staphylococcal endocarditis in particular may produce very small vegetations which are below the resolution of the technique. These vegetations are often quite difficult to see with the naked eye at post mortem.)

• In aortic stenosis a changing pattern of conduction and especially the development of first degree AV block strongly suggests an aortic root abscess.

• A fever as a result of antibiotic sensitivity may develop after a prolonged course of intravenous antibiotics (especially penicillins). This can lead to a false suspicion that the endocarditis is not successfully treated.

• Staph. aureus septicaemia should always be regarded as being consequent upon endocarditis.

• Right sided endocarditis is a disease characteristic of intravenous drug users. The condition may present with cardiac signs such as a murmur or evidence of tricuspid regurgitation on the JVP. However there may be few signs at the outset and the major abnormality may be on the chest X-ray, with areas of apparent consolidation suggestive of a bronchopneumonia. The condition may present with a "white out" of the two lung fields.

**Remember**

All patients with cardiac murmurs require antibiotic prophylaxis for dental procedures. For details consult British National Formulary

**GROUP 10:**

**ITEM 17:**

# Cardiology
# Cor pulmonale

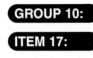

**Remember**

Patients with long standing lung disease may develop pulmonary hypertension.

Cor pulmonale is a term which refers to syndromes where the physical findings of heart failure are found in association with lung problems. A more stringent definition is that cor pulmonale is right ventricular hypertrophy due to structural or functional disease of the lungs (except where the lung disease is itself a consequence of left sided or congenital heart disease). This definition includes primary pulmonary hypertension and chronic pulmonary hypertension due to thrombo-embolism.

## CASE HISTORY 1

A 43-year-old woman has smoked since she was eight years old. Between the ages of 17 and 32 she also used intravenous heroin. Her alcohol consumption has also been very heavy over the years although she neither drinks nor uses illegal drugs now. She continues to smoke cigarettes although her consumption has fallen from over 40 per day to below 10.

She developed a persistent productive cough at the age of 38. In the last two years she has had eight admissions to hospital. She is cyanosed at rest and her best level of $PaO_2$ on air in the last 12 months is 8.2. She developed peripheral oedema needing diuretics one year ago. On her current admission, there was pulsation palpable to the left of the sternum and for four centimetres laterally to the sternum, the JVP was elevated to the angle of the jaw. She has not been able to use home oxygen because of her inability to give up smoking.

### Pathology

Cor pulmonale develops as a result of pulmonary arterial wall hypertrophy. This may be a direct effect of destructive lung diseases or may develop as a result of long standing alveolar hypoxia.

### Patho-physiology

Pulmonary hypertension leads to the elevation of right ventricular pressure and dilatation of both the right ventricle and the right atrium. This in turn may lead to the physical findings of peripheral oedema, raised JVP, hepatic enlargement (which may be pulsatile because of the tricuspid regurgitation) and ascites. In fact the cause of the fluid retention in cor pulmonale is still debated, since there is little evidence that it is truly due to haemodynamic dysfunction of the right ventricle. The most likely explanation is that hypercapnoea – an almost invariable feature of cor pulmonale – interferes with the humoral mechanisms controlling sodium and water balance leading to fluid retention.

In practice it is relatively common to encounter patients where there is evidence of fluid retention, right ventricular hypertrophy and evidence of left ventricular problems. Presumably this occurs because of coexistent primary problems such as ischaemic heart disease and hypertension.

## What are the causes?

**Table 10.17.1**

| Common | Other problems whose terminal event is commonly Cor Pulmonale | Diseases where Cor Pulmonale occasionally occurs |
|---|---|---|
| COPD | Pulmonary fibrosis | Asthma |
| Obstructive Sleep | Scoliosis and other chest wall deformities | Localised bronchiectasis Restrictive lung disease |
| Apnoea | Respiratory Muscle Weakness | such as Sarcoidosis |
| | Cystic Fibrosis | |
| | Generalised Bronchiectasis | |

### Investigations

• Arterial blood gases
• Plasma U & Es
• X-ray
• ECG – shows a frontal axis deviated to the right. In patients whose records contain a series of ECGs the rightward drift of the axis can be shown over time. This is diagnostic of pulmonary hypertension since the axis normally moves to the left over time.
• Echo

## How would you manage a case of Cor pulmonale?

In COPD an PaO$_2$ of less than 7.3 kP is an indication for home oxygen treatment. Oxygen is given for a minimum of 15 hours per day, usually by a home oxygen concentrator. This has been shown to reduce the level of pulmonary hypertension and should therefore both produce symptomatic relief and to improve prognosis.

Otherwise treatment of Cor pulmonale is symptomatic with diuretics for fluid retention and bronchodilators if they are indicated for the primary chest disease. There is no direct evidence of benefit from ACE inhibitors or other bronchodilators although many patients have co-existent LV dysfunction which may be presumed to benefit from ACE inhibitors.

## What is the prognosis?

In any lung disease the development of cor pulmonale is always a sinister sign. The prognosis of cor pulmonale in COPD without treatment is poor, the five year survival is about 30% compared with a five year survival of about 60% in otherwise comparable patients without cor pulmonale. Cor pulmonale is not an invariable feature of COPD, however in those with disease listed in the middle column of Table 10.17.1, cor pulmonale usually develops eventually and its diagnosis heralds the terminal phase of the illness.

**GROUP 10:**

**ITEM 18:**

# Cardiology
# Cardiomyopathy

### CASE HISTORY 1

A 50-year-old man is admitted with increasing breathlessness. There is no history of chest pain or palpitations but he has signs of pulmonary oedema.

### When should you consider a dilated cardiomyopathy (DCM)?

In a patient with features of cardiac failure:

**Remember**

• Cardiomyopathies are rare in acute medical practice but because of this they may be forgotten.

• Echocardiography is invaluable in defining the problem.

• Without a history of
  – hypertension
  – ischaemic heart disease
  – valvular heart disease
• With a history of
  – excess alcohol intake
  – a recent viral infection
  – late pregnancy or early postpartum
• With investigations showing
  – no frank infarction on ECG
  – global, rather than segmental, systolic dysfunction

### Learning points

The management of a DCM is similar to that of cardiac failure in general. The differences are:

• To define an aetiology if possible as this may be reversible e.g. alcohol excess
• To be sure that ischaemic heart disease has been excluded as secondary prevention would then be important. Coronary revascularisation has been proposed to improve the function of hibernating myocardium (see Group 10, Item 8)
• Some acute DCMs run an aggressive course with rapidly worsening ventricular function and transplantation may be required

## CASE HISTORY 2

A 35-year-old woman presented to the A&E department with palpitations and is noted to have a soft systolic murmur. Her ECG showed atrial fibrillation and marked left ventricular hypertrophy.

### Practice point

With the decline in rheumatic heart disease a hypertrophic cardiomyopathy (HOCM) has become a likely cause of a systolic murmur with atrial fibrillation.

### Differentiation of aortic stenosis and hypertrophic cardiomyopathy

|  | AS | HOCM |
|---|---|---|
| Murmur | Ejection systolic | Ejection systolic |
|  |  | May be additional mitral regurgitation murmur |
| Pulse | May be slow rising | Described as jerky |
| Additional sounds |  | 4th sound possible |
| ECG | Left ventricular hypertrophy in later stages | Left ventricular hypertrophy (including early stages) |
|  | May be normal even when severe | May be bizarre changes including large septal Q waves |
| CXR | Heart size may be normal even when severe | Heart size may be normal |
| Echo | Aortic valve thickened Gradient on Doppler across valve Left ventricular hypertrophy if severe | Characteristic 1. Asymmetric septal hypertrophy 2. Systolic anterior motion of mitral valve 3. Mid-systolic closure of aortic valve |

**⚠ Remember**

In heart failure with a normal size heart on CXR consider:
- Restrictive cardiomyopathy
- Constrictive pericarditis
- Aortic stenosis
- Mitral stenosis ("silent")

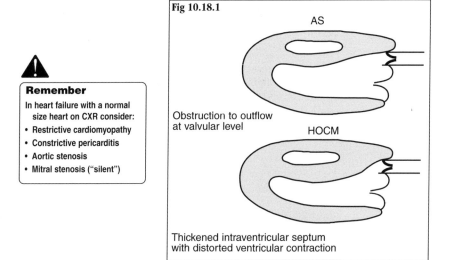

**Fig 10.18.1**

AS

Obstruction to outflow at valvular level

HOCM

Thickened intraventricular septum with distorted ventricular contraction

## Learning points

- A hypertrophic cardiomyopathy may be obstructive (HOCM) or non-obstructive (HCM)
- HOCM is the more troublesome and can be associated with sudden death
- Sudden death is more likely if there is a family history of HOCM and sudden death and/or if a 24-hour ECG tape shows episodic ventricular tachycardia
- Consider hypertension as causing left ventricular hypertrophy before diagnosing HCM
- Verapamil or a beta blocker are recommended in HOCM
- Amiodarone is advised if ventricular tachycardia is diagnosed
- Screen the family if HOCM is diagnosed

## CASE HISTORY 3

A 50-year-old woman presents with features of heart failure, normal blood pressure and heart sounds and has a small heart size on chest X-Ray. Investigations subsequently showed her to have cardiac amyloid.

Restrictive cardiomyopathy is rare, but may be due to:

- Amyloid
- Diabetes
- Sarcoid
- Haemochromatosis

**GROUP 10:**

**ITEM 19:**

# Cardiology
# Investigating hypertension (HT)

### CASE HISTORY 1

An anxious 38-year-old woman comes to A&E with a bad migraine. Her BP has been recorded as 165/110 on a number of occasions whilst she is waiting to be seen by the medical SHO. How will you assess her?

### What is the significance of the BP reading?

• Relevance of anxiety: raised BP is a common response to stress, more so in some individuals than in others
• Prior history of high BP: adds significance to present reading
• Presence of family history of hypertension: single most important determinant in essential HT
• Relationship to migraine: no direct link between this and HT has been established but beta blockers are good for both
• Relationship to age: BP does rise with age, but still carries an adverse cardiovascular risk. Current evidence suggests treatment of the elderly is probably more cost effective than the young.
• Relationship to lifestyle: high alcohol intake is a common contributory factor in high BP

### What should you be looking for?

• Clinical signs of end organ damage:
  – fundoscopy – hypertensive retinopathy grades I-IV
  – LVH – forceful/displaced apex beat, loud A2
  – proteinuria
• Causes of secondary HT:
  – coarctation aorta – have you felt the femorals?
  – renal disease – renal bruits/proteinuria/urea & electrolytes
  – Cushing's syndrome – obesity, striae; may have low $K^+$
  – Conn's – no signs; usually low $K^+$ and high normal $Na^+$
  – Phaeochromocytoma – presentation often atypical (e.g. acute pulmonary oedema, sweating attacks) rather than textbook flushing/palpitations.

Always exclude in young or unresponsive hypertensive. Measure 24-hour urinary excretion and plasma catecholamines.

### Assuming negative findings/investigations what will you do now?

• Identify whether this is sustained or 'white coat' HT:
  – further readings by GP/practice nurse probably most cost effective

• Home BP monitoring
   – automated BP machines now reliable enough to make this a good alternative for some patients
• Twenty-four hour BP monitor
   – now widely available and often eliminates 'white coat' hypertension
• Base line investigations
   – urea & electrolytes
   – ECG: a very insensitive detector of LVH, BUT when voltage criteria are present this carries considerable prognostic risk and should not be ignored. Fig 10.19.1 shows LVH with S in lead $V_2$ and R in $V_5$ more than 35mm.

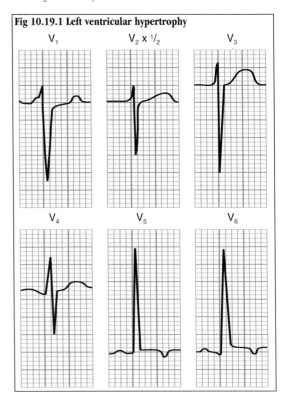

**Fig 10.19.1 Left ventricular hypertrophy**

**Information**

• Coarctation of aorta
   – a narrowing of the aorta at or just distal to the insertion of the ductus arteriosus
• Cushing's Syndrome
   – is caused by free circulating glucocorticoids
• Conns' Syndrome
   – is 1° aldosteronism due to adrenal adenoma or hyperplasia

– CXR: cardiomegaly when present is important, but rarely adds much to good clinical examination (rib notching exciting, but coarctation should not have been missed clinically!)
– Echo: a more sensitive indicator of LVH, but time consuming and operator dependent. Should be kept for difficult/borderline patients

## When should you look for secondary causes?

• Young patient (under 45) and no family history of hypertension
• HT resistant to treatment
• Those with accelerated HT

### Remember

• High BP is a significant risk factor for future cardiac events and should be followed up.
• Secondary causes apart from renal disease are rare – the average hospital consultant will probably see no more than two to three of each in a working lifetime.

## Investigations in this group include:

• Renal ultrasound: non-invasive, readily available, excludes major renal pathology
• Isotope renogram (+ captopril stress): reasonable screening test for renal artery stenosis, but not very sensitive (may miss some). Remember that significant radiation exposure (equivalent to barium enema) so caution in young people
• Renal angiogram: definitive diagnosis in renal artery stenosis
• Twenty-four hour urine collection: catecholamines & cortisol – these require separate bottles! Plasma catecholamines are most accurate for phaeohromocytoma if available
• CT/MRI abdomen: when adrenal disease suspected/confirmed + CT, MRI angiography for reno-vascular disease

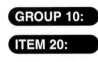

# Cardiology
# Drug treatment of hypertension

### Remember

The Hypertensive Crisis – recognising malignant (accelerated) HT – a rare problem with the earlier recognition and treatment of HT

### Investigations

- Renal function: renal impairment likely in severe HT and may be accompanied by electrolyte disturbance
- CT head scan: if focal signs present to exclude CVA

### Information

- Beware: Caution when reducing BP
- Lowering BP is crucial to the management of malignant HT, but should not be precipitant because of the risks of causing a stroke
- Very high BP readings can occur in an evolving stroke, and should be treated very cautiously because of the risk of extending the stroke

## CASE HISTORY 1

A 50-year-old man is visiting from Ghana and is brought to A&E by his relatives after behaving oddly. His BP is recorded by the nurses as 220/140 in both arms. This is accelerated hypertension.

### What is your immediate management?

Clinical assessment:

- CNS – orientation, focal neurological signs
  - differentiation of hypertensive encephalopathy and a small CVA may be difficult
- Fundoscopy – the presence of haemorrhages/exudates and/or papilloedema indicate accelerated hypertension
- LVH -clinical/ECG
  - most patients with severe HT have ECG evidence of LVH
  - look for secondary causes e.g. polycystic kidneys

### What drugs are available for treatment in this case?

- Oral:
  - beta blockers e.g. atenolol
  - calcium channel blockers e.g. nifedipine, diltiazem
  - diuretics
- Intravenous (only in a real emergency e.g. aortic dissection): labetalol, nitroprusside infusion
- In this man a reasonable approach would be 10mg capsule of nifedipine intrabuccally.

### Long-term treatment of hypertension

Current practice includes all major classes of antihypertensive drugs as first line therapy, but the only drugs shown to improve prognosis (as well as lower BP) are: diuretics, beta blockers and the older drugs such as methyldopa.

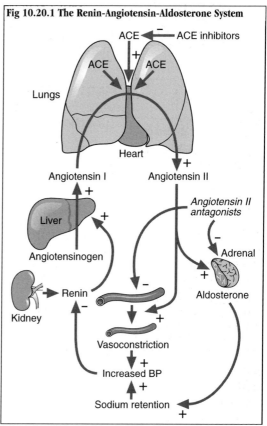

Fig 10.20.1 The Renin-Angiotensin-Aldosterone System

Redrawn from *Clinical Medicine*, 4th Edition, Kumar and Clark, 1998, by permission of the publisher WB Saunders

## Common side-effects of antihypertensive medication that may present acutely to hospital:

- Beta blockers:
  - asthma/bronchitis
  - bradycardia (especially in elderly)
  - cardiac failure
- Diuretics:
  - gout
  - hypokalaemia (if severe – < 2.5mmol/l – consider Conn's syndrome)
  - diabetes (often overlooked)
- ACE inhibitors:
  - cough (often overlooked)
  - hypotension/falls (especially in elderly)

– renal failure (especially in diabetics and claudicants where renal artery stenosis is more common)

• Calcium channel blockers:
  – ankle oedema (especially nifedipine, amlodipine)
  – constipation (especially verapamil)

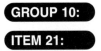

## Cardiology
## The swollen/ischaemic leg

Common causes of a swollen leg are:

• Deep venous thrombosis
• Acute rupture knee joint/Bakers cyst
• Trauma – e.g. rupture of tendon/muscle
• Infection – cellulitis, osteomyelitis

**Remember**

The diagnosis is usually straightforward in such a case, but studies show that in many situations, e.g. post operative, a DVT may be present without any physical signs, so a high degree of suspicion is necessary.

### CASE HISTORY 1

A 36-year-old woman on the oral contraceptive pill developed pain in her left calf 3 days ago; it had become increasingly swollen since. Examination revealed oedema of the lower leg without any change in colour or prominence of the veins; there was tenderness along the line of the deep veins. Doppler studies showed early thrombus in the popliteal veins. She was anticoagulated for six months and given alternative contraceptive advice.

The best way of making the diagnosis is currently a matter of debate:

• Venography
  – probably the gold standard, but may not be immediately available, and can be misleading if past history of venous thrombosis
• Doppler ultrasound
  – only detects clot reliably in popliteal/femoral vein, but not in calf veins
• Venous plethysmography:
  – may be viable alternative to ultrasound for femoral/popliteal veins but does not reliably detect thrombus confined to calf veins
• D-dimer assay
  – for detecting fresh thrombus – it has a high negative predictive value i.e. if negative, a DVT is unlikely

### Practice point

The importance of making a definitive diagnosis depends on the clinical scenario. In a young woman a precise diagnosis is essential as it will influence subsequent contraceptive advice and management of pregnancy. In a routine post operative DVT with no contraindications to anticoagulation, a clinical diagnosis is probably sufficient.

### Duration of treatment

Current recommendations of:

• Six months: proximal DVT +/− pulmonary embolus
• Three months: localised calf DVT. (Six weeks is probably enough for a 1st DVT with no persisting risk factors)

Target INR is 2.5

Note: Target values rather than ranges are now used. With recurrent DVT consider screening for thrombophilia

### Remember

**Ruptured knee joint** should be suspected if:
• The onset of symptoms is sudden
• There is a history of joint disease especially RA
• Knee effusions are present
• Any bruising is seen

## CASE HISTORY 2

A 56-year-old ex-rugby player developed a sharp pain in the leg on stepping off a bus. He went to his GP the next day when the whole calf was swollen and painful. The leg appeared inflamed and he was started on antibiotics with a provisional diagnosis of cellulitis. He attended A&E two days later when it was no better: the findings were of a diffusely tender and swollen calf with some ankle oedema but little residual erythema. A clinical diagnosis of DVT was made and intravenous heparin started. The following day there was extensive bruising around the ankle and dorsum of the foot. The registrar noted bilateral osteoarthritis of the knees with moderate effusions, and diagnosed a **ruptured knee joint**. This was confirmed by an ultrasound of the calf popliteal fossa.

**Remember**

Acute limb ischaemia
Usually embolic; seek cardiac source.

Early embolectomy may save a limb: IMMEDIATE surgical referral.

## CASE HISTORY 3

A 78-year-old man developed sudden pain and weakness of the left hand. The hand was cold and pulseless indicating **acute limb ischaemia**. He was in sinus rhythm but a systolic murmur was noted at the apex. Successful embolectomy was performed. Post operatively he had a low grade fever; blood taken at the time of admission showed anaemia (Hb 10.6g/dl) with normochromic picture and an ESR 76mm/hr. Blood cultures were negative. Echocardiography showed a mass in the left atrium which proved at surgery to be an atrial myxoma.

Common cause of embolisation:

• AF (even when paroxysmal) (see Group 10, Item 3)

Rarer causes of embolisation
• Bacterial endocarditis (see Group 10, Item 16)
• Atrial myxoma

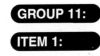

**GROUP 11:** Respiratory disorders

**ITEM 1:** Acute breathlessness

⚠️ **Remember**

Respiratory diseases can cause breathlessness within minutes or hours, or slowly over days, weeks or months.

### CASE HISTORY 1

You are bleeped by the nurses to see a 63-year-old man who has become breathless. As you are walking over to the ward you consider what the causes might be on this rather scanty history! The systems involved would most probably be cardiac (see heart failure Group 10, Item 14) or respiratory.

Go through this list as you walk to the ward

- If sudden – the causes may be
  - an inhaled foreign body
  - a pneumothorax
  - a pulmonary embolus
- If over a few hours
  - asthma
  - pneumonia
  - pulmonary oedema
  - respiratory muscle disease eg Guillain Barre
- If intermittent
  - asthma
  - pulmonary oedema
  - pulmonary emboli
- If over a few days
  - pleural effusion
  - carcinoma of the bronchus
  - pneumonia including pulmonary tuberculosis
- And lastly over months or years
  - idiopathic pulmonary fibrosis
  - COPD
  - chest wall or neuromuscular disease
  - occupational lung disease
  - non-respiratory causes    – anaemia, hyperthyroidism

Despite this long list, in this 63-year-old man, the chances are that it is COPD or heart failure, or if sudden, a pulmonary embolus.

### Basic examination is

- What does the patient look like?
- What is the severity of the problem?
- Tachypnoea?
- Using accessory muscles?
- Respiratory distress?

- Colour –? cyanosed
- Pulse – rate, type, volume?
- B.P.
- Then make a full cardiac and respiratory examination
- Evidence of D.V.T.

### Useful pointers to the diagnosis and management

**Is it acute asthma?**

Typical history.

- What is precipitating cause?

Assessment of severity:

- Tachycardia
- Tachypnoea
- Hyper-inflated, generally wheezy chest
- Difficulty speaking
- Low PEFR and low $FEV_1$

### Is it an acute exacerbation of COPD?

History of preceding COPD, precipitating causes

- Infection
- Onset of AF or LVF
- Sedatives
- Recent abdominal surgery

Check PEFR (or ideally $FEV_1$ and FVC, CXR, ECG, $O_2$ saturation using oximeter. Note an oximeter does NOT tell you about the carbon dioxide. Therefore, consider doing arterial blood gases as well if:

- Tachycardia >100
- Tachypnoea >25
- Confusion or agitation
- Raised JVP, gallop rhythm, evidence of low cardiac output

### Is it a Pneumothorax?

Confirm with Chest X-ray. If this is large – consider aspiration or tube if underlying lung disease.

Tension pneumothorax: **needs emergency $R_x$**

- Signs minimal if underlying lung disease
- Respiratory distress
- Contralateral mediastinal shift
- Hypotension and other signs of shock

### Is it a pleural effusion?

Confirm with chest X-ray, consider pleural tap. Signs:

**Remember**

Beware of the SILENT CHEST! If asthma is very severe air entry will be minimal and breath sounds quiet or absent.

• Stony dull percussion note
• Absent breath sounds

### Is it pneumonia?

Signs:

• Febrile / toxic
• Dull percussion note
• Bronchial breathing + crackles
• May be hypoxic – check by oximetry or ABG

### Is it a collapsed lung?

Confirm with chest X-ray. May require bronchoscopy eventually. Therefore, if acutely distressed call respiratory team.

Causes:

• Carcinoma of bronchus
• Inhaled foreign body
• Large sputum plug e.g. asthma or COPD

**Notable features**

• Ipsilateral mediastinal shift
• Dull percussion note
• Reduced or absent breath sounds – bronchial breathing
• Increased (or absent if bronchial obstr.) vocal fremitus

### Is it upper airways obstruction?

Often an emergency

• Stridor
• Respiratory distress
• Cyanosis +/– shock

**Causes of upper airways obstruction**

| | Action |
|---|---|
| • Anaphylaxis – laryngeal oedema | • Adrenaline IM/ hydrocortisone • $O_2$ |
| • Carcinoma of upper airway | • Call ENT for laryngoscopy |
| • Inhaled foreign body | • Heimlich manoeuvre (see box) then call ENT |
| • Tracheal compression eg bleeding post thyroidectomy | • Tracheal decompression eg release skin sutures |

⚠

**Remember**

The Heimlich Manouevre
Used to expel an inhaled foreign body

• Stand behind the patient
• Encircle your arms around the upper part of the abdomen just below the patientís rib cage
• Give a sharp, forceful squeeze, forcing the diaphragm sharply into the thorax. This should expel sufficient air from the lungs to force the foreign body out of the trachea

If this fails, urgent assessment by experienced ENT or cardiothoracic clinician required. Fibre optic or rigid bronchoscopy will be required if aspiration beyond vocal cords.

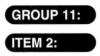

## Respiratory disorders
## Cough

Cough is common and may cause considerable fear and distress. Apart from the immediate discomfort of coughing, paroxysmal cough may interrupt sleep, provoke retching or vomiting and if severe result in rib fractures or syncope. Always enquire about sputum and its colour.

Cough is provoked by stimulation of mucosal irritant and stretch receptors of the lung. Accordingly it has a number of causes.

### Acute Cough

- Inhalation of direct irritants e.g. smoke, chlorine gas, ozone and other air pollutants
- In the asthmatic, inhalation of specific allergen e.g. pollen or non-specific low concentration irritants e.g. perfume, tobacco fumes
- Upper and lower respiratory tract infections (yellow/green sputum)

### Chronic Cough

- Large airway obstruction e.g. carcinoma of bronchus or inhaled foreign body (Note peanuts and other inhaled food will not be radiodense)
- Persistent bronchial inflammation e.g. asthma, bronchiectasis, COPD, smoking
- Persistent infection e.g. tuberculosis, lung abscess
- Interstitial lung disease e.g. pulmonary fibrosis, asbestosis
- Raised left atrial pressure e.g. mitral stenosis, left ventricular failure
- Gastro-oesophageal reflux (GORD) and bulbar dysfunction
- Iatrogenic e.g. ACE inhibitors, radiation pneumonitis

### Enquire about associated features such as

- Haemoptysis
- Pleuritic pain
- History of myocardial infarction (suggesting cough due to left ventricular failure)
- Breathlessness

### All patients with persistent cough should have a CXR

Other investigations will depend on likely cause e.g. serial peak flow in asthma, radio isotope contrast studies if gastro-oesophageal reflux or aspiration is suspected and sputum culture, including request for M. Tuberculosis isolation, if cough is productive.

**Respiratory disorders**

**Breathlessness and wheeze**

Asthma causes breathlessness, cough and wheeze. However, all that wheezes is not asthma. The following conditions need to be considered in differential diagnosis:

• COPD

   – patient usually > 40 years of age

   – heavy smoker > 20 pack years. (Note patients with asthma may also smoke)

   – history of variable wheeze. In patients with asthma, chest wheeze is usually worse at night and may only be episodic

• Upper airway obstruction

Stridor

   – occurs when there is a mechanical obstruction in the larynx or trachea

   – is heard during inspiration and expiration; but inspiratory sound when mouth open most typical

   – may be associated with vigorous accessory muscle activity and obvious distress

• Left ventricular failure

   – acute LVF may be difficult to differentiate from asthma

   – nocturnal symptoms common to both

## CASE HISTORY 1

A 24-year-old female was admitted with breathlessness for six hours. She has had a 'cold' for two days. Past history revealed her being 'chesty' as a child. It was noticed that she could not complete sentences easily. Heart rate was 126/min and respiratory rate was 30/min. There was expiratory wheeze over the lung fields.

This patient has acute severe asthma.

Fig 11.3.1 shows causes and triggers of asthma.

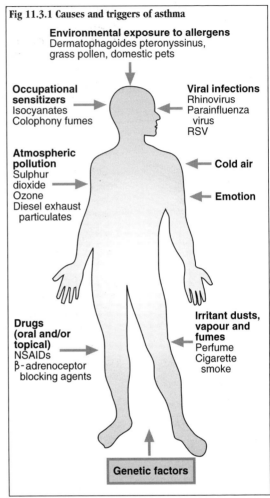

**Fig 11.3.1 Causes and triggers of asthma**

**Environmental exposure to allergens**
Dermatophagoides pteronyssinus,
grass pollen, domestic pets

**Occupational sensitizers**
Isocyanates
Colophony fumes

**Viral infections**
Rhinovirus
Parainfluenza virus
RSV

**Atmospheric pollution**
Sulphur dioxide
Ozone
Diesel exhaust particulates

**Cold air**

**Emotion**

**Drugs (oral and/or topical)**
NSAIDs
β-adrenoceptor blocking agents

**Irritant dusts, vapour and fumes**
Perfume
Cigarette smoke

**Genetic factors**

Redrawn from *Clinical Medicine*, 4th Edition, Kumar and Clark, 1998, by permission of the publisher WB Saunders

**Remember**

Acute Severe Asthma
• Increased Breathlessness
• Respiratory Rate > 25/min
• Heart Rate > 100/min
• PEFR <50% of best

### How would you manage this patient in A&E?

Immediate management should be:

• Reassurance that treatment will be effective
• Oxygen 40-60% (Keep $SaO_2$ > 90%)
• Systemic Corticosteroids
  − prednisolone 30–40 mgs daily or
  − I.V. Hydrocortisone 200 mg
• Nebulised $\beta_2$ agonist (Salbutamol 5 mg or Terbutaline 10 mg) with oxygen

Monitor

- $SaO_2$ by oximetry
- Do Arterial Blood Gases
  - initially if $SaO_2$ < 90% ?
  - recheck (two-hourly) if $PaO_2$ <8 kPa / $PaCO_2$ >5kPa until $SaO_2$ >90% and $PaCO_2$ is stable
- PEFR four-hourly. Note performing PEFR may be distressing for patient -do not demand unnecessary repeat testing
- Heart Rate

## Information

I.V. Aminophylline

- Ensure patient not on oral theophylline (DO NOT GIVE AMINOPHYLLINE IF THEY ARE)
- Monitor B.P. & heart rate
- Loading dose 250 mg over one-hour

Infusion:

- 1 mg/kg four hrs
- 0.5mg/kg thereafter
- 1 mg/kg if smoker
- Check aminophylline level at six to eight hours following start of infusion and adjust dose.

### Thirty minutes later there has been no significant improvement in her breathlessness and PEFR. What would you do next ?

Nebulise $\beta_2$ agonist with added Ipratropium (500 mcg). Repeat every 30 minutes if necessary.

Intravenous aminophylline infusion could be considered if patient does not respond to repeated nebulisation with $\beta_2$ agonist & Ipratropium. If oral aminophylline has been taken DO NOT USE.

Intravenous $\beta_2$ agonist is a better alternative in most cases.

### Life threatening features of asthma

- Silent chest, feeble respiration
- Bradycardia / Hypotension
- Exhaustion / Confusion
- PEFR < 33% of Best

### Indications For HDU or Intensive Care

Presence of life threatening features such as

- $PaO_2$ < 8 kPa on 60% oxygen
- $PaCO_2$ > 6 kPa
- Exhaustion, confusion or hypotension
- Previous history of IPPV

### There was improvement in PEFR and breathlessness with nebulised β2 agonist and Ipratropium. What treatment should be offered to her now?

Continuing management should be:

- Keeping $SaO_2$ > 90% with oxygen supplementation
- Cortico-steroids: Prednisolone 20-40 mg daily
- Two to four-hourly nebulised $\beta_2$ agonist therapy

### When could she be discharged?

The patient can be discharged when:

• Symptoms have improved, particularly nocturnal
• Ideally PEFR should be 75% of Best and diurnal variation (i.e. 'morning dips') < 25%. If patient is improving and compliance expected to be good an earlier discharge is reasonable.

### Twenty-four to 48 hours before discharge

• Add inhaled cortico-steroids to oral steroids
• Replace nebulised bronchodilators with inhalers
• Check inhaler technique (? may need spacer)
• Determine what was cause of this attack (non-compliance, infection, allergen exposure)

### Ask asthma nurse to see

At discharge, patient should have:

• Oral & inhaled cortico-steroids and, as required, inhaled $\beta_2$ agonist
• Peak flow meter and diary
• Management plan if condition deteriorates
Discharge letter to GP:
• Admission & discharge PEFR
• Recommended GP follow-up in one week
• Asthma clinic follow up preferably within four weeks

**GROUP 11:**

**ITEM 4:**

# Respiratory disorders
# Hyperventilation

### CASE HISTORY

A 15-year-old schoolgirl is brought by her teacher to the A&E department with dizziness and feeling faint. You notice that she is anxious, sighing and has erratic ventilation. There are no other physical signs on examination. Her teacher volunteered that the girl was anxious about impending examinations.

### What should you do?

Full examination and CXR, PEFR or spirometry and arterial blood gases (even if oximetry normal).

You have decided that her symptoms are due to hyperventilation. This should be confirmed by demonstration of a respiratory alkalosis with a normal A-a gradient. Reassure the patient and ask her to breathe into a closed paper bag: When settled she can be discharged with further reassurance. **Note**, mild asthma is a common provocative cause and may require further investigation.

**Hyperventilation syndrome** refers to a condition of recurrent attacks of anxiety, sometimes phobic in nature, provoking such profound hyperventilation to cause a reduction in arterial $pCO_2$ that tetany may occur. Other features include perioral parasthesia, carpopedal spasm, muscle weakness, dizziness and a sense of impending loss of consciousness or fear.

An attack of hyperventilation may be induced by a strong emotional experience in otherwise normal individuals e.g. witnessing an accident.

In many patients, the label of hyperventilation syndrome is inappropriately given when mild asthma, or other conditions such as heart failure, lie behind the respiratory sensation. Indeed, hypocapnia resulting from hyperventilation may further provoke bronchoconstriction.

Clinically obvious hyperventilation may also result from a metabolic acidosis and will be recognised by arterial blood gas analysis – a reduced pH and bicarbonate in contra distinction to the alkalosis of respiratory hyperventilation.

Tetany: see Group 14, Item 20.

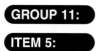

**GROUP 11:**

**ITEM 5:**

# Respiratory disorders
# Haemoptysis

**Remember**
- Chest x-ray may be normal eg pulmonary embolism
- Large opacity: consider malignancy or tuberculosis

Coughing up blood is a dramatic symptom and can be frightening to the patient and their family.

## Colour of blood
- Pink frothy sputum: Pulmonary oedema
- Rusty sputum: Pneumonia
- Make sure it is not haematemesis. This would be suggested by:
  History of retching
  Altered blood (resembling coffee grounds)
  Low pH

Enquire about epistaxis which may cause confusion. Blood stained saliva suggests bleeding from gums.

**Common conditions presenting with haemoptysis are**

- Carcinoma of the bronchus:
  - smoker
  - age > 40 years
  - usually abnormal chest X-ray
- Pulmonary embolism:
  - risk factors for DVT
  - chest X-ray often negative
  - history of acute breathlessness
- Pulmonary Tuberculosis:
  - more common in Asians, alcoholics, patients with HIV infection
  - age often < 40 years
  - chest X-ray usually shows patchy opacities in the upper lobes
- Bronchiectasis:
  - history of purulent sputum and/or possibly recurrent haemoptysis over years
  - cystic lesions on chest X-ray at lung bases in some but not all patients
  - CT scan of the lungs is diagnostic
  - bronchiectasis is a feature of Cystic Fibrosis

Less common causes of haemoptysis are

- Vasculitis:
  - Wegener's
  - microscopic vasculitis } (both ANCA positive)
- Pulmonary haemorrhage:
  - Goodpasture's syndrome
  - idiopathic Pulmonary haemosiderosis
- Chronic venous congestion of lungs:
  - mitral stenosis
  - left ventricular failure
- Aspergilloma:
  - seen in association with cavitatory lung disease

**Management**

This is of the underlying disease. Pulmonary embolism may require immediate treatment as will major haemoptysis (250 mls/24 hours).

**Management of massive haemoptysis**

As little as 250 ml can fill the bronchial tree and be life threatening. Happily it is uncommon but frightening for everyone involved.

- Monitor: oxygen saturation with oximetry, blood pressure and

pulse rate
- Exclude coagulation defects and perform CXR
- Endotracheal intubation and suction may be required
- Urgent bronchoscopy by an experienced doctor is sometimes required
- A balloon tipped arterial catheter may be employed to protect the unaffected lung. It is inserted into the bronchus over a guide wire via a bronchoscope
- Bronchial artery embolisation is highly effective if the bleeding vessel can be identified

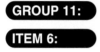

### Information

Massive haemoptysis can occur in the following conditions
- Tuberculosis
- Bronchiectasis
- Aspergilloma
- Carcinoma of the bronchus

### Beware

Only a minority of patients have a malignant cause of massive haemoptysis.

**GROUP 11:**

**ITEM 6:**

# Respiratory disorders
# Chest pain

Deciding the cause of chest pain is a common problem. It can be straightforward or take days to diagnose correctly. A careful history (eliciting site, character and radiation of the pain) is usually more important than tests.

- Exercise induced chest pain is usually cardiac in origin.
- Rest pain may be: cardiac, pleuritic, musculoskeletal, nerve root irritation, oesophageal, mediastinal or referred pain from abdomen.
- Lung diseases only cause pain if the pleura, mediastinum, intercostal nerves or bones are involved.

### Is it cardiac pain?

*(also look at Group 10, Item 6)*

Central chest  – radiates to arms and neck. Dull ache, severe 'constricting' character. May be associated with breathlessness.

### Typical angina

Occurs on exercise, and is eased by rest.

### Unstable angina

May give pain at rest or on minimal exertion

### Myocardial infarction

Severe with sweating, pain persists

### Pericarditis

Dull or sharp, central, eased by sitting forwards, may be worse with breathing.

### Aortic dissection

Severe sudden onset, may be described as 'tearing' pain in the back or anterior chest; patient often shocked

### Is it pleurisy?

Sharp pain in the sides of the chest which 'catches' with breathing. Often with fever, cough, sputum, haemoptysis, indicating underlying lung disease.

Think of:

• Pneumonia and pleurisy
• Pulmonary infarction
• Pneumothorax
• Malignant invasion of pleura

### Is it musculoskeletal?

• Trauma
  – rib fracture
  – 'point' tenderness
  – crushed vertebra
  – pain often referred around the chest
• Chronic pain
  – osteoarthritis. Long history with acute episodes. Look for spinal deformity.
  – rib or spine disease. May be metastatic cancer; local tenderness and swelling, lumps, history of cancer
• Muscles
  – Bornholm's disease. Follows an upper respiratory tract infection, a low grade fever can occur. Ache in muscles. May be tender. Definite cases rare
• Costochondral junction
  – Tietze's disease. Local pain on pressure over junctions. Also rare.

### Is it nerve root irritation?

Typically in a dermatome distribution around the chest may be unilateral.

Vertebral OA, osteomyelitis. prolapsed disc
Malignant nerve root compression
Herpes zoster (shingles) – is there a vesicular rash? (pain may precede rash)

### Is it oesophageal?

Reflux is retrosternal burning pain usually after food, worse lying flat and eased by antacid. Can be severe and mimic myocardial infarction.

### Oesophageal rupture

Central pain with shock. May have associated pleural effusion. Occurs after severe vomiting or more commonly endoscopy at which dilatation has been performed.

### Is it referred pain from outside the chest?

Diaphragm irritation may cause shoulder tip pain. Localisation may be difficult for the patient. Several abdominal emergencies may have chest pain with or without abdominal pain.

Think of:

- Acute cholecystitis
- Acute duodenal ulceration
- Sub-phrenic abscess
- Perforated bowel
- Peritonitis
- Pancreatitis

### Is it genuine?

Yes – nearly always – exclude organic disease in ALL cases.

A tiny minority may be attention seeking or have psychiatric disease. Even patients with Munchausen syndrome may have genuine disease.

### What tests do you need to do for chest pain?

After a good history and examination do (as a minimum):

- ECG
- CXR

Many diagnoses will now be obvious BUT remember:

- A normal ECG does not exclude cardiac pain
- A normal CXR does not exclude pulmonary embolism

**Remember**

If in doubt:
- Retake the history, re-examine the patient and consider unusual causes
- Is WBC or ESR raised?
- Is the patient pyrexial?
- Consider bone scanning/CT scanning for osteomyelitis if plain films normal and high clinical suspicion

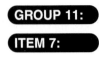

**GROUP 11:**

**ITEM 7:**

# Respiratory disorders
# Respiratory failure

Respiratory failure is a common medical emergency often presenting with non specific symptoms such as mild confusion or agitation. Recognition requires arterial blood gas (ABG) analysis – see below. Oximeters that estimate arterial oxygen saturation from the finger or ear lobe are useful in assessment or monitoring.

**Remember**

All breathless patients should have oximetry checked at triage in A&E.

Oximeters may be falsely reassuring in the patient breathing oxygen. Importantly they will not detect alveolar hypoventilation, producing high $pCO_2$.

Respiratory failure commonly results from either a problem with the respiratory pump or because of intrinsic lung disease.

**Remember**

All unconscious patients should have ABG analysis at initial assessment.

### With respiratory pump failure the arterial $PCO_2$ ($PaCO_2$) is raised (so-called Type II) you should consider

• Neurological depression – e.g. coma, sedatives
• Chest wall problem – e.g. flail chest, pneumothorax
• Neuromuscular disease – e.g. Guillain Barré, old poliomyelitis
• Severe air flow limitation – e.g. COPD

### In intrinsic lung disease (apart from COPD) hypoxaemia is often combined with a reduced PaCO2 (so-called Type I)

The hypoxaemia arises primarily from a mismatch of ventilation and perfusion in the pulmonary alveolar bed. Hypoxic stimulation of ventilation, coupled with abnormal respiratory sensation, then leads to a reduced arterial $pCO_2$ (alveolar hyperventilation). A raised $PaCO_2$ indicates impending respiratory arrest as it suggests either a reduction in ventilatory effort or failure of the respiratory pump.

### In hypoxaemia with reduced $PaCO_2$ consider

• Infection – e.g. pneumonia
• Shock – e.g. sepsis, hypovolaemia
• Allergy – e.g. asthma, allergic pneumonitis
• Cardiac disease – e.g. LVF, pulmonary hypertension
• Pulmonary embolism

### In respiratory failure arterial blood gas sampling is necessary to

• Assess severity
• Identify type ie alveolar hypo or hyperventilation
• Appreciate the degree of compensation

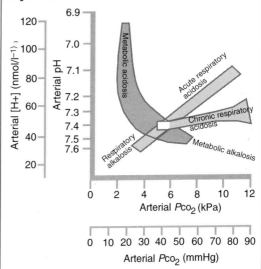

(i.e. the chronicity of the condition)

A co-existing metabolic acidosis commonly causes confusion and can be recognised by the base excess value (see below).

## Summary of Acid-Base changes (Fig 11.7.1)

**Fig 11.7.1 The Flenley Acid-Base Nomogram**
**The bands show the 95% confidence limits. The central white box shows the approximate limits of arterial pH and P$co_2$ in normal individuals**

Redrawn from *Clinical Medicine*, 4th Edition, Kumar and Clark, 1998, by permission of the publisher WB Saunders

### In a respiratory acidosis

Carbon dioxide clearance is reduced – there is alveolar hypo-ventilation. The Pa$CO_2$ and [H+] rise. The $HCO_3$ is also increased due to renal compensation.

Examples: flail chest injury, Guillain Barré syndrome, exacerbation of COPD.

### In a respiratory alkalosis

There is alveolar hyperventilation and both the Pa$CO_2$ and [H+] are decreased. The $HCO_3$ is slightly decreased.

Examples: acute asthma, anxiety attack

### In a metabolic acidosis

There is disturbance of bicarbonate regulation or excessive H+ production. The $HCO_3$ is reduced and the Pa$CO_2$ falls because of respiratory compensation.

Example: diabetic ketoacidosis, renal failure

### Information

The base excess value provided by the ABG analyser is calculated by back titration to normal values for PaCO2 and $HCO_3$.

### In a metabolic alkalosis

The $HCO_3$ is increased and relative hypoventilation leads to a small compensatory increase in the $PaCO_2$.

Example: excessive vomiting, profound hypokalaemia

Normal blood gas values: with $FiO_2$ 21%

> pH ~ 7.4
> *$PaO_2$ > 10.0 kPa
> ‡$PaCO_2$ 4.5 – 6.0 kPa
> $HCO_3$ 24 – 28 mmol/l

*To convert to mmHg multiply by 7.5

‡The pH changes by approximately 0.1 per 1kPa change in $PaCO_2$

### Common ABG abnormalities

Life threatening asthma

- pH 7.2
- $PaO_2$ 15.4
- $PaCO_2$ 5.5
- $HCO_3$ 16.2
- BE -7.3

Supplemental $O_2$ is being provided (note high $PaO_2$). There is a metabolic acidosis (note pH and BE) as a result of metabolic demands exceeding $O_2$ delivery and producing a lactic acidosis. Airflow obstruction limits the normal respiratory compensation to this profound acidosis.

### Acute on chronic respiratory failure in a patient with COPD

- pH 7.3
- $PaO_2$ 25.8
- $PaCO_2$ 12.6
- $HCO_3$ 42.1
- BE +4.3

Acute on chronic respiratory acidosis exacerbated by a high $F_iO_2$ using variable performance mask (40-60% $O_2$) (note high $PaO_2$). The high $HCO_3$ results from renal compensation.

### Severe pneumonia ($F_iO_2$ 60%)

- pH 7.15
- $PaO_2$ 4.8
- $PaCO_2$ 3.5
- $HCO_3$ 12.5
- BE -9.3

Despite high $F_iO_2$ this patient is hypoxaemic because of ventilation: perfusion mismatch. The profound associated metabolic acidosis indicates the need for urgent intubation and IPPV and is a reflection of circulatory failure resulting from septic shock.

## Management

Respiratory failure may be difficult to assess or manage. Discuss with your consultant or other more senior staff. If you feel that the situation is unstable, do not hesitate to call an anaesthetist. Semielective intubation is much preferred to a respiratory arrest. It should be performed in the ward before transfer of the patient to the ICU.

## How do I recognise impending respiratory arrest?

• Tachycardia > 120
• Tachypnoea, respiratory rate > 30
• Hypotension
• Sympathetic activation – pale and sweaty, agitation, confusion
• Progressive increase in $PaCO_2$ or fall in $PaO_2$
• Rapid desaturation on disconnection from $O_2$ eg when drinking or coughing

Evaluation is often an 'end of the bed' process. Be sensitive to subtle changes or a failure to improve.

## Treating the cause

• Individual causes will require different actions – for instance an intercostal drain for a tension pneumothorax or large pleural effusion (Group 11, Item 14)
• In neurological coma, intubation may be necessary for airway protection or to manage raised intracranial pressure by hyperventilation
• Drug induced respiratory failure may be confirmed by a therapeutic trial with a specific antidote i.e. a bolus injection of naloxone for opiates and flumazanil for benzodiazepines. However infusions will be required if a positive response is obtained
• Oxygen supplementation should be aimed at raising the $PaO_2$ to beyond the steep part of the oxygen dissociation curve (Fig 11.7.2). Very high $PaO_2$ values are unnecessary but controlled $O_2$ therapy via a fixed performance mask is only necessary in chronic respiratory failure resulting from COPD

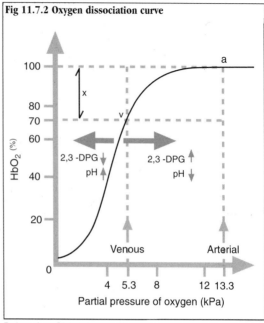

**Fig 11.7.2 Oxygen dissociation curve**

Redrawn from *Clinical Medicine*, 4th Edition, Kumar and Clark, 1998, by permission of the publisher WB Saunders

## CASE HISTORY 1

A 65-year-old with advanced COPD was admitted with a week's history of cough, breathlessness and purulent sputum. In the previous 24 hours he had become mildly confused. He was agitated with a respiratory rate of 35, BP 170/90, sweaty with an oximeter reading on air of 72%. There was widespread wheeze and coarse crackles suggestive of retained secretions. ABG analysis revealed pH 7.32, $PaO_2$ 5.8, $PaCO_2$ 8.1, and $HCO_3$ 29.

### What do these blood gases mean?

Hypoxaemia with mild acute respiratory acidosis. No evidence of chronic respiratory failure ie chronically elevated $pCO_2$ as $HCO_3$ normal.

The initial treatment in casualty was

- Nebulised bronchodilators
- 28% $O_2$ by controlled mask
- IV Amoxicillin
- IV Steroids (this is conventional treatment but there is limited evidence for effectiveness)
- Encouragement to clear secretions including sitting patient up and the attention of the physiotherapist
- CXR to exclude pneumothorax or demonstrate associated pneumonia

**Information**

Controlled oxygen via Venturi mask commonly leads to intermittent therapy as the mask is poorly tolerated by the agitated breathless patient. Oxygen via nasal prongs at 1 or 2 L/min may be more effective and continuous but is not "controlled".

Repeat ABG's were requested. pH 7.20, $PaO_2$ 6.5, $PaCO_2$ 12.5, $HCO_{30}$.

These results show further $CO_2$ retention and a deteriorating situation. Oxygen should not be removed -its removal will precipitate severe hypoxaemia. Alveolar ventilation must be increased. Despite using a nasal airway to stimulate cough and aid suction of respiratory secretions there was no improvement. Frusemide was given as co-existent LVF was difficult to exclude. Intubation was considered appropriate but a trial of non invasive ventilation (NIV) was first tried. On NIV the respiratory rate slowed and the acute respiratory acidosis resolved.

Non invasive ventilatory support employs a nose or face mask to provide ventilatory assistance to breathing (this is termed spontaneous pressure support) or timed breaths (pressure controlled ventilation). An exhalation valve reduces rebreathing. NIV is successful in approximately 70% of patients with respiratory failure resulting from COPD. It should not be employed if intubation would be more appropriate.

**Information**

Contraindications to NIV
- Unconscious or uncooperative
- Vomiting
- Large amount respiratory secretions
- Cardiovascularly unstable (beware hypotension)

## Mechanical Ventilation

In an unstable situation it is essential to maintain oxygenation. As intubation of an acutely unwell patient requires experience do not attempt this yourself. The laryngeal mask is increasingly being employed as insertion is easier than an endotracheal tube. It may replace the conventionally employed oropharyngeal (Geudal) airway and Ambubag in the future.

### Aims of intubation and mechanical ventilation
- Immediate correction of hypoxaemia
- Slower correction of hypercapnia
- Allow effective suctioning of respiratory secretions

### Hypotension after intubation is very common and relates to
- High airway pressures limiting venous return and causing a fall in cardiac output
- Vasodilation directly caused by sedatives
- A fall in sympathetic tone

For ventilatory techniques adopted in different circumstances *(see Service Based Learning for Anaesthesia)*.

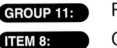

**GROUP 11:**

**ITEM 8:**

# Respiratory disorders
# Chest X-rays

A standard chest X-ray is taken P.A (PosteroAnterior) with the patient facing the X-ray plate – beam directed at the patient's back at a standard distance.

An emergency department film is often taken AP with the patient lying down (supine) on the X-ray plate – beam directed at the patient's front – the distance from X-ray source may vary.

In an AP

• Heart size and mediastinum are magnified
• May miss pleural effusion – lies along back of chest cavity when patient supine
• Film quality may be poor

Don't request an AP 'portable' film unless it would be unsafe for the patient to have a PA film

### CASE HISTORY 1

A 63-year-old male smoker presented with a four-month history of cough, recurrent small haemoptyses and exertional dyspnoea (Fig 11.8.1).

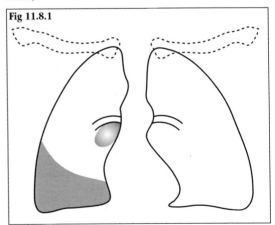

Fig 11.8.1

• Homogeneous opacity in right lower zone with meniscus rising in axilla
• Mass below right hilum
• Right diaphragm obscured

### Diagnosis

Right Pleural effusion. Probable underlying lung cancer.

## CASE HISTORY 2

A 70-year-old female smoker presented with cough, dyspnoea and weight loss (Fig 11.8.2).

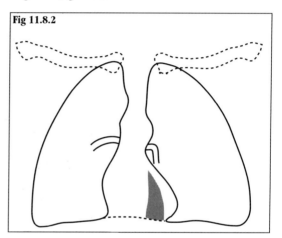

**Fig 11.8.2**

• There is a dense triangular opacity behind the heart
• The left pulmonary artery shadow is depressed
• Left diaphragm elevated
• Hyperlucent left chest
• Mediastinum shifted to left

### Diagnosis

**Left lower lobe collapse.** Possible lung cancer but could result from simple sputum retention.

Other lobar collapses look like this

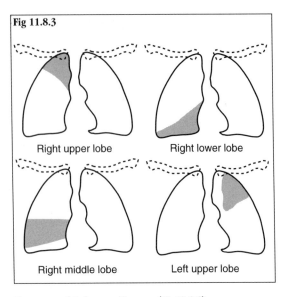

Fig 11.8.3

Right upper lobe

Right lower lobe

Right middle lobe

Left upper lobe

**Causes of lobar collapse** (Fig 11.8.3)

Think of

• Carcinoma of bronchus
• Inhaled foreign body
• Tenacious sputum causing bronchial obstruction

### CASE HISTORY 3

A 17-year-old presented with acute breathlessness, with sharp right sided chest pain.

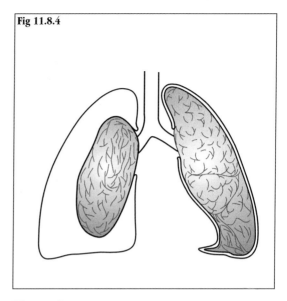

**Fig 11.8.4**

### Diagnosis

Right spontaneous pneumothorax (Fig 11.8.4) – Note absent lung markings on right side.

Two hours later his twin brother arrived in the accident and emergency department in respiratory distress (Fig 11.8.5).

### Remember

Tension pneumothorax
- Shift in mediastinum away from affected side
  THIS IS A MEDICAL EMERGENCY – DRAIN IMMEDIATELY
- Raised intrathoracic pressure limits venous return and impairs LV function resulting in tamponade and circulatory failure

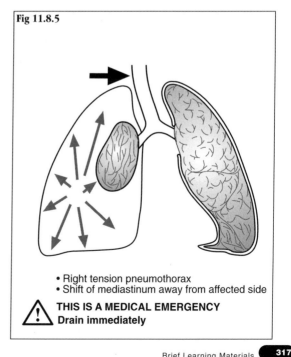

**Fig 11.8.5**

- Right tension pneumothorax
- Shift of mediastinum away from affected side

**THIS IS A MEDICAL EMERGENCY**
**Drain immediately**

### CASE HISTORY 4

A 35-year-old female had a two-day history of fever, productive cough and right sided pleuritic pain. CXR (Fig 11.8.6) showed:

- Homogeneous opacification of right upper lobe
- Air bronchogram indicates consolidation

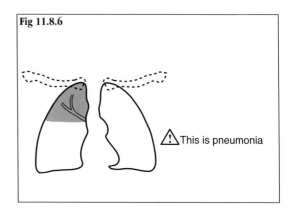

**Fig 11.8.6**

⚠ This is pneumonia

### Diagnosis

**Pneumonia.** If poor response to treatment; consider T.B. or atypical pneumonia

### CASE HISTORY 5

A 50-year-old diabetic male, recently arrived from Bangladesh, complained of loss of weight, night sweats and haemoptysis. CXR (Fig 11.8.7)

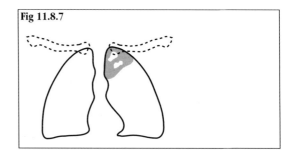

**Fig 11.8.7**

- Patchy opacification left upper lobe
- Two cavities

### Differential diagnosis

- Tuberculosis – most likely
- Staphylococcal pneumonia
- Klebsiella pneumonia

**Investigations**
- Send urgent sputum for AFB (smear and culture) and routine culture
- Isolate patient in side room

**Remember**

TB.

Urgent microcopy of sputum is performed by Auramine fluorescent dye testing and is much quicker than the Ziehl-Nielsen.

## CASE HISTORY 6

A 22-year-old West Indian female presented with painful lumps on the shins and breathlessness. BCG given at age 13. CXR (Fig 11.8.8)

- Fine nodular shadows (0.5 – 3mm) throughout lung fields
- The most likely diagnosis is sarcoidosis with erythema nodosum on the shins. The Heaf test was negative (due to decreased cell immunity) and non caseating granulomas were found on transbronchial biopsy.

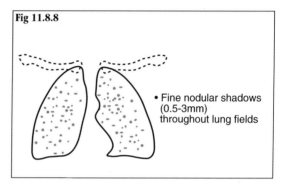

**Fig 11.8.8**

- Fine nodular shadows (0.5-3mm) throughout lung fields

### Diagnosis

**This is Sarcoidosis.**

The X-ray appearances on their own (without the above clinical scenario) could be due to:

- Miliary T.B.
- Extrinsic allergic alveolitis
  (ask about patient's occupation)
- Old chicken pox pneumonia – calcified spots
- Pulmonary metastases
- Pneumoconiosis
- Asbestosis
- Idiopathic pulmonary fibrosis

## CASE HISTORY 7

Your House Officer brings you a Chest X-ray and asks if he should drain the effusion. (Fig 11.8.9)

### Diagnosis

But when you look at the CXR it is a collapsed left lung.

Think of:
- Carcinoma of bronchus
- Retained sputum e.g. post-operatively
- Foreign body

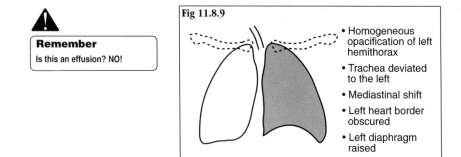

**Fig 11.8.9**

- Homogeneous opacification of left hemithorax
- Trachea deviated to the left
- Mediastinal shift
- Left heart border obscured
- Left diaphragm raised

⚠️ **Remember**
Is this an effusion? NO!

## CASE HISTORY 8

A man of 74 presented with a one month history of a productive cough with offensive tasting sputum, malaise and weight loss. His dentition was very poor. He had just stopped smoking. (Fig 11.8.10)

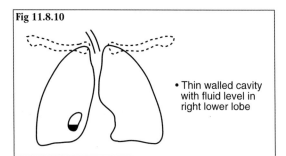

**Fig 11.8.10**

- Thin walled cavity with fluid level in right lower lobe

### Differential diagnosis
- Lung abscess
- Cavitating lung cancer
- Tuberculosis

Bronchoscopy showed thick secretions in right lower lobe. No bronchial obstruction. Cytology negative.

Patient responded to antibiotics and abscess resolved in six weeks. This probably resulted from aspiration with mouth anaerobes contributing to the unpleasant smell or taste of sputum.

### Diagnosis
**Pyogenic abscess.**

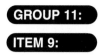

**GROUP 11:**

**ITEM 9:**

# Respiratory disorders

# COPD – acute exacerbation

### CASE HISTORY 1

A 63-year-old male ex-smoker has had a chronic productive cough for 20 years. For 10 years he has had gradually increasing exertional dyspnoea. His usual exercise tolerance is 200yds on flat. One week previously he became breathless on walking between rooms and his sputum became purulent. His normal medication is salbutamol and beclomethasone inhalers.

### The SHO decided not to admit him because

- He was able to cope at home with aid of his wife
- He was not cyanosed – oximetry showed $SaO_2$ 97%
- His general condition was good + he had a normal level of consciousness
- On examination his chest expanded poorly and he was wheezy, but there were no localising signs, no evidence of cor pulmonale or heart failure.
- His normal $FEV_1$/FVC was 1.9/3.2 (predicted 3.4/4.4) but on arrival was 0.9/2.6
- CxR showed no acute lesion

### He was discharged home with

- Amoxicillin 500mg x 3 daily for one week
- Prednisolone 30mg daily for two weeks
- advice to increase his inhaled bronchodilators to salbutamol four puffs, four-hourly via a spacer
- given follow-up appointment at chest clinic for two weeks

### Key points

- Patient did not need admission because
  - no evidence of respiratory failure
  - no evidence of cor pulmonale
  - able to cope at home
- Antibiotic was broad spectrum and, in particular, covered majority of H.Influenza organisms (the most common cause of acute exacerbation)
  - additional erythromycin unnecessary since Mycoplasma unlikely
- Oral steroids used as adjunct to antibiotics since patient already on inhaled steroids and possibly had a degree of steroid responsiveness. This is conventional treatment but limited evidence to support it
- Patient was given a spacer (and shown how to use it) in order to increase the lung deposition of aerosol

- Salbutamol dose increased and given 4 hourly since effect only lasts 4-6 hours and is partly dependent on dose
- Follow-up at chest clinic because patient had moderately severe COPD and had never been assessed

However, the GP, when seeing the patient one week later, cancelled the outpatient appointment believing it unnecessary. He wrote to the chest physician saying that he was able to manage the patient himself. He had a spirometer in the surgery and that when well the patient had an $FEV_1$ of > 50% predicated normal. Furthermore the GP said that the patient had

- A definite diagnosis
- Only moderately severe COPD
- No cor pulmonale
- No respiratory failure and did not need oxygen
- Did not have bullous lung disease
- Did not have a rapidly declining $FEV_1$

The GP was arranging to perform bronchodilator tests himself using a spirometer and checking the response to both salbutamol and ipratropium inhalers.

## CASE HISTORY 2

A 68-year-old female smoker with a chronic productive cough and five years of gradually increasing exertional dyspnoea had a usual exercise tolerance of 40 yds on flat and was breathless bending and washing. She was virtually housebound and lived alone. She developed a cough with purulent sputum and had been breathless at rest for two days. She was "blue-lighted" into A/E.

She was admitted immediately because she

- Showed signs of respiratory failure – drowsy and cyanosed, $CO_2$ flap
- Pulse 130/m atrial fibrillation, B.P. 100/60
- Cor pulmonale with tricuspid regurgitation
  - JVP up to the ear
  - midsystolic murmur at LSE
  - enlarged pulsatile liver
  - bilateral oedematous legs to knees
- Respiratory rate 30, shallow breaths using accessory muscles of respiration, generalised wheezing and bilateral basal crackles

### Remember

Spirometry is required to assess severity of COPD.

### Investigations

- Arterial blood gases pH 7.32, PaO2 5.6, pCO2 8.2 on air
- FBC Hb 17.8, Hct 54%, WBC 12.300
- Urea 9.0, K 3.5, creatinine 102
- ECG 130 (ventricular rate) Atrial fibrillation and right heart strain
- Chest X-ray: over inflated lungs with prominent pulmonary arteries (indicating pulmonary hypertension) and normal sized heart

### Key points

- Patient in respiratory failure with raised $PaCO_2$ give oxygen very carefully, continuously and monitor closely
- *Cor pulmonale* (right heart failure 2° to lung disease) is difficult to improve while the patient remains hypoxic

• *Atrial fibrillation* may only be secondary to hypoxaemia and may revert to sinus rhythm when $PaO_2$ improves

### Immediate treatment

• Oxygen at 2 litres/min via nasal spectacles and repeat gases in 30 to 40 mins. Consider fixed performance (Venturi) mask if significant rise in $PaCO_2$ (see later)
• Sit patient upright to help breathing
• Give nebulised bronchodilators
  – salbutamol 5.0 mg with ipratropium 0.5 mg four-hourly
  – air rather than high flow $O_2$ is safer for nebulising bronchodilators
  – oxygen continued via nasal spectacles
• Chest physiotherapy to help sputum expectoration
• Intravenous diuretics e.g. frusemide 40mg daily, (conventional treatment but fluid retention largely 'cosmetic' although associated LVF may be difficult to assess)
• Amoxicillin 500mg x 3 daily intravenous until condition improves and then oral for one week in total
• I.V. hydrocortisone 100mg x 2 daily until patient improves and then oral prednisolone 20 to 30mg daily for two weeks only
• Monitor oximetry + mental state, respiratory rate and pulse until improvement, and daily weights

### If no improvement consider

• Doxapram as a respiratory stimulant (1.5-4mg/min infusion) or
• Non-invasive intermittent positive pressure ventilation (NIV) (see Group 11, Item 7).

### Progress

• Patient more alert
• $PaO_2$ 7.0, $PaCO_2$ 9.0 on 2 litres nasal oxygen
• In sinus rhythm

### Key points

• Oxygen should be prescribed on treatment sheet and given continuously not "as required"
• Management of oxygen is the most important and difficult component of treatment
• Although oxygen by a Venturi mask gives a known concentration it is uncomfortable and claustrophobic. It has to be removed to eat, talk and cough and for nebulised Rx
• Oxygen by nasal spectacles is more comfortable and can be kept on continuously
• Nasal oxygen gives variable $FiO_2$ depending on pattern of breathing and flow rate between 24-35%. It worked on this patient but in many patients with COPD 24% oxygen via a mask is preferable when $PaCO_2 > 8.0kPa$

- It takes 30 to 40 minutes to equilibrate blood gases with any change in $FiO_2$ and blood gases should not be checked earlier
- It is unnecessary to get the $PaO_2$ normal – aim to get it at the top of the steep slope of the oxygen saturation curve (see Fig 11.7.2)
- If $PaO_2$ is >7.5kPa, a small fall in $PaO_2$ has little effect on $O_2$ saturation – this is safe.

If $PaO_2$ is 6.5 or less, a small fall produces a dangerous fall in $SaO_2$. (Note, Sigmoid shape of oxygen dissociation curve. See Item 7 Respiratory Failure)

- Increasing the inspired oxygen may cause small rise in $PaCO_2$ (mostly because of relaxation of hypoxic vasoconstriction in relatively poorly ventilated alveoli). A pH change of < 0.1 or $PaCO_2$ < 1kPa is not significant, so do not reduce or remove the oxygen
- If, on increasing $F_iO_2$, this patient had not clinically improved and ABGs showed $PaO_2$ 6.8, $PaCO_2$ 12.0,
  – action – patient still needs oxygen but at a more controlled concentration. Use 24% $O_2$ via Venturi mask
  – consider a respiratory stimulant
  – get help from senior, preferably from respiratory team and consider transfer to HDU for non invasive ventilation or to
- ITU for ventilation
- Over the next few days the patient improved and felt well by one week. His Hb came back as 18g, Hct 55. What would you do now?

## Action

Venesect cautiously under Haematology guidance. Three to four units venesected over next few weeks starting before discharge aiming for a Hct of 50. Continue bronchodilators as inhalers via spacing device, oral steroids continued for two weeks and diuretics continued.

## Key points

Before discharge Blood gases checked on air. $PaO_2$ 7.0, $PaCO_2$ 6.3. Respiratory nurse visited to:

– discuss disease/risk factors especially to urge to stop smoking
– mechanism of action of drugs
– teach use of aerosol devices and spacers
– give chest clinic follow-up for two weeks

### Follow-up in chest clinic

- To optimise bronchodilator treatment
- Monitor for polycythaemia and cor pulmonale
- Assess for long term domicilary oxygen (indication $PaO_2$ < 7.3 on 2 occasions 3-4 weeks apart when patient stable)
- Consider obstructive sleep apnoea (see Kumar & Clark Clinical

Medicine 1998 4th Ed page 781) in view of marked
polycythaemia

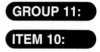

**GROUP 11:**

**ITEM 10:**

# Respiratory disorders
# Pneumonia

### CASE HISTORY 1

A 33-year-old female non smoker was admitted with a two-day
history of fever, sweating and cough, productive of yellow, lightly
bloodstained sputum. She had pleuritic pain in the left axilla.
There were signs of consolidation in the left lower lobe and herpes
labialis.

This is typical of community acquired pneumonia

### Signs

• Fever T39°C
• Respiratory rate 28/min
• Dullness to percussion left lung base
• Bronchial breathing left lung base
• Tactile vocal fremitus ↓ left lung base

### Investigations

• Chest X-ray
• Arterial blood gases
• Blood count, WBC + diff
• Urea and electrolytes
• Urinalysis for sugar (is patient diabetic?)
• Blood and sputum culture
• Blood for viral serology and Legionella/mycoplasma
• Serology for pneumoccocal antigen
• Rapid urine test available for Legionella

### Likely infecting organisms

• Strep pneumoniae – the most likely cause
• H. Influenzae (especially in smokers with COPD)
• Mycoplasma (four-yearly epidemics)
• Legionella (ask for foreign travel)
• Staph. aureus
• Viral-Influenza
• Chlamydia psittaci

### How ill is this patient?

The following indicate **increased risk** in pneumonia.

**Bedside assessment**

• Hypoxaemia $PaO_2 < 8kPa$
• Age > 60 years
• Respiratory rate > 30/min
• Confusion
• Atrial fibrillation
• Diastolic B.P. < 60 mm Hg or systolic <90mm Hg
• Underlying disease present

**Investigation results**

- CXR Multi-lobar involvement
- Urea > 7mmol/l
- WBC < 4000 or > 20,000
- Bacteraemia

This **patient** is young, previously fit, not breathless or shocked. Only the left lower lobe is consolidated and WBC is 11,500. Normal urea. PaO2 10.5kPa. (Chest X-ray – see Group 11 Item 8).

- The pneumonia is not severe
- The patient can be treated with oral antibiotics and can be discharged in 24 to 48 hours
  (see Antibiotic choices later)

## CASE HISTORY 2

A man of 73 is brought to A&E by his very anxious wife. He has had winter bronchitis for the last five years and is a current smoker of 20 cigarettes/day. One week ago he had "the flu" and this morning became increasingly breathless, sweaty, pale and confused. He had angina diagnosed two years ago.

### Investigations show

CXR (Fig 11.10.1)
   – diffuse opacification in both lungs
   – ring opacities in right lung
Urea 9mmol/l
WBC 28,000
ABG $PaO_2$ 9.0 kPa, $PaCO_2$ 5.3 kPa, on $FiO_2$ 40%

**i**

### Information
Bedside assessment
- **73 year old**
- **RR > 30/min**
- **Confusion. Dehydrated**
- **Pre-existing COPD**
- **Pre-existing angina**
- **B.P.110/40**

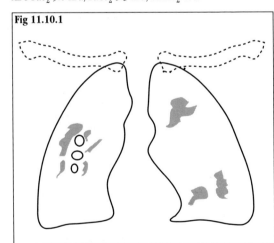

Fig 11.10.1

This is a high risk case. He has influenza and a superinfection with staph. aureus causing **severe pneumonia** with early abscess formation. (Ring opacities on the CXR)

**i**

**Information**

**Indication for intensive care monitoring and assisted respiration**

- PaO$_2$ < 8 kPa on 60% O$_2$
- PaCO$_2$ > 6.4 kPa
- Patient exhausted, drowsy or unconscious
- Shock
- Hypotension or circulatory failure

He needs

- Rehydration – intravenous fluid
- Intravenous antibiotics. See Antibiotics below
- Pulse oximetry. Give O$_2$ to try to keep O$_2$ sat > 90%
- Nursing where he can be easily observed or in an HDU (Hourly B.P., pulse, RR)
- To be watched for respiratory failure – IPPV may be needed
- Physiotherapy if difficulty coughing up sputum

**Antibiotic choices**

Consult your Hospital Formulary or select from below.

**Uncomplicated non-severe pneumonia**

- Treat for five days with oral medication unless patient not swallowing or not absorbing
- Oral amoxycillin 500mg x3 + erythromycin 500mg x4 daily. For poor absorption I.V. amoxycillin 500mgs x3 or I.V. benzylpenicillin 1.2g 6 hourly + erythromycin 500mgs x4 daily For penicillin allergic patients erythromycin 500mgs x4 daily oral/i.v.

**Non-severe pneumonia in penicillin allergic patient with underlying lung disease (H Influenza suspected)**

- Clarithromycin 500mg x2 daily

**Severe pneumonia**

- i.v. antibiotics until significant improvement
- antibiotics for up to 10 days erythromycin and ampicillin 1g x4 with flucloxacillin 2g x4 or erythromycin with cefuroxime 750mg x3 daily (NB dose reduction if renal impairment [creatinine clearance < 20ml/min])

**Staphylococcal pneumonia**

- Treat for 10 to 14 days
- Flucloxacillin 2g x4 I.V. + fusidic acid 0.5-1g x3 or gentamicin 3.0-5.0mg/kg daily as single dose (check gentamicin levels pre 2nd dose)

**Legionnaire's disease**

- Treat for three weeks
- Clarithromycin 500mg x2 daily (for severe cases i.v.)

**Mycoplasma pneumonia**

- Treat for two weeks
- Erythromycin 500mg x4 i.v. or oral daily
- If allergic to erythromycin, tetracycline 500mg x3 or ciprofloxacin 500mg x2 daily

**Q fever and psittacosis**
– tetracycline 500mg x3 daily for 10 days

**Aspiration pneumonia**
• Amoxicillin 500mg + metronidazole 400mg x3 oral or if
severe/unable to swallow i.v. amoxicillin 500mg +
metronidazole 500mg x3 daily or IV co-amoxiclav +
metronidazole

## CASE HISTORY 3

A 24-year-old male, recently arrived in the UK from East Africa,
presented with breathlessness of two weeks' duration, gradually
increasing in severity with a dry cough and sweats. He had a
diarrhoeal illness six months ago and has recently noticed swollen
glands in his neck.

**Bedside assessment**

• Looks worried
• RR 34/min
• Tachycardia 120 bpm
• Temperature 41
• No abnormal signs in chest
• Pre-existing illness – HIV infection

**Investigations**
• CXR (Fig 11.10.2)
 – ground glass appearance of
 lung fields
 – bilateral and perihilar
 shadowing

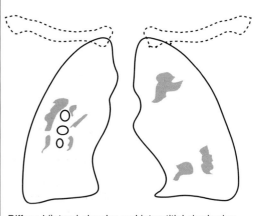

Fig 11.10.2

Diffuse bilateral alveolar and interstitial shadowing

**ABGs** PaO$_2$ 9.0 kPa   on F$_1$O$_2$ 60% PaCO$_2$ 3.2 kPa

WBC 2,300

Normal urea

You should think of HIV infection with a Pneumocystis carinii pneumonia (PCP) because of country of origin, six-month history of illness, lymphadenopathy, low white cell count and appearance on CXR. (Fig 11.10.2)

## Other unusual pneumonias

• Alcoholics – inhalation pneumonia (gram negative organisms)
• Drug addicts – 'dirty' drugs and syringes, infected emboli to lungs (*staphylococcus aureus*)
• Remember Tuberculosis – a sputum smear for AFB is quick and easy to do. Can co-exist with other pneumonias
• Cytomegalovirus
• Fungal – aspergillus, candida albicans

These latter two are seen in immunocompromised patients viz

   – HIV infection
   – leukaemia and lymphoma patients
   – patients on chemotherapy
   – transplant recipients
   – patients on steroid drugs
   – chronic renal failure patients

### Treatment should start in this patient for PCP

• High dose I.V. co-trimoxazole
• Add I.V. cefuroxime and erythromycin if in doubt as to cause of the pneumonia
• If in doubt also consult HIV team or Microbiologist
• May need high dose steroids I.V. if deteriorates
• Give O$_2$ to keep O$_2$ sat > 90%
• Arrange for induced sputum collection next day
• Consult HIV team for further management

## CASE HISTORY 4

A 68-year-old female smoker was admitted by the surgical team 9 days previously with intestinal obstruction. A laparotomy showed severe diverticulitis with a pelvic mass; a defunctioning colostomy was performed. She has been very slow to mobilise post operatively and has had a troublesome cough. Two days ago she developed a fever and has now become breathless, tachycardic and has right sided pleurisy.

## Investigations

- CXR  Patchy opacification R lung base
- ABG  PaO$_2$ 7.3 PaCO$_2$ 4.6
- WBC  16,000
- Urea  10mmol/L
- ECG  sinus tachycardia

### Bedside assessment

- Looks ill
- RR 24/min
- Pulse 112 bpm regular
- Temp 40°C
- Coarse crackles right lung base, patchy bronchial breathing
- Pleural rub
- No evidence of DVT
- Has vomited recently
- Recent surgery
- The surgeons gave her five days of I.V. Amoxicillin post op

### What is the diagnosis?

- Severe hospital acquired (nosocomial) pneumonia – most likely
- DVT with pulmonary emboli may coexist
- Patient may have inhaled vomit
- Previous antibiotics may have selected out Gram -ve organisms
- Intravenous cannulae can become infected
- May have pre-existing lung disease  – smoker

### Bacteriology in nosocomial pneumonia

Wide range of possible organisms

- Gram-negative bacilli 50%
  - *E. Coli*
  - Proteus
  - Klebsiella
  - Pseudomonas
- Gram positive cocci
  - *Staph aureus*
  - *Strep pneumoniae*
  - *H. Influenzae*
- Anaerobes
  - Bacteroides
  - Clostridia

### Management

- Give O$_2$ to raise O$_2$ saturation to > 90%
- Rehydrate intravenously
- Give I.V. antibiotics to cover wide spectrum
  - cefuroxime 1.5g I.V. x3 daily
  - metronidazole 500mg x3 daily I.V.
- If improving after 48 hrs and able to swallow change to
  - oral Cefuroxime 500mg x2 daily and
  - oral Metronidazole 400mg x3 daily

- Patient is at high risk of pulmonary emboli
  – heparinise intravenously or daily fractionated Heparin s.c.
- Watch for deterioration (see indications for ITU – box Case 2)
- Ask for surgical review
- Physiotherapy to encourage cough

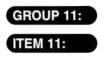

# Respiratory disorders
# Tuberculosis

### CASE HISTORY 1

An 18-year-old man who came to this country two years ago from the Indian sub-continent presented with general malaise, photophobia, unproductive cough, weight loss and night sweats. On examination his temperature was 39.5º C. He looked unwell and appeared rather vague. Investigations revealed Na 120, K 2.6 and urea 2.8, Hb 10.4 & WBC 6.4. ALT and Alkaline Phosphatase were slightly raised. Portable AP chest film was considered to be normal. He was admitted with the diagnosis of pyrexia of unknown origin. He had blood and urine cultures and CSF examination. CSF showed an increased cell count, mostly lymphocytes, raised protein and low glucose. No organisms were seen but cultures sent. A departmental PA chest X-ray was done after two days and showed miliary mottling.

This patient has miliary tuberculosis with meningitis. It carries a high morbidity if not treated early. The hyponatraemia is dilutional secondary to inappropriate ADH secretion

### CASE HISTORY 2

A 50-year-old alcoholic man, living rough was brought to A&E "collapsed". He had stopped drinking alcohol one week previously because he was too unwell to collect his "giro". He was confused and hallucinating and coughing.

### On examination

He was unkempt and emaciated, confused and jaundiced.
T = 37.9, P = 100, B.P. 100/60. OE upper chest bronchial breathing + coarse crackles on the right; trachea deviated to the right.
Liver enlarged 3cm below costal margin. Ascites

### Investigations

- Hb 10.8 MCV 106 WBC 8,500
- Urea 1.3 K 3.5
- Creatinine 60 Na 126
- Bilirubin 40 Alk phosphatase ALT raised
- Chest X-ray: patchy opacification with cavitation at right upper lobe. Trachea deviated to right (Fig 11.11.1)

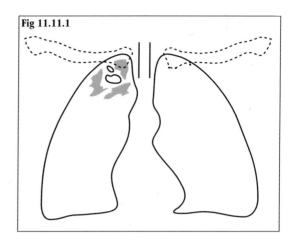

Fig 11.11.1

A provisional diagnosis was made of

- Delirium tremens
- Pulmonary tuberculosis
- Alcoholic liver disease

Next most useful investigation is urgent sputum sent for culture + sensitivity and particularly for AFB – if no organisms found send at least 3 more good sputum specimens

### Risk factors for developing post-primary pulmonary TB

- Alcohol or other drug abuse
- Diabetes mellitus
- Malnutrition
- Immunosuppression (any cause including steroid tablets)

### Management

- Isolate patient
- Treat delirium tremens. (Group 5 Item 7). Note: always also give thiamine
- Start anti-TB (see end of this Item) as soon as possible
- Notify patient and contact TB health visitor to do contact tracing
- He will almost certainly need directly observed treatment since it is unlikely that he will comply with treatment otherwise
- Refer to Respiratory Team

## CASE HISTORY 3

A 64-year-old white male smoker was treated for bronchitis three months ago by his general practitioner. His cough did not resolve and he was admitted one week ago. Initial assessment showed a right upper lobe pneumonia and he was treated with oral Amoxicillin and erythromycin. Blood and sputum cultures were negative. He had a persistent low grade fever, and the chest X-ray still showed patchy right upper lobe consolidation. You have been called to see him because he has just had a haemoptysis.

### Why is this pneumonia slow to resolve?
**Consider**

- Obstructing carcinoma of right upper lobe bronchus
  – is there a hilar mass?
  – should he be bronchoscoped?
- Unusual infecting organism

### Further history

- Always worth retaking the history
- His mother was treated for pulmonary tuberculosis in 1941. He was seen in a chest clinic as a child but does not think that he had drug treatment. He has no recall of having BCG.
- Pulmonary TB is a possible diagnosis
- Look carefully at a new PA chest X-Ray (Fig 11.11.2)

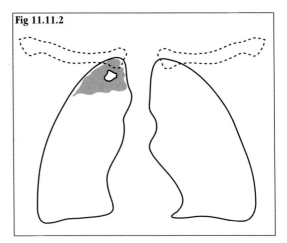

Fig 11.11.2

There is right upper lobe consolidation and there is a small apical cavity – probably obscured by the clavicle on previous chest X-ray.

### Action

This is TB until proved otherwise.

- Send urgent sputum for Auramine or ZN staining and TB culture
- Send at least 3 sputum specimens
- Check blood count, liver function, renal function

**Result**

The microbiologist calls you urgently.

- The patient has AAFB seen on sputum smear
- Sputum is being cultured for TB
- Culture results will be available in six to eight weeks
- Sensitivities perhaps not for 12 weeks

**Action**

- Isolate the patient in side room
- START TREATMENT FOR TB (see below)
- TB is a notifiable disease and allows contact tracing to be initiated.

## CASE HISTORY 4

A Ugandan 34-year-Old refugee presented to A&E with high fever, diarrhoea and weight loss. She omitted to inform the casualty staff that she had been found to be HIV positive six months previously (with a CD count of 250) and had declined further investigation or treatment at that time.

On examination she appeared unwell, cachetic and was coughing continuously.

- CXR Rt lower lobe shadowing and possible Rt hilar lymphadenopathy
- Hb 7.5, WBC 4.2, L 0.8, Plat 156
- Na 128, K 2.5, Urea 118, Alb 18

Blood, stool, sputum and urine cultures were taken and she was admitted to the general ward and commenced on Amoxicillin and Erythromycin. She failed to improve and after 3 days the antibiotics were changed to Ciprofloxacin although sputum culture was unhelpful. On day five the microbiologist was consulted: examination of sputum for AFB was positive and subsequently Mycobacterium TB was isolated from blood and stool.

**Key points**

- Many patients may not volunteer their HIV status
- You must indicate that Mycobacterium TB is a possibility when requesting sputum examination
- Atypical radiological changes are common in TB in the immunocompromised
- Both Mycobacterium intracellulare avium and Mycobacterium tuberculosis may be isolated from stool and blood
- A patient from Africa with pneumonia should be admitted to a side room until TB has been excluded
- The risk of TB developing in those infected (i.e. disease reactivation) increases when CD count < 200

### Treatment

Drug Therapy In Tuberculosis

- Rifampicin
  - body weight < 50 Kg : 450 mg daily
  - 50 Kg : 600 mg daily.
- Isoniazid : 300 mg daily
- Pyrazinamide: 25 mg/Kg
- Ethambutol : 15 mg/Kg
- Give all drugs together once daily with breakfast
- All four drugs for two months followed by Rifampicin & Isoniazid for four months (having checked the sensitivities)
- Tuberculous Meningitis: Recommended duration 12 months
  - Four drugs three months; Rifampicin+Isoniazid nine months
  - Cortico-steroids are indicated in tuberculous meningitis, pericarditis and spinal tuberculosis with neurological compression

### Monitor

- Liver biochemistry
- Patient compliance with medication

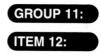

**Respiratory disorders**
**Pleural effusion**

### CASE HISTORY 1

A 63-year-old man presented with a two month history of increasing breathlessness and could only walk at a slow pace on the level.

### Examination

• Reduced chest movement on the right
• Stony dullness to percussion
• Absent breath sounds
• Apex beat in anterior axillary line

### Chest X-Ray (Fig 11.12.1)

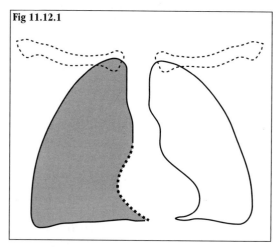

Fig 11.12.1

**CXR** – Right homogeneous opacity; absent heart border and hemidiaphragm obscured. Heart shifted to left

### Extra signs to look for

• Clubbing – suggests malignancy
• Glands in neck
• Wasting
• Enlarged liver

### What do you do next?

Diagnostic aspiration
• 20mls of fluid (syringe + green needle) for:

- protein
- cell count
- culture including TB
- cytology for malignant cells

## Result

• Fluid is blood stained
• Fluid protein is > 30g/litre indicates exudate
• Few white cells and mesothelial cells
• Cultures sterile
• Malignant cells – probably squamous origin

## Diagnosis

• Malignant pleural effusion
• Underlying squamous cell carcinoma of bronchus
• If the diagnosis was not obtained on the aspirate, a pleural biopsy and a larger volume pleurodesis with cytological examination of the spun cellular debris may be performed

## What next?

• The patient has inoperable lung cancer (malignant cells in fluid)
• Treatment should be aimed at relieving symptoms

Drain the effusion with an intercostal drain placed ideally over the top of the diaphragm.

An ultrasound to guide placement is useful. Use 24 to 28 gauge to reduce risk of kinking or blocking. Alternatively cut additional holes in the drain to reduce risk of tube obstruction. This may allow a smaller tube to be used which is more comfortable. Clamp intermittently and limit flow to 1 litre in the first hour to reduce the risk of re-expansion pulmonary oedema or discomfort from mediastinal shift. Re-expansion pulmonary oedema occurs much more commonly following re-expansion of the collapsed lung associated with a pneumothorax. It relates to endothelial dysfunction and is not therefore hydrostatic. Diuretics are not helpful and may exacerbate any tendency to hypovolaemic hypotension.

## Consult

Chest specialist about further management e.g. pleurodesis with tetracycline, – Oncologist or Palliative Care Team.

## CASE HISTORY 2

A 43-year-old woman developed increasing breathlessness and malaise after treatment for pneumonia two weeks previously at home with oral cefalexin. She is febrile T 39°C, flushed and anorexic with signs of a left pleural effusion.

**Fig 11.12.2: Chest X-Ray (PA) + left lateral of an empyema**

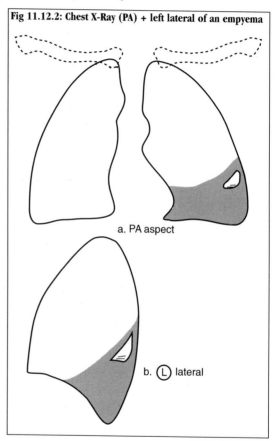

a. PA aspect

b. (L) lateral

**PA**

**CXR** – Homogeneous shadow rising into the axilla
Fluid level indicates air/fluid interface
= gas forming organisms in the pleural space
**Left, lateral view**
This is an empyema – pus in the pleural space.
You cannot aspirate this with a 'green' needle!

### What should you do?

• Drain the empyema by placing an intercostal drain size 24 to 28. The fluid may be thick and require suction applied to the drain bottle, 10cm of water pressure should be enough

- Start antibiotics (after taking blood and fluid cultures), either cefuroxime 1.5g I.V. three times daily + metronidazole 500mg I.V. three times daily or Co-Amoxiclav 600mg I.V. three times daily + gentamicin 3-5mg/kg once daily I.V.
- Consult chest team for advice about increasing drainage by instilling Streptokinase
- Consult chest physician/surgeon early if drainage is incomplete. Decortication of the lung or a rib resection and wide bore drain may be needed.
- Bronchoscopy should be performed to exclude bronchial obstruction. CT scanning may be helpful to assess presence of underlying lung abscess.

### Causes

- Malignancy
- Mesothelioma (incidence increasing)
- Metastatic cancer – breast, bowel
- Lymphoma
- Pneumonia
- Tuberculosis
- Heart failure
- Nephrotic syndrome
- In association with intra-abdominal sepsis or pancreatitis

**Remember**

If in doubt:
- Consult a more senior colleague
- Learn under supervision

### Check your practical skills!

Can you perform the following safely?

- Chest aspiration
- Pleural biopsy
- Place an intercostal drain
- Manage an underwater seal drainage system

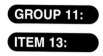

**GROUP 11:** Respiratory disorders

**ITEM 13:** Pulmonary embolism

The diagnosis of pulmonary embolism may be difficult for a number of reasons:

- It is often not present when thought of
- It is present when not thought of
- Presumptive treatment is not without risk
- Proving the diagnosis may be difficult

## CASE HISTORY 1

Joan was 24 years old. She had been getting breathless for three months when referred. Asthma seemed unlikely and the CXR was normal. A short pulmonary diastolic murmur was noted and a cardiology opinion sought. Spirometry was normal but CO gas transfer was reduced ($TL_{co}$ 60% predicted). The echocardiographic appearances were normal.

About two weeks later Joan was admitted in cardiogenic shock. The ECG showed acute Rt heart strain ($S_1$, $Q_3$, $T_3$ with dominant R waves in $V_{1-3}$) and the pulmonary artery diastolic pressure was calculated to be 25 cm $H_2O$ plus the Rt atrial pressure (by doppler echocardiography of the tricuspid regurgitant wave). Joan was managed on the CCU with daily intravenous Alteplase for three days and the echocardiogram used to monitor response. A subsequent VQ scan revealed the typical multiple patchy perfusion abnormalities of recurrent minor pulmonary embolism. It has remained abnormal and Joan continues to be breathless. Leiden factor V deficiency was discovered and the oral contraceptive stopped. She has been advised to remain on life long warfarin.

The source of dislodged thrombus is most commonly the pelvic or femoral veins with the classical triad of stasis, hypercoagulopathy or trauma being present in most patients. In some circumstances air, amniotic fluid, infected clot and even sheared off intravenous catheter material may be causal.

### The most common clinical scenarios you will meet are

- Acute minor pulmonary infarction producing pleuritic chest pain and possibly haemoptysis
- Episodic non specific symptoms in the post operative patient (such as palpitations and anxiety attacks) possibly followed by a cardiac arrest when at toilet
- Chronic minor thrombo-embolism leading to established pulmonary hypertension
- Acute life threatening major embolism with cardiogenic shock

Venous thrombosis occurs in 10% of hospitalised patients and was much more common on surgical wards before routine prophylaxis was introduced. Patients with malignancy, advanced cardio-respiratory disease or a past history of venous thrombosis are most at risk. Risk calculation should now guide prophylaxis which should include pressure stockings as well as heparin.

Simple investigations are usually only helpful when the diagnosis is clinically obvious. The ECG or CXR may however reveal evidence of alternative causes such as myocardial infarction, pneumothorax or aortic dissection

**Look for DVT** Doppler ultrasound and venous plethysmography are replacing contrast venography and have sensitivities of 90% and 70% respectively for proximal thrombus.

The value of V/Q scanning for PE *(see Kumar & Clark 4th ed, p720, 761,)* can be summarised as follows:

- A normal scan excludes PE
- It is of most value in the ambulatory relatively low risk patient
- It is most often of intermediate diagnostic value in the patient with underlying cardiac or obstructive lung disease
- It is unnecessary when clinical suspicion is high and venous plethysmography positive
- A scan of high diagnostic certainty makes angiography unnecessary

**Spiral CT Scans** with IV contrast show good sensitivities and specificities for medium sized PEs.

### The echocardiogram can be very useful

- It may show RV dilation with paradoxical septal wall movement; pulmonary artery pressure may also be estimated
- It may exclude or confirm an alternative diagnosis e.g. cardiac tamponade, LVF.
- RV clot is occasionally imaged and is an adverse prognostic sign with 10% mortality risk

### Pulmonary angiography

Should be performed more frequently given the serious implications of thromboembolism in terms of immediate therapy and long term management. Only 60% of patients with high clinical suspicion of PE have the diagnosis confirmed at angiography. It is not universally available but you should discuss with your consultant the need for a pulmonary angiogram especially if there is a relative contra-indication to anticoagulation or thrombolysis. Spiral CT scanning is increasingly employed in many institutions as an alternative to angiography.

**Information**

90% of patients have chest pain and/or breathlessness as the major complaint

**Information**

An undetectable plasma D-dimer level (reflecting fibrin activation) essentially excludes significant thrombo embolism but a raised value is non specific

## Treatment

In the original trials of I.V. heparin in patients with obvious clinical venous thrombosis and pulmonary embolism, treatment with heparin reduced mortality from 40% to 7%.

- Heparin requirements (to prolong the APTT~ 200s) are greater in the initial 24 hours and monitoring is essential when using unfractionated heparin
- Treatment prevents further clot formation whilst endogenous clot lysis or organisation and fixation of thrombus may lead to a resolution of acute RV failure
- Low molecular weight heparin is now licensed for use in DVT and patients with minor PE e.g. pulmonary infarction may be treated without admission if the necessary organisation is available in the out patients
- Warfarin can be initiated and heparin discontinued after one week in uncomplicated cases
- Three months warfarin is adequate therapy and six weeks may be sufficient in patients with surgery as the provoking factor and no underlying coagulopathy

*i*

### Information

Thrombolysis should be considered in all patients with cardiogenic shock or those most at risk from further PE e.g. advanced cardiorespiratory dysfunction. You should discuss with your consultant before treating.

There is increasing experience of thrombolytic therapy in major pulmonary embolism. Although evidence of reduced mortality is lacking, faster and more complete resolution of echocardiographic abnormalities or V/Q defects have been demonstrated.

- 1.5 million units streptokinase followed by an infusion for 24 to 48 hours or Alteplase 100mg bolus, 50mg over four hours and repeated at 24 hours
- Both carry a higher risk of bleeding than heparin (~ 5% major) with a 1% risk of fatal intracerebral haemorrhage

If thrombolysis is contra indicated (recent major surgery, active peptic ulcer disease, stroke or danger of significant chest trauma following CPR) transvenous placement of venocaval filters should be considered. Emergency embolectomy is rarely a possibility – it can only be performed in cardiothoracic centres. Transvenous embolectomy has been described and may be an alternative in the future.

## Respiratory disorders
## Pneumothorax

### CASE HISTORY 1

A 23-year-old man presented to the A&E Department with sudden onset of chest pain worse on deep inspiration associated with acute breathlessness. This started at rest and was not associated with cough. There were no pre-existing medical problems and no other symptoms.

### Key points

Common causes of pleuritic chest pain and dyspnoea:

– pneumothorax, pulmonary embolism, pneumonia with pleurisy

### On examination

Healthy young man – afebrile, not cyanosed, no signs of DVT

- Pulse rate 100/min Respiratory rate 30/min
- Trachea central
- Chest movement reduced right side
- Percussion note hyperresonant right side
- Breath sounds reduced right side

### Diagnosis

Right sided spontaneous pneumothorax

- Key investigation Chest X-ray (Fig 11.14.1)

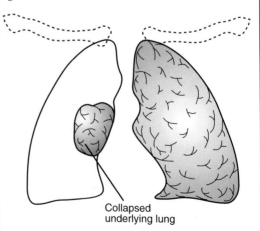

**Fig 11.14.1**

Collapsed underlying lung

**CXR findings**

Pneumothorax = 1/2 hemithorax

## Management of pneumothorax

nil if small   – Discharge and review next day
↓ aspirate    – Admit/discharge and review next day
↓ drain       – Admit

This man was symptomatic and had a moderate sized pneumothorax. Aspiration is the first choice

• Technique for simple aspiration
  – infiltrate with local anaesthetic down to pleura in 2nd intercostal space in midclavicular line using FG16 cannula (or less ) at least 3cm long
  – once in pleural space, remove needle
  – connect cannula via 3 way tap to chest, 50ml syringe.
  – stop aspirating when resistance felt, or patient coughs or complains of discomfort, or when 2.5 litres aspirated
• Patient re X-rayed: the lung was completely re-expanded

## Further management

• Patient was discharged home taking his discharge X-ray
• Instructed not to fly or deep sea dive until seen
• Given follow-up appointment in chest clinic for one week
• Instructed to re-attend (bringing X-ray) if he became breathless.

## CASE HISTORY 2

A 69-year-old man with long-standing COPD and an exercise tolerance of 100yds on the flat became acutely breathless at rest. On examination he was distressed and cyanosed:

• Using accessory muscles of respiration
• Respiratory rate 40 per minute. Pulse 120 B.P. 100/60
• Barrel-shaped chest with poor expansion
• Hyper-resonant chest with almost inaudible breath sounds

## Main differential diagnoses

• Acute exacerbation of COPD but no obvious infection + symptoms very acute
• Pulmonary embolism
• Pneumothorax
• Acute myocardial infarction with LVF

## Action

• Urgent chest X-ray, arterial blood gas

**Diagnosis was tension pneumothorax = life-threatening**

• Emphysematous lungs with mediastinal shift to the right and complete left pneumothorax

**Management**

• Controlled oxygen as per blood gases
• Urgent insertion of intercostal tube

**Management of intercostal tube**

### Insertion of tube

• Explain and reassure patient throughout
• Premedicate with opiate and atropine to prevent reflex bradycardia, particularly if patient anxious but care in patients with pre-existing lung disease
• Double check the side of pneumothorax
• Site – 4-6th intercostal space in ant-axillary line – mark with pen + position patient supine with head at 30° and arm abducted to 90°
• Wear sterile gloves
• Drain 20-24 FG (adult). Check assembly and tight connection and that underwater seal is ready
• Local anaesthetic
   – intradermal bleb in appropriate intercostal space
   – infiltrate deeper with blue, then green needle to parietal pleura at upper surface of rib: NB neuro-vascular bundle runs along lower surface
   – use 5 to 10ml 1% lignocaine
   – check intermittently if in pleural space (air aspirated into syringe)

### Insertion of drain

   – 1 to 2cm incision in skin + subcutaneous fat
   – Insert 2 horizontal sutures across incision (leave loose for subsequent sealing of wound on drain site)
   – wide tract made through intercostal muscles down to and through pleura by blunt dissection with forceps (not sharp trocar)
   – insert trocar + drain assembly without force
   – withdraw metal trocar 5cm and advance tube in apical direction
   – remove trocar and connect tube to underwater seal
   – secure tube firmly with one of two 2 sutures (1 loop through skin + 4 times round tube). Purse string suturing is no longer advised as it leaves unsightly scarring.
   – loop tube + secure to skin with plaster (NB no kinks)
   – prescribe adequate oral/i.m. analgesia

**Removal of tube**
- Leave tube draining until no further bubbling + then re X-ray (X-ray earlier if in doubt about site or efficacy of tube)
- Note, if level not swinging tube blocked. Clear or replace if lung not re-expanded
- Some patients need premedication for tube removal
- Remove holding suture + withdraw while patient's breath-holds in expiration
- Seal wound with 1 of original sutures
- Observe overnight + if no recurrence of pneumothorax (clinical + X-Ray) discharge with Chest Clinic appointment in seven to 10 days. Patient keeps last X-ray to bring to appointment or to A&E in emergency

**GROUP 11:**

**ITEM 15:**

# Respiratory disorders
# Carcinoma of the bronchus

**Information**

Carcinoma of the Bronchus
- Most common form of cancer in both sexes
- Non-small cell
  - squamous cell carcinoma (39%)
  - adenocarcinoma (10%)
  - large cell carcinoma (25%)
  - alveolar cell carcinoma (2%)
- small cell (20–30%)

### CASE HISTORY

A 53 year old male presents with a history of having coughed up blood a few hours ago. He has been smoking 20 cigarettes a day for the past 30 years. On examination there is diminished breath sounds at the right upper chest anteriorly.

### What is the most likely diagnosis and why?

Carcinoma of the bronchus
- Cigarette smoking is the most common risk factor
- It is a common cause of haemoptysis in smokers > 40 years of age
- Physical sign of diminished breath sounds suggests bronchial obstruction

### What are the important diagnostic investigations?

- Chest X-ray
- Sputum cytology
- Bronchoscopy for histological diagnosis

If histological diagnosis is not made on bronchoscopy, CT guided percutaneous needle biopsy should be considered

The commonest chest X-ray presentation is a hilar shadow. Other presentations are:

- Consolidation / collapse of part or whole of lung
- Pleural effusion (see Group 11, Item 12)
- Cachexia or metastatic disease
- Raised hemi-diaphragm due to phrenic nerve palsy

### Management

For practical purposes carcinoma of the bronchus can be divided as:

Small cell lung cancer (SCLC). It is rarely operable.

Non-small cell lung cancer (NSCLC)

### What treatments can be offered to a patient?

**Surgical Resection**

– all patients with NSCLC should be assessed for surgical resection as it is the only curative treatment

**Chemotherapy**

– this mode of treatment should be offered to patients with SCLC

– its role in NSCLC is not well established. Recent meta-analysis has shown a significant advantage in favour of platinum containing chemotherapy regime. Opinion of an experienced specialist should be sought

**Radiotherapy**

– radical radiotherapy is useful in selected patients with NSCLC

– has an important role in palliation of symptoms

– addition of thoracic irradiation to chemotherapy in limited SCLC disease reduces the rate of recurrence

– adjunctive treatment with chemotherapy or radiotherapy is increasingly employed in peri-operative management of NSCLC

**Palliative Therapy**

– all patients should be offered palliative therapy for symptoms
- Breathlessness
  – treat cause if possible, e.g. Pleural effusion, tracheal or large airway obstruction
  – opiates
- Severe pain
  – potent analgesics e.g.– opiates, including Fentanyl
- Bone pain
  – NSAID's
  – local radiotherapy
- Nerve root pain
  – amitriptyline
  – carbamazepine

*i*

**Information**

SCLC Limited Disease
– Tumour confined to one hemithorax and ipsilateral supraclavicular node

Extensive Disease
– Involvement of any site outside the hemithorax

## Management of major complications
**Hypercalcaemia** (Group 14 Item 9)
- intravenous fluids 3-4 L
- diuretic : Frusemide 40 mg I.V. (ensure adequately rehydrated).
- intravenous Pamidronate – treatment of choice

### Weakness of legs
This suggests spinal cord compression and is a medical emergency especially with bladder or bowel dysfunction
- start Dexamethasone 4 mg x three times daily.
- MRI scan of the spine and referral for radio-therapy/surgery.

### Stridor
This is due to obstruction above the level of carina (demonstrated in a flow volume loop)
- start Dexamethasone 4 mg x three times daily
- urgent bronchoscopy followed by CT scan of the chest/neck
- intraluminal growth: referral for laser therapy / stenting
- extrinsic compression: referral for radiotherapy / stenting

### Superior vena-caval obstruction
- start on dexamethasone 4 mg x three times daily
- refer for radiotherapy
- consider heparin or thombolysis

## Management of patients with neutropenia following chemotherapy
Indications for Antibiotic Therapy
- Absolute Neutrophil Count < 1.0 / Total white cell count < 2.5
- Pyrexia.

## Recommended antibiotic regimes
- I.V. Gentamicin (3-5mg/kg IV once a day. Monitor trough levels) and an ureidopenicillin (Azlocillin)
- In presence of severe renal insufficiency, replace Gentamicin with I.V. Ceftazidime 1-2 g x three times daily or Ciprofloxacin 400 mg x two times daily
- Continue antibiotics for five days or until white cell counts are in normal range and symptoms have remitted

## If no improvement after 48 to 72 hours of antibiotic therapy
- Repeat blood and urine cultures and chest X-ray
- Consider the following infections
  - fungus: Blood & urine cultures
  - start Fluconazole &/or Amphotericin

### Investigations
- Blood (preferably two samples from two different sites) and urine cultures
- Chest X-ray
- Culture from any suspected site of infection e.g. cannula exit site, sputum

• Protozoa: Broncho-alveolar lavage
• Virus: Viral serology
• Resistant Staphylococcus:
  – more common with central venous catheter
  – treat with Vancomycin

**Indications for Filgrastim (G-CSF):**
  – absolute neutrophil Count 0.2.
  – persistent neutropenia (< 1.0 for more than 48 hours)
  – stop therapy when absolute neutrophil count is 1.5 or more

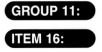

**GROUP 11:**

**ITEM 16:**

# Respiratory disorders
# Sarcoidosis

### CASE HISTORY

You are phoned up by a GP who has a 28-year-old woman with tender, bluish lumps on front of her legs in the surgery. She also complains of stiffness of the ankles and a temperature. He thinks that this is erythema nodosum but would like another opinion.

### Is this erythema nodosum (EN)?

From his description this sounds very likely and you ask him to send the patient up to outpatients when you will arrange for a CXR to be performed. (Fig 11.16.1)

**Fig 11.16.1 – CXR showing bilateral hilar and paratracheal lymphadenopathy**

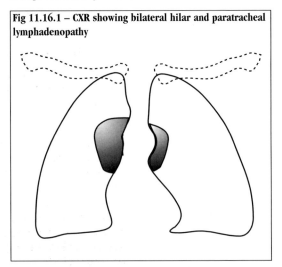

EN with lymphadenopathy on CXR is a characteristic presentation of Sarcoidosis. Along with her arthritis and fever the syndrome is called **Lofgren's syndrome**. In outpatients the patient poses several questions for you on hearing her diagnosis.

### What is sarcoidosis?

You explain that this is a well recognised disorder for which no cause is known. You emphasise, however, that in her case the skin rash (EN) will subside within two months but the CXR may take up to a year to revert to normal. No treatment is required other than pain relief.

The chances of further trouble are negligible.

You discuss this later with your consultant who reminds you of the extrapulmonary manifestations which can be troublesome.

- Skin and ocular lesions are most common.
- Skin lesions (10%) of cases. Apart from EN, a chilblain-like lesion (lupus pernio) and nodules are seen.
- Eye involvement (5%) Anterior uveitis (misting of vision, pain, red eye) is common. Posterior uveitis may present with a progressive loss of vision. Conjunctivitis and retinal lesions are seen. Asymptomatic uveitis may be found in 25% of patients.
- Metabolic Hypercalcaemia is found in 10% but it is rarely severe
- CNS involvement is rare (2%) but can lead to severe neurological disease.
- Bone and Joint involvement Arthralgia without EN is seen in 5% of cases.
- Cardiac involvement is rare (3%) clinically although seen in 20% of post mortems. Ventricular arrhythmias, conduction defects and cardiomyopathy with CCF are seen. The serum ACE is insensitive in cardiac sarcoid and echocardiography should be performed in chronic sarcoidosis.

## CASE HISTORY 2

You are contacted by the ENT registrar because he has seen a patient with nasal stuffiness and a blocked nose. He had also noted some blood-stained nasal discharge. An X-ray of the patient's sinuses shows destruction of the nasal bones. He wants you to see the patient as he found out that this man has had longstanding pulmonary sarcoidosis. As you walk to the ENT ward you think over your knowledge of sarcoidosis remembering that patients with upper respiratory tract involvement usually have pulmonary disease.

On arrival on the wards you retake the history – he has been breathless for years and tells you that all his numerous CXRs show that his lungs are "full of sarcoid". He has not been on steroids because of its lack of efficacy and side-effects which have made him non-compliant.

## Investigations

- CXR
- FBC – shows:
  - a mild normochromic normocytic anaemia.
  - low lymphocyte count +/–
  - low neutrophils
  - thrombocytopenia
- Blood gases $PO_2$ 6.8 kPa, $PCO_2$ 4.3 kPa

On examination he is noticeably breathless and cyanosed. Chest examination shows widespread crackles.

You arrange to give the patient oxygen by ordinary face mask 4 L/min.

The next morning you return with your consultant having obtained the patient's old notes.

You note multiple CXRs showing widespread pulmonary infiltration with no hilar lymphadenopathy. The latest CXR also shows a rounded opacity in the right apex – thought to be an aspergilloma.

Fibre optic bronchoscopy with transbronchial biopsies was performed 10 years ago. This showed epithelial and giant cell granulomas. (This test has a 90% sensitivity with pulmonary infiltration.)

### Lung function tests showed

- Reduced total lung capacity (restrictive ventilatory capacity)
- Impaired gas transfer (TLCO)
- Low compliance
- Serum ACE levels – this had been done a few years back and was found to be raised.

## Remember

Serum ACE levels raised in only 30 to 50% of patients with untreated sarcoidosis. Persistently raised levels are a poor guide to clinical activity.

Review of his past treatment shows that he has been given steroids on many occasions and azathioprine and methotrexate as steroid sparing agents.

Your consultant congratulates you on your review of the notes which is crucial for the future management of this case. He suggests you start high dose steroids and suggests that cyclosporin has been shown to be of some benefit.

Progressive respiratory failure is well recognised in sarcoidosis. Unfortunately recurrence in the transplanted lung (as well as limited availability of organs) has led many centres to not consider transplantation for end stage pulmonary fibrosis. Lung transplantation may be indicated if this patient fails to improve.

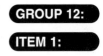

**GROUP 12:**

**ITEM 1:**

# ITU
## Shock

**Remember**

- Shock is a life threatening condition in which the patient is hypoxic
- Oxygen must be given immediately to all haemodynamically unstable patients
- Establish clear airway

### CASE HISTORIES 1 AND 2

On your medical take you are called to A&E to see two patients in neighbouring cubicles. Case 1 is a 60-year-old bank manager with crushing central chest pain. The other (case 2) is a 50-year-old man with painless haematemesis. Both patients are reported to be tachycardic at 120 bpm and to be hypotensive (90/60) on non-invasive blood pressure measurement.

The bank manager is cold and clammy to touch. The second patient admits to a previous hospital admission with cirrhosis of the liver and oesophageal varices. He is sweating profusely with visible shaking of his extremities.

These two patients are shocked but for different reasons. From the information given we cannot be completely sure of the cause of the shocked state and further questioning and investigation is required after the institution of emergency measures.

### Physiology

Shock is 'inadequate tissue oxygenation' where there is failure of the circulatory system due to

- Failure of the heart to maintain an adequate cardiac output eg myocardial infarction
- Reduction in the volume of blood within the circulation eg haemorrhage
- Loss of vascular tone within the circulatory system eg septicaemia
- Obstruction to the circulation eg pulmonary embolism

**Remember**

A patient may have more than one of the above eg case 2 may have a cardiomyopathy (pump failure) as well as his haematemesis (decreased volume).

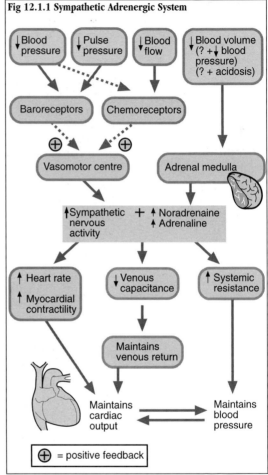

Fig 12.1.1 Sympathetic Adrenergic System

Redrawn from *Clinical Medicine*, 4th Edition, Kumar and Clark, 1998, by permission of the publisher WB Saunders

### Causes of shock

- **Cardiogenic** – myocardial infarction, tam-ponade, aortic dissection, pulmonary embolism, tension pneumothorax.
- **Sepsis** – infective causes eg pneumonia, urinary or meningococcal septicaemia or the so-called "systemic inflammatory response syndrome" (SIRS) resulting from trauma, post surgery or anaphylaxis.
- **Hypovolaemia** – profound dehydration, haemorrhage.

### Is the shock state in case 1 due to myocardial infarction, an obstructed circulation or other shock-inducing factors?

A history in a shocked patient of pain in the chest associated with ECG evidence of myocardial ischaemia would probably be the true cause of a shocked state. Caution is necessary, however, since ECG changes involving tachyarrythmias and ST segment changes characteristic of myocardial ischaemia may occur in hypovolaemic shock.

## Is the shock state in case 2 due to fluid loss? If so, what fluid and from where?

In this case the blood loss is obvious ie haematemesis. Try and estimate from the patient how much was lost. In other cases blood loss might be concealed eg fractured femur where up to two litres may be lost from the circulation.

### Investigations

- Haemoglobin and haematocrit, U&Es, LFTs
- ECG and monitor
- Central venous pressure see Group 9 Item 1
  - If the CVP is low (< 5 cm water) fluid replacement is necessary
  - If 10cm or more fluid replacement is not required.

## Clinical examination

In assessing the shocked patient the following indices should be monitored

- Pulse rate
- Peripheral venous filling/capillary filling
- Limb temperature
- Arterial blood pressure
- Urinary output
- Mental state

**Case 1** – the bank manager – has a problem with the circulatory pump and needs no extra intravascular fluid administration.

**Case 2** – the haematemesis patient – has lost circulating volume with a low central venous pressure. His problems are with the plumbing circuit not the heart pump and his condition may be compounded by coagulation and biochemical disturbances consequent upon concomitant hepatic insufficiency.

- Arterial blood gas analysis. In hypovolaemic shock (as in all shock states) there is a metabolic acidosis with a high hydrogen ion concentration and low bicarbonate concentration. In cases with respiratory complications the $pO_2$ and $pCO_2$ values will help indicate the need for ventilatory support.
- Lactate levels. Blood lactate levels rise approximately in proportion to the severity of the shock.
- X-rays. These are usually of little value in the acute stages of shock management. A CXR will exclude any treatable pathology such as a pneumothorax or haemothorax complicating insertion of monitoring lines.

### How would you treat?

Both patients should be admitted to high dependency nursing units.

## CASE 1

In cardiogenic hypotension, key issues are pain relief, arrhythmia management and treatment of pulmonary oedema. Pain relief by incremental doses of intravenous opiates will aid reduction in myocardial oxygen consumption. Correcting electrolyte disturbances, hypoxia and controlling angina pain may assist in arrhythmia management. Temporary transvenous pacing may be required for significant bradycardia. Continuous infusion of vasodilators plus diuretics may be needed for pulmonary oedema. Acute revascularisation (thrombolysis, angioplasty, coronary artery bypass grafting) may also be indicated. In the context of persistent hypotension infusion of inotropic agents such as dobutamine may be necessary whilst correctable abnormalities are sought eg acute mitral regurgitation following papillary muscle rupture or the development of an ischaemic ventricular septal defect. Percutaneous insertion of an intra-aortic balloon counterpulsation pump may be considered for refractory cardiogenic hypotension following transfer to a specialist centre as a prelude to surgical intervention.

## CASE 2

In hypovolaemic hypotension the principle issues are the reduction in further fluid loss whilst simultaneously restoring fluid volumes via wide bore intravenous cannulae. Infusion of red cells provide sufficient oxygen transport capacity (a target of 8 to 10 g/dl is broadly accepted). Fresh frozen plasma (for example to obtain a target INR of < 1.5) may be necessary. At the earliest opportunity the patient with haematemesis will require endoscopy to find the bleeding lesion. (see Group 5, Item 5)

## CASE HISTORY 3

On take you are called to see a patient in A&E. Mr B is 68. He is pyrexial at 39°C, BP 90/40 HR 120 bpm, tachypnoeic with a distended and silent abdomen.

### What is the cause of shock in this patient?

Mr B has septic shock probably secondary to intra-abdominal sepsis. He will need fluid resuscitation and urgent laparotomy.

### How would you manage this case?

Immediate action

- Correct hypoxaemia – high flow $O_2$
- Determine cause – examination, chest and abdominal x-ray, ECG, ABGs, FBC, U&Es , Blood cultures.
- Initiate treatment – IV fluid resuscitation, inotropes.

---

## $i$

### Information

Patients at risk of further deterioration may have one or more of the following vital signs which might suggest **transfer to an Intensive Therapy Unit**

- Heart Rate > 120 bpm
- Heart Rate < 40 bpm
- Systolic blood pressure > 200 mmHg
- Systolic blood pressure < 80 mmHg
- Respiratory rate > 30 breaths per minute
- Respiratory rate < 8 breaths per minute
- Oxygen saturation < 90%
- Glasgow coma scale < 8
- Core temperature > 39C
- Core temperature < 35C
- Urine output less than 0.5 ml/kg/hr for two consecutive hours.

Shock is a medical emergency. The longer it persists the lower the chance of recovery as secondary injury, from co-existent hypoxaemia and delayed reperfusion, is now recognised to cause further cytokine activation and the development of multiple organ dysfunction syndrome (MODS) or multiple organ failure (MOF).

Clinical point – the medical records of many patients admitted to the ICU from the ward show progressive evidence of impending doom – increasing heart rate, oliguria, tachypnoea or confusion. **Act before shock has become established!**

**Pathophysiology of Septic Shock.** In sepsis, hypotension primarily results from impaired vascular tone. Sympathetic activation often leads to a high cardiac output with a low systemic vascular resistance. Hypovolaemia may occur from interstitial fluid losses due to endothelial dysfunction which is widespread, and reduced venous tone. In more profound sepsis, myocardial depression also occurs due to circulating cytokines such as TNF.

### Further Management
- Central line for CVP measurement
- Titrate fluid resuscitation to provide adequate cardiac output.
- Inotropic support. Think of giving a vasoconstrictor eg noradrenaline (norepinephrine) if vasodilated
- New agents (Dopexamine) yet to show clinical benefit compared with adrenalin
- CPAP, NIV or intubation and IPPV depending on situation.
- Reducing fever – important in limiting metabolic oxygen demands.
- Seek surgical opinion for treatment of abdominal condition.
- Novel therapies
  - Cytokine inhibitors continue to be developed and tested but are "two-sided weapons" – immune modulation awaits better methods to characterise the immune deficient from the hyperimmune state.
  - Antioxidant therapy has a theoretical basis in sepsis by scavenging oxygen free radicals that are implicated in tissue injury.
  - Bicarbonate haemofiltration when lactic acidosis prevents the use of lactate solutions.
  - Glutamine, and other non-essential amino acid in nutritional suplementation, may have an immunomodulatory role and limit muscle catabolism.

### Summary
Timely intervention in patients with sepsis may prevent the development of shock. Fluid resuscitation and treatment aimed at the primary cause should be instituted rapidly and high flow oxygen given to limit regional hypoxaemia. Prognosis is dependent on cause and response to treatment. For instance, mortality from urinary sepsis has a better prognsis than a similar clinical situation resulting from peritonitis.

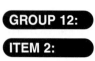

## ITU
## Acute lung injury

### CASE HISTORY

You are called urgently to the receiving room when on take. A 35-year-old known drug abuser has been blue lighted into the hospital having been found unconscious. The Glasgow Coma Score (GCS) is 5, BP 100/60 with a respiratory rate of 20 and $SaO_2$ on high flow $O_2$, 85%.

**What are possible causes of depressed consciousness and what are your immediate actions?**

• You need to consider intoxication, hypoglycaemia, respiratory failure, head injury or a post ictal state.

• Look for evidence of focal neurological signs, pinpoint pupils, trauma to the head or evidence of seizures such as tongue laceration, incontinence.

• Ensure airway not obstructed, establish IV access, take blood gases, blood glucose and blood and urine for toxicology and give Nalorphine.

• ABG analysis reveals pH 7.2, $paO_2$ 6.4, $pCO_2$ 2.5.

**What do these results indicate?**

• Acute type I respiratory failure with a metabolic (lactic) acidosis.

• There is vomitus around the mouth and on his clothing. The chest x-ray shows patch shadowing at the right base.

• Following Nalorphine he becomes agitated, moving all limbs but does not respond purposely to command.

**What is the immediate management?**

Respiratory failure is probably related to aspiration of vomitus. Intubation and IPPV is indicated. CPAP or non-invasive ventilation (NIV) is contra-indicated because of danger of further vomiting and lack of co-operation.

He is transferred to the ICU. On the post take ward round next morning, ventilatory pressures are high for standard tidal volumes and he remains hypoxic on $FiO_2$ 100%. Your consultant suggests you make a short presentation on acute respiratory distress syndrome (ARDS) to the students at the lunch-time meeting.

## Key features

- Pulmonary infiltrates-due to an increase in lung interstitial fluid not related to heart failure; by definition pulmonary artery capillary wedge pressure < 18 cmH$_2$O
- A reduction in pulmonary compliance, i.e. stiff lungs, resulting in high inflation pressures.
- Profound gas exchange abnormalities defined as PaO$_2$ mmHg/FiO$_2$ < 300 for Acute Lung Injury (ALI) or < 200 for ARDS
- A cause other than primary pneumonia.

## Causes

- Severe sepsis e.g. peritonitis, septicaemia
- Pulmonary aspiration
- Multiple trauma and massive transfusion
- Post cardiac bypass
- Pancreatitis
- Toxic fume exposure including smoke inhalation
- Cerebral injury e.g. subarachnoid haemorrhage
- Pneumocystis pneumonia

## Pathophysiology

- Profound hypoxaemia results from venous admixture or shunting of deoxygenated blood through poorly or unventilated lung units. This arises because:
- Endothelial dysfunction leads to widespread interstitial oedema and impaired alveolar capillary perfusion
- The stiff (low compliance) lungs results in reduced tidal volume and reduced end expiratory lung volume – this then causes small airway collapse-once collapsed Laplace's law explains why it is difficult to re-expand the airway (consider the difficulty in initially blowing up a balloon)
- Additional small airway pathology particularly with direct lung injury, e.g. smoke inhalation
- The lung may be likened to a wet sponge – the dependent sponge is waterlogged and the air spaces collapsed. Only the non-dependent areas of the lung may be contributing to gas exchange. The additional component of airway inflammation in some causes of ARDS may explain the high mortality associated with direct lung injury (>60%).

## Management

The high mortality of ARDS is critically dependent on resolution of the primary cause. Treatment of the lung is essentially supportive. Avoidance of further injury by employing permissive hypoxaemia (aiming to limit oxygen toxicity by FiO$_2$<70%) and hypercapnia (limiting tidal volume to avoid barotrauma – over-distension of functioning lung and risk of pneumothorax).

Ventilatory techniques include:
• Deep sedation and neuromuscular paralysis to increase chest wall compliance
• Small tidal volumes and prolonged inspiration to limit airway pressure
• Use of PEEP (positive end-expiratory pressure) to recruit lung units
• Prone positioning to improve $\dot{V}/\dot{Q}$ matching and clearance of lung secretions

### Experimental methods include:
• Inhaled nitric oxide to overcome hypoxic pulmonary vasoconstriction and improve $\dot{V}/\dot{Q}$ matching and reduce pulmonary hypertension
• Steroids to limit the proliferative fibrotic process of lung repair
• High frequency or liquid ventilation
• Extra corporel membrane oxygenation

### Outlook
Mortality from ALI/ARDS remains high (overall 40 to 50%). Lung remodelling may, however, result in considerable eventual recovery. Progress of the underlying disease, nosocomial infection or the development of cardiogenic shock, secondary to right ventricular failure, are critical in determining survival.

## CASE HISTORY (CONTINUED)

The patient developed multi-organ dysfunction with impaired hepatic synthesis including coagulopathy, cholestatic jaundice and acute tubular necrosis requiring haemofiltration. Antibiotic therapy initially was Cefuroxime and metronidazole, but subsequently Pseudomonas was cultured from respiratory secretions. A week later a tracheostomy was performed and ventilatory support was progressively weaned over the next three weeks. He was discharged from hospital six weeks after admission.

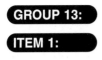

## Poisoning
## Self poisoning

This is a common problem leading to over 100,000 hospital admissions in England and Wales per annum.

### General points
• 80% will be conscious
• There is poor correlation between history of amount, type and timing of poisons consumed and blood toxicology
• Frequently more than one drug will have been consumed
• Alcohol is the most commonly consumed second agent

### What particular points do you need to assesss on physical examination?
• Assess and record conscious level using Glasgow Coma Scale
• Document respiratory rate and cyanosis
• Measure blood pressure and pulse
• Record pupillary size and reactivity to light
• Measure temperature – rectally if unconscious
• If depressed consciousness check for co-existent head injury
• Look for needle tracks or signs of drug abuse – may help with opiates

### CASE HISTORY

A 25-year-old woman is admitted semi-conscious, smelling of alcohol having taken an indeterminate amount of an unknown drug at some point earlier that evening.

On examination she has depressed consciousness (Glasgow coma Scale of 11), respiratory rate of 12 per minute, blood pressure of 95/70 mm Hg and small reactive pupils.

### What should you do?
• Baseline Full blood count, urea and electrolytes, liver function
• Paracetamol and salicylate levels at four hours or thereafter post overdose.
• Blood and urine samples for toxicology particularly useful in seriously ill with altered consciousness
• $O_2$ saturation, arterial blood gases if depressed respiration

### General management of self-poisoning
Take advice of 24-hour poisons information service in all serious overdoses particularly, in case there are advances in management of the specific poisoning under your care.

Some common drugs used for overdose exhibit delayed action eg aspirin, paracetamol, tricyclic antidepressants, iron (commoner in children), diphenoxylate and atropine, paraquat and all modified release preparations.

## General

- Nurse in left lateral position
- Clear mouth of vomitus, debris, obstructing objects
- Catheterisation of bladder may be unnecessary as gentle suprapubic pressure can empty bladder
- IV cannula
- Nursing care of mouth and pressure areas

## Respiratory support

- Protect airway as vomiting is a risk. Vomiting is particularly associated with opiates, benzodiazepines, alcohol, tricyclic antidepressants or phenothiazines.
- Give oxygen – start with 60% humidified $O_2$
- Loss of gag or cough reflex is the prime indication for intubation.

## Cardiovascular support

- Watch for Hypotension (systolic BP below 80 mmHg):
  - mild – raise end of bed
  - severe – use IV volume expanders eg dextran
  - very severe – insert CVP line to monitor fluid replacement
  - Measure Urine output – aim for 0.5 ml/kg/hour. Urine output is an important guide to the adequacy of the circulation.
- Monitor ECG for arrhythmias

## What other problems might occur?

### Blood pressure

- watch for hypotension (see above). Avoid vasopressant drugs as these may interact adversely with the poison.
- less commonly transient hypertension may be seen with amphetamine and cocaine.

### Arrhythmias

- may arise from hypoxia or metabolic acidosis.
- ventricular and supraventricular tachycardias may occur due to theophyllines, tricyclic antidepressants/phenothiazines (due to prolonged QT interval) cocaine and amphetamine.

### Hypothermia

- may occur due to unconsciousness especially with phenothiazines and barbiturates. Measure temperature rectally.
- nurse under space blanket with warming if needed using water bottles.

## What specific management procedures are there for overdoses?

### Reducing absorption
• Gastric lavage or induced emesis.
• Gastric lavage after four hours of overdosage is still useful for salicylates and tricyclics.
• Avoid lavage if corrosives, paraffin or petrol taken because of risk of inhalation. Always intubate if the patient is unconscious.
• Induced emesis – use ipecacuanha only if fully conscious.
• Activated charcoal binds drugs in the intestine and is most effective for aspirin, tricyclic antidepressants and theophylines. Particularly useful if lavage or emesis are contraindicated.

### Active elimination
• Repeated doses of charcoal may enhance elimination even after the drug has been absorbed. This works for aspirin,barbiturates, quinine, theophyline and carbamezepine.
• Alkaline diuresis for salicyclate poisoning is rarely indicated.
• Haemodialysis helps in severe salicylate poisoning, barbiturates, ethylene glycol, alcohol and lithium poisoning.
• Haemoperfusion involves passing heparinised blood across absorbents such as charcoal. Works for barbiturates and theophylline.

### Antagonising the influences of poisons
• Methionine or N-acetylcysteine replenish cellular glutathione stores in paracetamol poisoning.
• Ethanol is a competitive inhibitor of alcohol dehydrogenase and is given in ethylene glycol (anti-freeze) poisoning. Fomepizole is also useful.
• Naloxone and opiates compete at the same receptor.

**Paracetamol** is consumed in 45% of overdoses.

As little as 7.5 to 15 gms (15-30) tablets may cause severe hepatic necrosis.

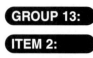

**GROUP 13:**

**ITEM 2:**

# Poisoning
## Paracetamol poisoning

### CASE HISTORY

A 23-year-old girl was brought into A&E by her boyfriend who had found her drowsy. There was an empty bottle of paracetamol tablets and half a bottle of wine by her. They had had a fight the previous night and she had threatened suicide. He thought that she had taken the tablets six hours ago. On examination she had a GCS of 13. There were no other physical signs.

### Investigations

- Baseline urea and electrolytes
- Liver function (including INR) and biochemistry
- Paracetamol and salicylate levels at four hours or thereafter post overdose. Her paracetamol level was 160 mg/L. Salicylates <10 mg at six hours post overdose.

### Points to remember

- Nausea and vomiting in first 24 hours
- Abdominal pain 24 hours plus
- Persistent nausea with subcostal pain usually indicates significant hepatic necrosis
- Remember paracetamol is a constituent of co-proxamol or co-dydramol with opiate.
- Chronic alcohol excess or other enzyme inducing drugs are important

### Physical examination (Fig 13.2.1)

- Later – Liver flap and altered consciousness may develop three days plus
- Check respiratory rate in case compound preparation consumed

### Management – The problems

Paracetamol may cause hepatic necrosis with maximum damage sustained 72 to 96 hours after ingestion. Renal damage occurs even without major liver damage.

### How should you manage this patient?

For general management see Group 13, Item 1

The treatment nomogram (Fig 13.2.1)

There are two lines on the nomogram – the normal and the high risk treatment lines.

The high risk treatment line should be used for patients who are likely to be glutathione deplete eg the malnourished or HIV positive patients.

Chronic alcoholics or those on enzyme inducers eg phenytoin, rifampicin, carbamezepine are also at high risk from lower levels of paracetamol.

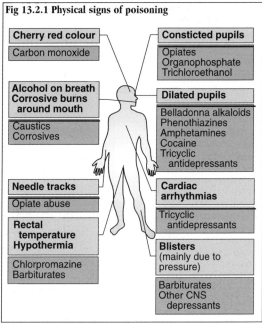

Fig 13.2.1 Physical signs of poisoning

**Cherry red colour**
Carbon monoxide

**Consticted pupils**
Opiates
Organophosphate
Trichloroethanol

**Alcohol on breath**
**Corrosive burns**
**around mouth**
Caustics
Corrosives

**Dilated pupils**
Belladonna alkaloids
Phenothiazines
Amphetamines
Cocaine
Tricyclic
  antidepressants

**Needle tracks**
Opiate abuse

**Cardiac**
**arrhythmias**
Tricyclic
  antidepressants

**Rectal**
**  temperature**
**Hypothermia**
Chlorpromazine
Barbiturates

**Blisters**
(mainly due to
pressure)
Barbiturates
Other CNS
  depressants

Redrawn from *Clinical Medicine*, 4th Edition, Kumar and Clark, 1998, by permission of the publisher WB Saunders

This patient required treatment (see below) due to her high paracetamol levels at six hours.

### The antidotes – regime for treatment

• N acetylcysteine by infusion
  – N-acetylcysteine 150 mg/Kg in 200mls of 5% glucose over 15 minutes.
  – Then 50 mg/kg in 500 ml 5% glucose over four hours. Followed by 100 mg/Kg in l litre over 16 hours.

• Oral methionine – only useful outside hospital
  – Methionine may be given orally if charcoal has not been administered.
  – Dosage is 2.5mg followed by three further doses of 2.5mg at eight-hour intervals.

### What are the adverse reactions to N-acetylcysteine?

• Local itching and rashes at infusion sites.
• Systemic effects include nausea, flushing, angioedema, bronchospasm and hypotension.

• Bronchospasm and hypotension may be treated with

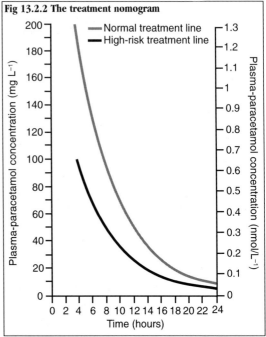

**Fig 13.2.2 The treatment nomogram**

From BNF with permission

discontinuation of the infusion and an antihistamine.

Once resolved then the infusion may be resumed at 100mg/Kg in 1 litre over 16 hours (even if another dose level is begun).

Opiates were suspected in this patient and naloxone 0.8-2mg IV was also given. As she responded to this a naloxone infusion was started at a dose of 2mg diluted in 500 mls rate adjusted to clinical response as an IV naxolone stat dose only lasts 30 minutes.

Intubation and ventilation was considered but pulse oximetry showed no impaired oxygenation.

### Summary

### How would you treat a paracetamol overdose?

*If presentation within eight hours (as in this case)*

- Gastric lavage or emesis up to 4 hours post ingestion.
- Use treatment nomogram at 4 hours or later to guide use of N-acetylcysteine.
- If there is doubt about the timing or more than 12 gms ingested then treat with N-acetylcysteine immediately.
- If the 4 hour paracetamol level is below the treatment line discontinue N-acetyl cysteine except where the patients are at high risk (see above).

## *i*

### Information
**Important points**
- Severe liver or renal damage – seek specialist advice.
- Contact liver unit if INR greater than 3.0 or alanine aminotranferase greater than 1000 U/litre, evidence of acidosis, encephalopathy or hypotensive with systolic less than 60 mm Hg.
- Hypoglycaemia may develop in first 48 hours.
- Alert renal physicians if abnormal creatinine develops.
- There is evidence that administration of N-acetylcysteine in patients with established hepatic encephalopathy may improve the prognosis.

- If methionine or N-acetylcysteine is started within 8 hours the prognosis is good and patients can be considered for discharge at the end of the infusion if blood tests are normal.
- Prior to discharge check the INR and plasma creatinine are normal
- Advise patient to return if vomiting ensues.
- Ensure that liaison with psychiatric services occurs.

*If a patient presents at eight hours – 24 hours post ingestion.*

Patients presenting greater than 8 hours post ingestion are at greater risk of hepatotoxicity – the efficacy of treatment with N-acetylcysteine declines but still give it.

Individual response to paracetamol overdose may be variable and the validity of the treatment line beyond 15 hours post ingestion is not clear.

If there is doubt about the timing of overdose or more than 12 gms have been consumed then treat with N-acetyl cysteine immediately.

At the end of the infusion check the INR and plasma creatinine are normal. If so, risk of damage is negligble and discharge can be planned.

If INR or creatinine are abnormal or patient develops symptoms continue to monitor these blood tests till normal.

*If a patient presents 24 hours plus post ingestion*

The treatment remains controversial but there is evidence of benefits of N-acetylcysteine in those who develop hepatic encephalopathy.

All should have INR, creatinine, and arterial pH monitored.

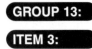

**GROUP 13:**

**ITEM 3:**

# Poisoning

## Salicylate, benzodiazepine and tricyclic antidepressant overdose

### SALICYLATE OVERDOSE

- Aspirin is rapidly absorbed – usually peaks at four hours.
- 10-20 gms will cause moderate to severe toxicity
- Beware modified release formulations which prolong absorption.
- Aspirin itself may delay gastric emptying.

#### Clinical features

- Early features include nausea, vomiting, tinnitus or deafness (severe overdose), sweating and hyperventilation.
- Later features include Kussmaulís respiration, confusion, coma, fits and renal impairment.

#### Management – The problems

- Aspirin delays gastric emptying
- People who appear well may have very high levels.
- Early hypokalaemia and respiratory alkalosis may be replaced after 4-6 hours by metabolic acidosis due to salicylate.
- Hypo-prothrombinaemia may occur.

#### Investigations

- **Baseline urea and electrolytes, liver function**
- **Paracetamol and salicylate levels at four hours or thereafter post overdose**
- **Blood gases if severe poisoning is suggested by levels**

#### Treatment

- Gastric lavage up till 12 hours
- Repeated doses of charcoal may enhance elimination.
- Intravenous fluids with potassium supplements to correct dehydration, hypokalaemia and improve urine flow.
- Forced alkaline diuresis is rarely indicated and can be dangerous. Only consider if salicylate level is 500mg per litre or above.
- The latest protocol for forced alkaline diuresis should be established with the poisons unit.
- Haemodialysis should be considered above 700 mg per litre.

### BENZODIAZEPINE OVERDOSE

40% of all overdoses

#### Clinical features

- Drowsiness, ataxia, slurred speech, coma
- Respiratory depression and hypotension may occur

## Management – The problems

Respiratory depression or in combination with alcohol – vomiting and aspiration.

## Treatment – supportive

• Protect airway and neurological observations.
• Flumazenil is a benzodiazepine antagonist which may be used in severe overdose with marked respiratory depression only.
• Beware – seizures have followed flumazenil administration.
• Patients are usually fit to be discharged at 24 hours.

## TRICYCLIC ANTIDEPRESSANT OVERDOSE

Rarer since the selective serotonin reuptake inhibitors became available (much safer). Features of overdose are mainly due to anti-cholinergic and alpha blocking adverse effects

Arrhythmias may occur due to prolongation of the QT interval

### Clinical features

• Drowsiness, confusion but rarely unconsciousness
• Blurred vision due to fixed dilated pupils
• Sinus tachycardia with long QT interval
• Ventricular arrhythmias
• Hypotension
• Hypothermia
• Hyper-reflexia and extensor plantars may occur

• Agitation, visual and auditory hallucinations are common during recovery

### Treatment – supportive

• Gastric lavage up to 4 hours post ingestion
• Activated charcoal reduces absorption of -tricylics, anticholinergic action delays gastric emptying
• Cardiac monitor and watch for hypotension
• Neurological observations
• Seizures may require IV diazemuls 10 mg
• Ventricular arrhythmias due to prolonged QT interval should not be treated with anti-arrhythmics but with under drive or over drive temporary pacing
• Rarely heart block and electrical mechanical dissociation have occurred
• Occasionally metabolic acidosis ensues -this should be corrected if pH of 7.0 or less develops using 1.4% sodium bicarbonate

### References

Bialas, M.C, Evans, R.J. Hutchings, A.D., Alldridge, G., Routledge, P.A. The impact of nationally distributed guidelines on the management of paracetamol poisoning in accident and emergency departments. J Accid Emerg Med 1998; 15:13-17.

Keays R., Harrison P.M., Wendon J.A., et al. Intravenous N-acetylcysteine in paracetamol induced fulminant hepatic failure – a prospective controlled trial. BMJ 1991; 303:1026-1029.

**GROUP 13:**

**ITEM 4:**

# Poisoning
# Anaphylactic shock

Typically follows second or third challenge.

### History
- Exposure to Insect bite, bee or wasp sting, seafood, nuts, drugs e.g. penicillin, NSAIDs and contrast media.
- Dizziness, wheeze and facial swelling
- Past history of allergy

### Examination
- Facial oedema
- Tachycardia, hypotensive
- Stridor due to laryngeal oedema
- Bronchospasm

### Immediate management
- Ensure clear airway and establish large bore venous access.
- Oxygen 35% unless hypoxic.
- If there is serious hypoxia and stridor tracheostomy may be required.
- Lie flat and elevate legs.
- Cardiovascular observations.
- Administer 1 mg epinephrine (adrenaline) intramuscularly (not IV) to create depot support for the circulation.
- Repeat after 20 minutes if still hypotensive.
- Follow with antihistamine – chlorpheniramine 10 mg IV.
- Then hydrocortisone 100 mg IV.

### Further management
- If persistent hypotension infuse plasma expander e.g. 1 litre of haemacel.

– Salbutamol 2.5mg-5mg nebulised or IV may be needed for bronchospasm or continued shock.
– Consider an aminophylline infusion for continuing bronchospasm
– Always identify precipitant.
– Advise on medic-alert bracelet.
– Prescribe adrenaline minijet 0.3mg with tuition to inject in thigh in the event of exposure to allergen. This should be carried with the patient at all times.

# Notes

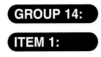

**GROUP 14:**

**ITEM 1:**

# Endocrinology and diabetes
# New diagnosis of diabetes mellitus

These cases illustrate the importance of distinguishing Type 1 from Type 2 diabetes.

## CASE HISTORY 1

You are called by a GP who has seen a 50-year-old man in his surgery who complains of thirst and polyuria. His BM stix was 30mmol/l. He is otherwise well.

### What are the key difficulties in this case?

• Does this patient need admission?
• Does he need insulin?
• What is the immediate management ?

The likelihood is that this patient has **Type 2 diabetes** (see table 14.2.1), and that he can be managed on diet alone.

The risk of ketoacidosis is small and he will not need admission unless he either is ketotic (ketonuria 3+) or is very dehydrated. He should be advised to avoid sweet drinks (especially sweetened canned drinks and Lucozade) and sent an appointment to attend the next diabetic outpatient clinic. Contact the diabetic liaison sister in your hospital and arrange for the patient to be seen.

### Indications for admission

• Severe dehydration (may have hyperosmolality)
• 3+ ketonuria
• Air hunger (acidotic breathing which is deep but may have a normal rate)
• Tachycardia or tachypnoea

## CASE HISTORY 2

You are called by a GP who has seen a 17-year-old man in his surgery who complains of thirst and polyuria. His BM was 30 mmol/l.

The key difficulties in this case are identical to the previous case:

• Does this patient need admission?
• Does he need insulin?
• What is the immediate management ?

### Information

Possible secondary causes of diabetes (always Type 2 diabetes)

• Drugs: Steroids, beta agonists
• Cushingís syndrome
• phaeochromocytomas
• thyrotoxicosis
• cystic fibrosis
• mumps
• chronic pancreatitis

This patient is much more likely to be presenting with early **Type 1 diabetes** and may not be ketotic yet because he may be in the honeymoon phase of his diabetes. Again assessment of ketosis, acidosis and dehydration must be made to determine whether he needs admission. He should be seen within 24 hours either by the diabetic liaison sister or in hospital to commence insulin. If there is any doubt, the patient should be seen in A&E.

**Table 14.1.1**

| Type 1 (IDDM) | Type 2 (NIDDM) |
|---|---|
| Young | Old |
| Thin | Obese |
| Risk of ketoacidosis | Risk of severe dehydration and hyperosmolality |
| Usually symptomatic | May not report symptoms |
| Acutely ill | Slow insidious onset of illness |
| Other autoimmune diseases | |
| Dependent on insulin | Diet alone may be sufficient but insulin or hypoglycaemic agents may be necessary to control hyperglycaemia and/or symptoms. |
| Severe acidosis may cause loss of consciousness | Severe dehydration may cause loss of consciousness |

**GROUP 14:**

**ITEM 2:**

# Endocrinology and diabetes
## Diabetic ketoacidosis

### CASE HISTORY

A 21-year-old girl presents to A&E shocked. She has been generally unwell for two weeks and was treated for a urinary tract infection by her GP. Examination reveals severe dehydration, a tachycardia of 120 and a blood pressure of 90/50. The nurses have checked her BM and found it to be 30 mmol/l.

### How do patients present with ketoacidosis?

- Unwell ± intercurrent illness (e.g. bacterial or viral infection)
- Polyuria and polydipsia
- Hyperventilation or dyspnoea
- Vomiting ± abdominal pain
- Coma

Patients known to have diabetes most commonly develop ketoacidosis when insulin is omitted because of missed meals

**𝑖**

**Information**

90% of patients presenting with diabetic ketoacidosis are known to have insulin dependent diabetes. The remaining 10% are newly diagnosed cases. It does not occur in Type 2 (NIDDM) diabetes.

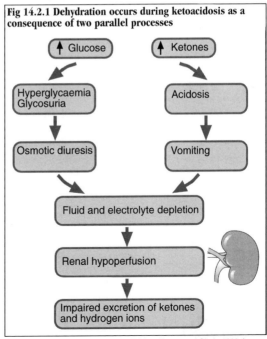

**Fig 14.2.1 Dehydration occurs during ketoacidosis as a consequence of two parallel processes**

Redrawn from *Clinical Medicine*, 4th Edition, Kumar and Clark, 1998, by permission of the publisher WB Saunders

### Investigations

- Blood glucose
- Arterial blood gases
- Urea and electrolytes
- Urinalysis (ketones strongly positive +++)
- Full blood count
- Blood ± urine cultures

### Information

Calculation of osmolality

$2 \times (Na^+ + K^+) + glucose$

Normal range 285 – 295 mosmol/kg

during an intercurrent illness (e.g. gastroenteritis). Patients become rapidly dehydrated (Fig 14.2.1) and acidotic (over hours). Kussmaul respiration (a deep sighing respiration) is prominent with the smell of ketones on the breath. It is the fall in pH which causes coma.

The blood glucose may not be particularly high, and severe acidosis may be present with glucose values as low as 10mM/l. This may be due to recent self administration of insulin, which is insufficient alone to correct the acidosis in the presence of dehydration.

### Assessment of severity

Poor prognostic features include:

- pH < 7.0
- Oliguria
- Osmolality can be measured directly or calculated (from blood levels) as is usual in diabetic ketoacidosis (see Information Box)

  (note that urea does not contribute to osmolality as it freely diffuses into cells)
- Low potassium at presentation

### Management

#### General treatment measures

- Rehydration and insulin therapy are the mainstays of treatment
- Site the IV cannula away from a major vein in the wrist. This may be required for an AV fistula in patients subsequently developing diabetic nephropathy
- Insert a central line in patients with a history of cardiac disease/autonomic neuropathy or the elderly. Avoid excessive fluid
- Consider inserting an arterial line to monitor ABG's and plasma potassium
- Nil by mouth for at least six hours
- Nasogastric tube: If there is impaired conscious level to prevent vomiting and aspiration
- Urinary catheter if oliguria is present or serum creatinine is high
- Heparin (5000 U) s.c x3 daily as prophylaxis for deep vein thrombosis
- The use of bicarbonate is controversial. If the pH < 7.0, isotonic (1.26%) sodium bicarbonate given at a maximal rate of 500 ml (i.e. 75 mmol) over one hour is safe and probably appropriate. Faster infusion rates have been shown to cause a paradoxical intracellular acidosis. If the pH> 7.0, bicarbonate need not be given.

**Fluid replacement**

As with any shocked patient, colloid should be given to restore circulating plasma volume.

The following guidelines are applicable to the young.

- 1 litre N/Saline over the first 30 minutes then
- 0.5-1 litre N/saline with potassium each hour for four hours then
- 1 litre N/saline (with potassium) every four hours until rehydrated (~24 hours).
- When blood glucose is less than 10 mmol/l, commence a 5% dextrose infusion. This will enable the insulin infusion to be continued. Continued insulin is required to inhibit ketoacid production. The intravenous insulin infusion should be continued until four hours after the patient is commenced on subcutaneous insulin because the half life of intravenous insulin is only 3.5 minutes.

Total body potassium can be depleted by approximately 1 mole and the plasma potassium falls rapidly as potassium shifts into the cells under the action of insulin. Use less potassium in patients with renal impairment or oliguria.

**Insulin Regimen** (Table 14.2.1)

Add 50 units of soluble insulin to 50 ml 0.9% saline and administer by intravenous infusion. This equates to 1 U/ml. In patients with Type 1 diabetes, the insulin should never be stopped however low the glucose as ketosis will recur. Glucose must be administered to prevent hypoglycaemia and the insulin infusion rate should be continued at a minimum of two u/hour.

**Table 14.2.1**

| Level of Blood Glucose (measured hourly) | Insulin infusion (units per hour) |
| --- | --- |
| 0 – 10.0 mmol/l | 2 (lowest infusion rate in type 1 DM) |
| 10.1 – 15.0 mmol/l | 3 |
| 15.1 – 20.0 mmol/l | 4 |
| 20.1 – 30.0 mmol/l | 6 |
| > 30.1 mmol/l | call DOCTOR |

**Assessment during treatment**

- Remember the role of insulin is primarily to suppress ketogenesis rather than to lower blood glucose
- As a general rule, rapid normalisation of biochemistry can be detrimental in any patient. It is wiser to be cautious and sub-optimal, than enthusiastic and supra-optimal
- Blood glucose (BM stix every hour, laboratory blood glucose four-hourly)

- Plasma potassium every four hours. The main risk is hypokalaemia
- ABG's four-hourly, until persistent improvement or normalised. Venous blood gases or calculated anion gap (needs chloride estimation) may be adequate for monitoring
- Plasma osmolality four-hourly. Sudden shifts in plasma osmolality or in pH may precipitate cerebral oedema

**Table 14.2.2 Examples of blood values**

|  | Severe Ketoacidosis | Non-ketotic hyperosmolar coma |
|---|---|---|
| $Na^+$ (mmol/l) | 140 | 155 |
| $K^+$ (mmol/l) | 5 | 5 |
| $CI^-$ (mmol/l) | 100 | 110 |
| $HCO_3^-$ (mmol/l) | 5 | 30 |
| Urea (mmol/l) | 8 | 15 |
| Glucose (mmol/l) | 30 | 50 |
| Arterial pH | 7.0 | 7.35 |

The normal range of **osmolality** is 285 to 300 mOsmol/kg. It can be measured directly, or can be calculated approximately from the formula:

Osmolality = $2(Na^+ + K^+)$ + glucose.

For example, in the example of severe ketoacidosis given above:

Osmolality = $2(140 + 5) + 30 = 320$ mOsmol/kg

and in the example of non-ketotic hyperosmolar coma:

Osmolality = $2 (155+s) + 50 = 370$ mOsmal/kg

The normal **anion gap** is less than 17. It is calculated as $(Na^+ + K^+) - (CI^- + HCO_3^-)$. In the example of ketoacidosis the anion gap is 40, and in the example of non-ketotic hypersomolar coma the anion gap is 20. Mild hyperchloraemic acidosis may develop in the course of therapy. This will be shown by a rising plasma chloride and persistence of a low bicarbonate even though the anion gap has returned to normal

Reprinted from *Clinical Medicine*, 4th Edition, Kumar and Clark, 1998, by permission of the publisher WB Saunders

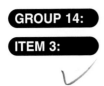

**GROUP 14:**

**ITEM 3:**

# Endocrinology and diabetes
# Hyperosmolar non-ketotic coma

## CASE HISTORY

A 60-year-old lady is referred to A&E following a collapse. She has been generally unwell for the last year. Her husband confirms that she has had polyuria and polydipsia with nocturia of three to four times every night. Over the last month, she has started using lucozade to build herself up as she has been losing weight.

Examination reveals an extremely dehydrated woman with increased tissue turgor. Pulse 100 regular, BP 100/60. JVP was not visible.

Investigations revealed:

Na 165, K 5.9, U 24.7 Cr 170 Bicarb 20 Glucose = 64 mmol/l

pH 7.31 pCO2 = 4.7 kPa pO2 = 11.2 kPa

Plasma osmolality: $2 \ (165+5.9) \ +64 \ = \ 405$ mOsmol/kg (see Information box in Item 14.2)

### How should this patient be managed ?

**Hyperosmolar non-ketotic coma** occurs in elderly patients with Type 2 diabetes. It is characterised by a very high glucose, a relatively normal acid base balance, and high plasma osmolality. These patients are also at increased risk of venous and arterial thromboses. The mortality is very much higher than for ketoacidotic coma. The patient's biochemistry has been slowly getting worse over many weeks, so normalisation must be equally slow.

### How do patients present?

• Insidious onset of polyuria and polydipsia
• Severe dehydration
• Impaired conscious level
• A diagnosis of diabetes is not usually known, and the patient is elderly
• Respiration is usually normal
• The patient may rarely present with a CVA, a fit or myocardial infarction

### Diagnosis and investigations

• Plasma glucose (usually >40mmol/l)
• U&E (dehydration causes a greater rise in urea than creatinine (normal ratio of creatinine:urea up to 20:1 (µMoles:mMoles). Significant hypernatraemia may occur, but may be hidden by

the high glucose. The hypernatraemia may appear to worsen as the glucose falls
* Arterial blood gases (relatively normal)
* Plasma osmolality >350 mosm/kg
* FBC (may show polycythaemia (dehydration) or a leukocytosis of infection)
* ECG looking for myocardial infarction or ischaemia
* CXR looking for signs of infection
* Urine for urinalysis, microscopy and culture. Remember that ketones may occur in any starved person. The presence of blood and protein on urinalysis may indicate urinary tract infection

### Assessment of severity

* The degree of consciousness correlates most closely with plasma osmolality. Coma is usually associated with an osmolality of greater than 440 mosmo/kg
* A coexistent lactic acidosis considerably worsens the prognosis

### Management

### General Treatment Measures

* Rehydration and insulin therapy are the mainstays of treatment. Be much more cautious in the elderly. Avoid fluid overload
* Site the IV cannula away from a major vein in the wrist. This may be required for an AV fistula in patients subsequently developing diabetic nephropathy
* Central venous line in all patients
* Nil by mouth for at least six hours
* Nasogastric tube: If there is impaired conscious level to prevent vomiting and aspiration
* Urinary catheter if oliguria is present, or serum creatinine is high
* Intravenous heparinisation with 12,000 units every 12 hours by infusion as prophylaxis against venous or arterial thrombosis, maintain the APTT (or PTTK) at between 60 and 100 seconds. Alternatively, low molecular weight heparin eg enoxaparin should be used

### Fluid Replacement

Caution must be exercised as elderly patients tolerate fluid shifts badly.

* 1 litre N/Saline over the first 60 minutes then
* 1 litre N/saline with potassium (unless anuric) over four hours then
* 1 litre N/saline (with potassium, as in DKA) every six hours until rehydrated (~48 hours)
* Normal saline has a sodium concentration of 150 mmol/l. Normal saline is safe even in very hypernatraemic patients. The

measured sodium may appear to climb as the blood glucose falls. This is because the sodium level is artificially lowered by the high glucose level. The corrected sodium level can be calculated by adding a third of the blood glucose to the sodium level. Thus a fall in glucose by 30 mmol/l will be associated by an apparent rise in sodium by 10 mmol/l from say 155 mmol/l to 165 mmol/l

- When blood glucose is less than 10 mmol/l, commence a 5% dextrose infusion, and consider stopping insulin therapy and commencing oral hypoglycaemic agents or diet alone

- The insulin regimen for a patient with Type 2 diabetes is similar to that for Type 1 diabetes, but as the patient is not dependent on insulin to suppress ketogenesis, insulin infusion can be stopped when glucose levels are normal (Table 14.3.1)

**Table 14.3.1**

| Level of glucose (hourly) | Insulin infusion rate (units per hour) |
|---|---|
| 0 – 5 | 0 |
| 5.1 – 7 | 1 |
| 7.1 – 10 | 2 |
| 10.1 – 15 | 3 |
| 15.1.- 20 | 4 |
| 20.1 – 30 | 6 |
| >30.1 | Call doctor |

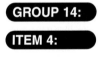

**GROUP 14:**

**ITEM 4:**

# Endocrinology and diabetes
# Hypoglycaemic coma

### CASE HISTORY

A 25-year-old known Type 1 diabetic is brought to A&E. He is aggressive and irrational and punching the staff. He is held down by the staff and a BM stick reads "LOW".

### How would you manage this patient?

All unconscious patients should be assumed to be **hypoglycaemic** until proved otherwise. Always check a blood glucose using a glucostix (or BM stix) immediately, and confirm with a laboratory determination. Occasionally the glucostix is incorrect. The most common cause of coma in a patient with diabetes is hypoglycaemia due to drugs. The long acting sulphonylureas such as chlorpropamide or long acting insulins such as ultratard are more prone to do this. Patients who are NOT known to have diabetes, but who are hypoglycaemic should have a laboratory determined blood glucose, and blood saved (serum) for insulin and C-peptide determination (insulinoma or factitious drug administration).

## How do patients present?

| Sympathetic Overactivity | Neuroglycopenia |
|---|---|
| (average glucose < 3.6 mmol/l) | (glucose < 2.6 mmol/l) |
| • Tachycardia | • Confusion |
| • Palpitations | • Slurred speech |
| • Sweating | • Localised neurological impairment |
| • Anxiety | • Coma |
| • Pallor | |
| • Tremor | |
| • Cold extremities | |

Patients with long-standing diabetes even if now well controlled have often had frequent episodes of hypoglycaemia, and can become desensitised to sympathetic activation. These patients may develop neuroglycopenia before sympathetic activation and complain of "loss of warning". Use of ß blockers may also minimise the warning signs of hypoglycaemia by abrogating the features of an activated sympathetic nervous system. Conversely patients with poorly controlled diabetes develop sympathetic signs early, and avoid these by running a high blood glucose. They may complain of "being hypo" when their blood sugar is normal or high. They do not require glucose.

### Information

Patients with Type 2 diabetes who are on diet alone or metformin (but no insulin or sulphonylureas) CANNOT become hypoglycaemic.

### Assessment of severity

• Patients with pancreatitis or following pancreatectomy are more liable to severe attacks because they have no glucagon
• A lab glucose of less than 2.2 mmol/l is defined as a severe attack. The clinical effects of such hypoglycaemia can vary from mild sweating in patients who have chronic hypoglycaemia, to severe adrenergic symptoms in patients who normally have a high glucose. Coma usually occurs when the blood glucose has fallen below 1.5 mmol/l

### Investigations

• Blood glucose (glucostix)
• Blood glucose (laboratory)
• Urea and electrolytes (hypoglycaemia is more common in diabetic nephropathy because the kidney is one of the sites of insulin metabolism)
• Save serum (prior to glucose administration) for insulin and C-peptide (send directly to the lab for immediate centrifugation) if indicated

### Management

In a patient who has unexplained hypoglycaemia, it is important to take blood immediately for insulin, C-peptide and glucose before administering glucose. Twenty ml of clotted blood should suffice for serum insulin and C-peptide levels. This blood should be sent directly to a laboratory for centrifugation and separation of the serum. A low C-peptide and high insulin level indicate exogenous insulin. A high C-peptide and insulin level indicate that the insulin is coming from the patients own pancreas. This can occur either following surreptitious drug (sulphonylurea) ingestion or rarely because of an insulinoma.

- If patient is conscious and co-operative, give 50g oral glucose or equivalent
- 50ml of 20% dextrose IV (50% dextrose is unnecessarily toxic to the veins) if patient is unable to take oral fluids
- Admit the patient if the cause is a long acting sulphonylurea or a long acting insulin, and commence a continuous infusion of 10% glucose (e.g. 1 litre 8 hourly) and check glucose hourly or two-hourly
- If IV access is impossible, give 1mg of glucagon IM. Then give the patient some oral glucose to prevent a hypoglycaemic episode an hour later

Patients should regain consciousness or become coherent within 10 minutes although complete cognitive recovery may lag by 30 to 45 minutes. Do not give further boluses of IV glucose without repeating the blood glucose. If the patient does not wake up after 10 minutes or more, repeat the blood glucose and consider another cause of coma. Patients on sulphonylureas may become hypoglycaemic following a CVA or receive a head injury during their confused state. Recurrent hypoglycaemia may herald the onset of diabetic nephropathy, since it may decrease insulin requirements: Insulin is partly degraded by the kidney.

### Other causes of hypoglycaemia

- Drugs
  - surreptitious insulin or sulphonylurea ingestion
  - ethanol
  - salicylates
  - quinine
  - pentamidine
  - disopyramide
  - ß blockers
  - consider prescription errors e.g. chlorpropamide for chlorpromazine (ask for all drugs to be brought in)
- – insulinoma
- – tumours. Retroperitoneal sarcomas and other malignancies can secrete IGF-2
- liver dysfunction
- hypopituitarism, causing ACTH, GH and TSH deficiency
- myxoedema

**GROUP 14:**

**ITEM 5:**

# Endocrinology and diabetes
## Sick diabetic patient

### CASE HISTORY

A 40-year-old man with a 15-year history of Type 1 Diabetes Mellitus (IDDM), and previously documented proteinuria, is referred from A&E with vomiting and feeling generally unwell. Glucose was 20mmol/l, electrolytes were normal and blood gases did not support Diabetic Ketoacidosis (pH 7.4 bicarbonate 20mmol/l). ECG performed routinely shows evidence of evolving anterior M.I.

This is the typical presentation of a "silent M.I.", chest pain is frequently atypical in diabetes due to small fibre neuropathy. The other major causes of this type of non-specific presentation are occult infection and uraemia.

**Investigations**
- FBC
- Urea and electrolytes
- ABG
- CXR
- MSU
- ECG
- Blood cultures

Other investigations to consider later if occult infection is suspected:
- Abdominal USS or abdominal CT scan
- Tc bone scanning
- Labelled white cell scan

### Management of Type 1 diabetes in hospital

Type 1 diabetic patients can become ketotic in a matter of hours. Insulin should be administered by continuous infusion until eating and drinking has resumed (see table 14.2.1). Insulin treatment has been proven to improve outcome in diabetic subjects in the immediate period after myocardial infarction.

Once eating and drinking, the patient can be converted back to their usual insulin regimen, or if tight glycaemic control is essential, on to 4 x daily insulin (see below).

### Protocol for converting diabetics from intravenous to subcutaneous insulin

- Calculate total dose over last 24 hours
- Give 50% of total as soluble insulin (e.g. Actrapid) 30 minutes before each meal (i.e. three times daily)
- Give 50% of total dose as intermediate acting insulin (e.g. Insulatard) at 10pm
- Monitor blood glucose fasting and 2 hours post prandial – each BM stix measures the adequacy of the previous dose
- Aim for glucose < 10mmol/l post prandial and < 8mmol/l fasting
- Do not discontinue IV insulin until at least 4 hours AFTER s/c insulin is administered. IV insulin has a half life of only 3.5 minutes, so ketogenesis can rapidly occur if insulin levels fall

**⚠ Remember**
Always carefully inspect feet in unwell diabetic patients

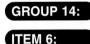

# Endocrinology and diabetes

## Management of Type 2 diabetes mellitus

### CASE HISTORY

You are asked to see a 50-year-old man with no previous history of diabetes who is admitted for CAVG and found to have a blood glucose of 13mmol/l – the anaesthetist has asked for a medical opinion.

### How would you manage this patient?

- Ask about typical symptoms
- Ensure a lab glucose has been sent
- Screen for microvascular disease (inspect fundi and check urine for albumin) – 20% of NIDDM patient have retinopathy at diagnosis
- Start insulin by continuous infusion from 6am on the day of surgery (see Table 14.3.1) with 5% dextrose + 20mmol KCL 8 hourly
- Ensure close supervision of blood glucose post op as for Type 1 diabetic patient

⚠️

**Remember**

Good glycaemic control aids recovery (lucozade does not)

### Who needs insulin perioperatively?

- All Type 1 diabetic patients
- All acute surgical emergencies (Type 1 and 2)
- All patients undergoing major surgery (Type 1 and 2)

In other words – all diabetic patients should receive insulin except Type 2 diabetic subjects undergoing minor surgery.

### Regular checks for patients with Diabetes

These items are modified from those set out in The European Patients' Charter published by the St Vincent Declaration Steering committee of the WHO. The charter sets out goals for both the healthcare team and the patient.

### Checked at each visit

- Review of self-monitoring results and current treatment
- Talk about targets and change where necessary
- Talk about any general or specific problems
- Continued education

### Checked at least once a year

- Biochemical assessment of metabolic control (e.g. glycosylated Hb test)
- Measure bodyweight
- Measure blood pressure
- Measure plasma lipids (except in extreme old age)
- Measure visual acuity
- Examine state of retina (ophthalmascope or retinal photo)
- Test urine for proteinuria
- Test blood for renal function (creatinine)
- Check condition of feet, pulses and neurology
- Review cardiovascular risk factors
- Review self-monitoring and injection techniques.
- Review eating habita

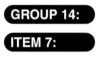

**GROUP 14:**

**ITEM 7:**

# Endocrinology and diabetes
# Diabetic foot

### CASE HISTORY

The chiropodist in the diabetic clinic asks you to review an 84-year-old lady who is complaining of severe pain in her big toe. She had attempted to cut a toe nail a week ago and the toe had become painful and infected. She is known to have Type 2 diabetes for which she takes glibenclamide 10mg daily. She does not have regular supervision of her diabetes.

### What further points would be helpful in the history?

- Is there a previous history of foot problems?
- Does she regularly inspect and wash her feet? Is she careful about buying shoes of the correct size?
- How good is her sight?
- Does she live alone? Does she have any help?
- Is there any suggestion of peripheral vascular disease e.g. intermittent claudication?
- Is there any suggestion of peripheral sensory problems? Does she complain of numbness in her feet?

### What particular points do you look for on examination?

- Inspect the lesion. There is a 2cm deep ulcer with pus. You take a swab for culture.

**Remember**

50% of patients have no previous history of neuropathy or peripheral vascular disease.

- Look for signs of neuropathy:
  - dry skin
  - evidence of sensory loss to pin prick/light touch/vibration
  - check ankle jerks
- Look for signs of vascular insufficiency:
  - check peripheral pulses
  - are the toes cold?

### Pathogenesis of foot ulcers

- Most ulcers occur as a result of trauma
- Neuropathy causes:
  - reduced sensitivity
  - altered proprioception with 'high pressure' on parts of foot
  - autonomic dysfunction leading to dry skin with cracks and fissures
- Peripheral vascular disease:
  - very common
  - leads to ischaemic ulcers (pure ischaemic ulcers in 10%)

90% of ulcers are due to neuropathy alone or a combination of neuropathy and ischaemia

### Management

- Admit patient if possible
- Early effective antibiotic treatment is essential
  - use broad spectrum antibiotic until cultures back e.g. ciprofloxacin
- Ask diabetic team to fully assess her and arrange for future follow-up care

### Remember

- Many foot problems are avoidable. Older diabetic patients must be taught good foot care and should not cut their own toe nails.
- Diabetic foot problems can occur in both Type 1 and Type 2 diabetics.

| Meggitt-Wagner classification of diabetic foot ulcers | |
| --- | --- |
| Grade 0 | High-risk foot with no ulcers |
| Grade 1 | Superficial ulcer |
| Grade 2 | Deeper ulcer infection/cellulitis. No bone involvement |
| Grade 3 | Osteomyelitis and foot ulceration |
| Grade 4 | Localised gangrene (toes, forefoot or heel) |
| Grade 5 | Gangrene of entire foot |

**GROUP 14:**

**ITEM 8:**

# Endocrinology and diabetes
# Urgent surgery in patients with diabetes

Surgery requires patients to fast for several hours. In addition a general anaesthetic and surgery produces significant stresses on an individual. The hormonal response to stress involves a significant rise in counter-regulatory hormones to insulin, in particular cortisol and adrenaline. For this reason, patients with diabetes under going surgery will require an increased dose of insulin despite their fasting state. Long acting hypoglycaemic agents must be stopped the night before surgery as hypoglycaemia may otherwise occur. In case of an emergency operation where the patient has taken a long acting insulin, an infusion of 10% dextrose can be used, (usually with potassium) together with a controlled infusion of insulin.

- Always try to put the patient first on the list. Inform the surgeon and anaesthetist early. Discontinue long acting insulin or sulphonylurea the night before surgery if possible
- Commence an infusion of 10% dextrose with 20 mmol/l of potassium. Infuse at 100ml/h. Commence an intravenous sliding scale of insulin. Measuring the glucose from fingerprick hourly will avoid hypoglycaemia. Use the table 14.2.1 for Type 1 diabetics and the table in 14.3.1 for Type 2 diabetics.
- If the patient has Type 1 (insulin dependent) diabetes, the infusion must be continued until he has his second meal with his normal subcutaneous dose of insulin. At no time must the patient be without insulin. Since intravenous insulin has a very short half life (3.5 minutes), this must be continued until the patient's subcutaneous insulin is being absorbed. An overlap of 4h is recommended.
- If the patient's diabetes is normally managed with oral hypoglycaemic agents, these can be started once the patient is eating normally. The sliding scale can be tailed off starting 4h later.
- If the patient's diabetes is normally managed on diet alone, the sliding scale will automatically be reduced as the patient's glucose falls after surgery. The patient should be continued on insulin intravenously for 24h following surgery.

**GROUP 14:**    Endocrinology and diabetes

**ITEM 9:**    Diabetes in pregnancy

### CASE HISTORY 1

You are called to see a 28-year-old lady who is 18 weeks pregnant who has been complaining of polyuria and polydipsia. She is found to have a blood glucose of 10 mmol/l.

### How should this patient be managed?

The patient should be taught to monitor her blood glucose levels and be advised on diet. Blood glucose levels should be measured one hour after each meal. If blood glucoses are below 7 mmol/l, then insulin is not required. Oral hypoglycaemic agents are contraindicated in pregnancy, so that if glucose levels are above 7mmol/l, insulin therapy is required. High levels of glucose are associated with risk of neonatal macrosomia and postnatal hypoglycaemia. Thus the patient should be commenced on soluble insulin with each meal and a long acting insulin at night.

### CASE HISTORY 2

You are called to the labour ward to see a patient who is on insulin and in labour. She has been on actrapid (soluble insulin) 12 units three times daily and insulatard 18 units last thing at night with very good control of her blood sugars. She is now in labour and is nil by mouth.

### How will you manage this patient?

It is essential to determine whether the patient had Type 1 diabetes before pregnancy (in which case insulin should never be stopped) or whether she has gestational diabetes, when insulin therapy can be stopped after delivery. The placental progesterone results in profound insulin resistance, and after the third stage of labour, gestational diabetes may disappear.

An intravenous sliding scale must be commenced as in the management of DKA (Table 14.2.1) if the patient previously had Type 1 diabetes. Poor diabetic control is associated with neonatal hypoglycaemia and it is important to check the neonatal blood glucose one and two hours postpartum.

If the mother has Type 1 diabetes, she can be commenced on her pre-pregnancy dose of insulin when she is eating. Intravenous insulin must be continued until four hours after the first dose of subcutaneous insulin.

| GROUP 14: | # Endocrinology and diabetes |
|---|---|
| ITEM 10: | # Emergency management of Cushing's syndrome |

### How would it present?

The metabolic effects of corticosteroids can occasionally present as a metabolic emergency. Patients with excess endogenous cortisol from for example ectopic ACTH, have particularly high cortisol levels, which may result in excess of both cortisol and mineralocorticoid action. Patients may have had undiagnosed Cushing's syndrome for some time, and present due to metabolic decompensation either due to hypokalaemia, which can be severe, or due to glycosuria and resultant dehydration.

Other complications follow rapidly, including secondary infection, bruising and bleeding, uncontrollable hypertension and fractures.

### CASE HISTORY

A 55-year-old doctor known to have a pancreatic endocrine gastrinoma with liver metastases presents with features of Cushing's syndrome. Her gastrinoma has been well controlled with omeprazole, and but she now presents to A & E dehydrated and hypotensive, having previously been hypertensive. She is found to have 4+ glycosuria and a blood glucose of 30mmol/l.

- Arterial blood gases reveal
  - pH 7.60
  - $pO_2$: 12.0kPa
  - $pCO_2$: 4.4 kPa

This patient has a metabolic alkalosis, which is likely to be caused by chronic hypokalaemia. Electrolytes come back from the lab, confirming your suspicions

- Na 145
- K 2.7
- U 15.0
- Cr 120

### How would you manage this patient?

The hypokalaemia and the glycosuria need urgent but cautious treatment. Total body potassium is likely to be extremely low, and as potassium is replaced, the initial effect will be to reduce the bicarbonate rather than to increase the extracellular (serum) potassium.

- Start potassium replacement both orally and intravenously with as much potassium as you dare! Monitor $K^+$ carefully

**Information**

Causes
(percentages in brackets refer to proportions of endogenous Cushing's syndrome)
- Excess corticosteroid administration
- Pituitary dependent Cushing's disease (85%)
- Adrenal adenoma (10%)
- Ectopic ACTH (5%)

- Rehydrate the patient with saline with potassium chloride (40 mmol per litre) added to each bag
- Start an intravenous infusion of insulin at four units per hour. This will further exacerbate the fall in serum potassium
- Use potassium sparing drugs to control any hypertension (amiloride, spironolactone, triamterine, ACE inhibitors)
- Measure the plasma cortisol and ACTH to confirm the diagnosis. Refer to an endocrinologist for dexamethasone suppression tests. This patient is likely to have ectopic ACTH secretion from her gastrinoma
- Commence medical management of the hypercortisolaemia with ketoconazole and/or metyrapone. In patients who are nil by mouth or on intensive care, intravenous etomidate can be used

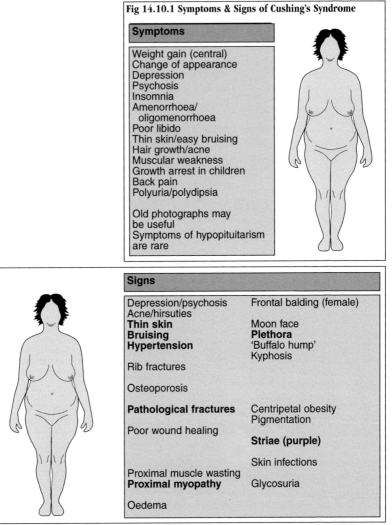

### Fig 14.10.1 Symptoms & Signs of Cushing's Syndrome

**Symptoms**

Weight gain (central)
Change of appearance
Depression
Psychosis
Insomnia
Amenorrhoea/
 oligomenorrhoea
Poor libido
Thin skin/easy bruising
Hair growth/acne
Muscular weakness
Growth arrest in children
Back pain
Polyuria/polydipsia

Old photographs may
be useful
Symptoms of hypopituitarism
are rare

**Signs**

| | |
|---|---|
| Depression/psychosis | Frontal balding (female) |
| Acne/hirsuties | |
| **Thin skin** | Moon face |
| **Bruising** | **Plethora** |
| **Hypertension** | 'Buffalo hump' |
| | Kyphosis |
| Rib fractures | |
| | |
| Osteoporosis | |
| | |
| **Pathological fractures** | Centripetal obesity |
| | Pigmentation |
| Poor wound healing | |
| | **Striae (purple)** |
| | |
| | Skin infections |
| Proximal muscle wasting | |
| **Proximal myopathy** | Glycosuria |
| | |
| Oedema | |

Redrawn from *Clinical Medicine*, 4th Edition, Kumar and Clark, 1998, by permission of the publisher WB Saunders

# Endocrinology and diabetes
# Thyrotoxicosis

## CASE HISTORY 1

A 65-year-old woman presents with atrial fibrillation and breathlessness. Thyroid function tests reveal a Free T4 of 45 pmol/l (NR 13-30). ie Hyperthyroidism.

### What should you do?

Determine the cause of the hyperthyroidism. (See below).

Check the patientís electrolytes, and exclude hypokalaemia.

Control the heart rate using beta blockers (propranolol 40 mg every 8 hours)

Treat heart failure if needed with diuretics.

Anticoagulate the patient (heparin and warfarin).

Beta adrenoreceptors are sensitised to normal circulating catecholamines by high levels of thyroxine and thus the first line treatment of hyperthyroidism is beta blockade. Propranolol is used in high doses (40 mg every 8 hours) because it crosses the blood brain barrier, as it is lipid soluble.

### Why is beta blockade used particularly in thyroid heart failure?

Heart failure is caused by a lower cardiac output than the patient requires. In most cases of heart failure that you see in A&E, the patients mount a tachycardia (up to a heart rate of 150) to increase their cardiac output. The cardiac output is maximised at a heart rate of around 150. A faster heart rate reduces cardiac output, as the diastolic filling time is reduced. When heart failure is due to thyrotoxicosis, it is a rate dependent failure, with a rate of say 170 bpm. Betá blockade to slow this rate down to 150 will increase cardiac output and will therefore treat the heart failure.

### What should I do in a patient who is known to have congestive cardiac failure who also develops hyperthyroidism.

It depends on the patient's heart rate. It should not occur if patients are carefully managed. If the rate is very high, you can be confident that slowing their rate down to 150 bpm will improve their cardiac output. If the rate is only 130 bpm, then beta blockade e.g. bisoprolol may still be helpful (Group 10 Item 14).

**Remember**

WEIGHT LOSS without obvious cause always requires a TSH.

**Table 14.11.1 Characteristics of thyroid function tests in common thyroid disorders**
(the clinically most informative tests in each situation are shown in **bold**)

| | TSH (0.3–3.5 mU/l) | Total T$_4$ (60–160 mmol/l) | Free T$_4$ (13–30 pmol/l) | T$_3$ (1.2–3.1 nmol/l) |
|---|---|---|---|---|
| Thyrotoxicosis | **Suppressed (<0.05 mU/l)** | Increased | **Increased** | **Increased** |
| Primary hypothyroidism | **Increased (>10 mU/l)** | Low/ low-normal | Low/ low-normal | Normal or low |
| TSH deficiency | Low or normal or subnormal | Low/ low-normal | **Low/ low-normal** | Low/ low-normal |
| T$_3$ toxicosis | **Suppressed (<0.05 mU/l)** | Normal | Normal | **Increased** |
| Compensated euthyroidism | **Slightly increased (5–10 mU/l)** | Normal | **Normal** | Normal |

Reprinted from *Clinical Medicine*, 4th Edition, Kumar and Clark, 1998, by permission of the publisher WB Saunders

## CASE HISTORY 2

A 37-year-old female was referred up to General Medical outpatients with weight loss, general malaise and apathy. Clinical examination was unremarkable except for a mild tachycardia of 100bpm. You sent off routine investigations, including thyroid function tests (Table 14.11.1), and have now been telephoned by the biochemist with the following results:

- fT$_4$   56pmol/l   (NR: 13-30)
- TSH   < 0.1mU/l   (NR: 0.3-3.5)

Typical thyrotoxic presentations are easy to spot, but elderly patients may have atypical features. Treatment of these patients is very worthwhile.

### Some presentations of thyrotoxicosis in the elderly

- Weight loss
- Atrial fibrillation
- Lethargy in the elderly
- Proximal myopathy

### Causes of thyrotoxicosis

**Common:**

- Graves' disease
- Multinodular goitre
- Toxic nodule
- Viral thyroiditis
- Amiodarone induced

### Investigations

Thyroid antimicrosomal autoantibodies and antithyroglobulin antibodies (in the serum) – positive in up to 90% of patients with Graves' disease

⚠️

**Remember**

Agranulocytosis occurs in 1:1000 patients with antithyroid drugs. All patients prescribed antithyroid drugs should be warned to report severe mouth ulcers or sore throats immediately, and should have an urgent full blood count if symptoms are experienced.

**Rare:**
- TSH secreting pituitary adenoma
- Choriocarcinoma
- Factitious (self-medication)

## Tests in patients with Goitres

- Thyroid ultrasound scan – to confirm clinical impression of multinodular goitre
- Technetium pertechnate uptake – to distinguish a "hot nodule" from Graves' disease (uniform uptake) and from viral thyroiditis (zero uptake)
- Fine needle aspiration (FNA) should be performed in any solitary nodule or a dominant nodule in a multinodular goitre to diagnose malignancy.

## Drug treatment in thyrotoxicosis

- Rapid symptomatic treatment (if necessary)
  - propranolol 40-80mg eight hourly
- Control thyroid overactivity
  - carbimazole 20-60mg daily in divided doses, or
  - propyl thiouracil 200-600mg daily in divided doses

Both drugs inhibit the formation of thyroid hormones.

Primary treatment of toxic nodules and Grave's disease with radioiodine is safe provided the patient is adequately $\beta$ blocked.

## CASE HISTORY 3

You have been telephoned by a GP who has received the results of some thyroid function tests (TFT's). The blood test report showed a high free T4: 45pmol/l (13-30) with a suppressed TSH (< 0.1mu/l). On further questioning it transpires that the test was performed in a patient who was unwell with a painful neck. You arrange for the patient to come to outpatients in two weeks.

When you see the patient he complains of severe tiredness and repeat TFT's are as follows:

free $T_4$: 7pmol/l, TSH 25 mU/l i.e. hypothyroid but the initial biochemistry unequivocally demonstrated thyroid overactivity

This presentation is typical of viral thyroiditis (De Quervains). A short course (but not lifelong) of thyroxine may be of benefit. Autoantibodies may be positive because the viral damage to the thyroid results in autoimmunisation with thyroid microsomes and thyroglobulin. Viral thyroiditis does not require treatment; hypothyroidism is usually transient.

Follow up TFTs and a radioiodine or Tc 99m Tc pertechnetate scan are necessary.

### Features of viral (De Quervains) thyroiditis

• Neck discomfort or pain on swallowing
• History of viral illness
• Thyrotoxicosis (usually one month followed by hypothyroidism), followed by resolution
• Disparity between clinical features and biochemistry
• High ESR
• Reduced uptake on radio Iodine uptake scan
• Weakly positive anti thyroid antibodies

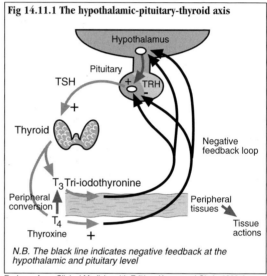

**Fig 14.11.1 The hypothalamic-pituitary-thyroid axis**

N.B. The black line indicates negative feedback at the hypothalamic and pituitary level

Redrawn from *Clinical Medicine*, 4th Edition, Kumar and Clark, 1998, by permission of the publisher WB Saunders

**GROUP 14:**

**ITEM 12:**

# Endocrinology and diabetes
# Thyroid storm

This is a rare medical emergency. It should not occur if patients are carefully managed. It is a clinical diagnosis and is defined as being present in a patient with hyperthyroid biochemistry who has any two of the following.

- Tachycardia > 145 beats per minute ± atrial fibrillation
- Any other arrhythmia
- Hyperpyrexia > 41°C
- Rate dependent heart failure
- Jaundice
- Psychosis

Patients who have two or more of the above have a 50% mortality. Other patients have a very low mortality even if untreated. Symptoms can also include vomiting, diarrhoea, seizure and coma. It can be precipitated by thyroid surgery, the administration of radioiodine, the withdrawal of antithyroid drugs and in acute illnesses.

## Treatment
- Cool the patient with tepid sponging and a fan. Do not use aspirin which is contra-indicated in thyroid storm. (It displaces thyroxine from its binding globulin and increases the free T4)
- Beta blockers (propranolol 5 mg IV then 40 mg 8 hourly orally) unless contraindicated by asthma. (Heart failure is not a contraindication to beta blockers [see Group 10 Item 14]
- Fluid replacement. This needs careful assessment with central venous monitoring. Heart failure will rapidly come under control once the patient's heart rate is lowered
- Hydrocortisone 100mg IV six-hourly. This blocks T4 to T3 conversion
- Propylthiouracil 250mg four-hourly
- Potassium iodide 60 mg eight-hourly. This must be given at least one hour after the propylthiouracil, which blocks iodine incorporation, but not uptake (Group 14 Item 13)

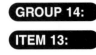

# Endocrinology and diabetes
# Amiodarone and thyroid function

Patients with thyroid disease often present with atrial fibrillation to the cardiologists who may commence intravenous amiodarone before getting the thyroid function results. Amiodarone contains an enormous amount of iodine. Amiodarone is very lipid soluble and has a half life of about a month. Thus amiodarone behaves like slow release iodine. You may be called to interpret the thyroid function tests after amiodarone has been given. Proceed as follows:

**Remember**

Amiodarone can cause both hyper- and hypo-thyroidism

- Ask the laboratory to check the thyroid function on an initial blood sample taken for electrolytes when the patient was admitted. It is likely that someone will have checked the patient's potassium
- Find out how long the patient has been on amiodarone. In patients who have silent nodules, thyrotoxicosis may be precipitated. In others, the Wolff-Chaikoff* effect may result in hypothyroidism. Amiodarone also blocks T4 to T3 conversion. This conversion is also blocked within the pituitary gland. Amiodarone always therefore causes a rise in TSH although it usually remains in the normal range
- Re-examine the patient to find out if he is clinically thyrotoxic
- If both the T4 and the T3 are low, start thyroxine replacement. Unlike in normal hypothyroidism, one would pay relatively little attention to the TSH, which may be high. Once on replacement, the free hormone levels are the least poor markers of replacement
- If the patient is clinically and biochemically thyrotoxic, commence carbimazole and consider discontinuing the amiodarone. Because amiodarone contains large amounts of iodine, radioiodine cannot be used until 6 months after amiodarone has been discontinued

**Information**

*Wolff and Chaikoff* first noted that excessive iodine suppresses thyroid function and causes short term atrophy of the thyroid gland. Surgeons use this effect by administration of potassium iodide for 10 days before surgery. This is also why we use potassium iodide in thyroid storm.

**GROUP 14:**

**ITEM 14:**

# Endocrinology and diabetes
# Hypothyroidism

The textbook presentation is now something of a rarity. Hypothyroidism is diagnosed by a multitude of practitioners e.g.

| | | |
|---|---|---|
| 1. | Lipid clinic | cause of hypercholesterolaemia |
| 2. | Psychiatrists | organic psychosis or depression |
| 3. | Neurologists | ataxia |
| 4. | ENT surgeons | dysphonia or deafness |
| 5. | Cardiologists | during follow up on amiodarone treatment |
| 6. | Dermatologists | dry skin or hair |
| 7. | Gynaecologists | oligo or amenorrhoea, infertility |
| 8. | Geriatricians | screening test/hypothermia |
| 9. | Diabetologists | screening test in Type I Diabetes |

In primary hypothyroidism the TSH will ALWAYS be elevated and usually above the assay limit.

For practical purposes in the Western world, adult onset primary hypothyroidism is due to autoimmune disease, unless:

• Patient on amiodarone
• Previous thyroid surgery
• Previous radioiodine treatment
• Viral thyroiditis

**Remember**

When replacing hypothyroid patients with thyroxine aim for TSH 1.0mu/l

### What dose do you start on?

If the patient is otherwise fit and not at risk of ischaemic heart disease, then start on 100mcg thyroxine daily

### And then . . . ?

It takes about six weeks for a steady state to be reached. Aim to increase the thyroxine dose in 25mcg increments every three to four weeks until the TSH is within or just below the normal range (0.4-4 mu/l). Occasionally patients require only 50 to 75 mcg daily.

### THINK ABOUT associated autoimmune diseases

• $B_{12}$ deficiency
• Myasthenia gravis
• Addison's disease
• Other organ specific autoimmune diseases
• The association of Addison's disease with primary

hypothyroidism was described by Schmidt in 1926 and is known as Schmidt's syndrome

### And if they have angina?

Be very careful indeed. Many clinicians start at 25mcg o.d. but you cannot go too slowly

### What is compensated hypothyroidism?

Early in the course of hypothyroidism the TSH is elevated (4-20mU/l) but $T_4$ and $T_3$ are normal. Opinion differs as to the need for treatment. Most endocrinologists replace with thyroxine:

• If autoantibodies are present
• If the patient has typical symptoms of hypothyroidism
• In the presence of a high cholesterol
• TSH > 10mU/l (NB mU/l = milliunits/l)

Note: TRH tests are obsolete in modern practice since new TSH assays are very sensitive.

**GROUP 14:**

**ITEM 15:**

# Endocrinology and diabetes
# Difficult thyroid function tests

Since TFTs are now so commonly performed, patients who apparently have no features of thyroid disease are referred with abnormal tests.

### High free $T_4$ High/Normal TSH

• Early in the treatment of hypothyroidism
• Familial dysalbuminaemic hyperthyroxinaemia: causes a spuriously high free and total $T_4$
• Thyroid hormone resistance ( high levels of $T_4$ is required because of defective thyroid hormone receptors)
• TSH secreting pituitary adenoma

The first step is to establish whether the patient is thyrotoxic clinically. SHBG (Sex Hormone Binding Globulin) is an occasional useful assay of thyroid activity, but should not replace clinical assessment. Hypothyroidism increases the rate of conversion of androstenedione to oestrogens which increase SHBG.

**Low free T$_4$ Low/Normal TSH**
- Sick euthyroid syndrome
- Recovery from thyrotoxicosis
- Early after radioiodine
- Hypopituitarism/hypothalamic disease

**Fig 14.15.1 – Interpretation of thyroid function tests**

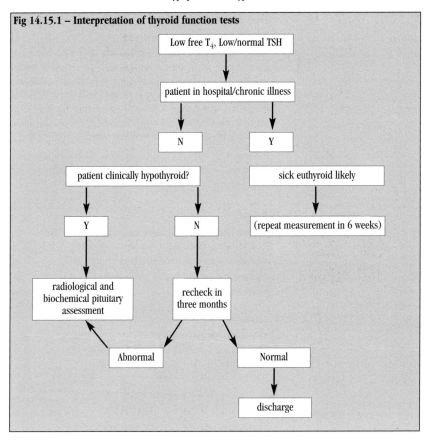

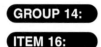

**GROUP 14:**

**ITEM 16:**

# Endocrinology and diabetes
# Addison's disease

(Also applies to patients on steroids for surgery and unwell patients on steroids)

Presentation may vary from a gradual course over days to months in otherwise well individuals, who then present with cardio-vascular collapse, usually in association with infection, trauma or surgery. Crisis may also occur in patients with known Addison's disease on replacement hydrocortisone during relatively trivial stressful episodes such as a viral infection. For this reason patients are advised to increase the dose of hydrocortisone during illness.

Patients who are on long term steroids for inflammatory conditions such as asthma may also have pituitary adrenal suppression.

### Acute
- Hypotension (may be severe (shock) or postural) and cardiovascular collapse
- Faintness (particularly on standing)
- Nausea and vomiting
- Hyponatraemia
- Dehydration (thirst may not be apparent because of the low sodium)
- Diarrhoea in 20% of cases

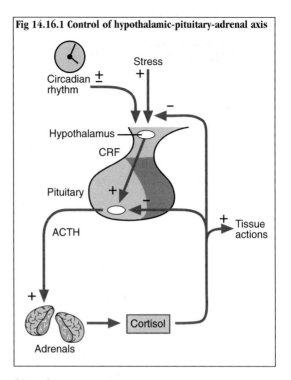

**Fig 14.16.1 Control of hypothalamic-pituitary-adrenal axis**

### Chronic

- Weight loss
- Fatigue
- Weakness
- Hyperpigmentation
- Other features include fever, asthenia, arthralgia, myalgia and anorexia. Psychiatric features are common and include depression, apathy and confusion. Treatment with glucocorticoids reverses most psychiatric features

### Causes

- Autoimmune adrenalitis (note associated endocrinopathies)
- Tuberculosis of the adrenals (ask re symptoms of TB)
- Malignant secondaries in the adrenal glands are present in half of patients with lung disseminated cancer, breast tumours and malignant melanomas. Adrenal failure will only occur when over 90% of the gland is replaced by metastases however and therefore occurs late in the course of disease
- Adrenal haemorrhage
- Hypopituitarism (because there is no mineralocorticoid deficiency, the salt and water loss and shock are less profound than in primary Addison's disease)

## Investigations

- U&E (hyponatraemia, hyperkalaemia (rarely>6.0 mmol/l, low bicarbonate)
- FBC (anaemia, normochromic normocytic)
- Glucose (hypoglycaemia)
- Calcium (may be high)
- Short synacthen test (see note 2) for cortisol
- ABG's (acidosis)
- CXR (TB, carcinoma)
- AXR (adrenal calcification)
- SXR (if indicated, e.g. empty sella of hypopituitarism)

- Drugs
  - metyrapone (inhibits 11 ß-hydroxylase)
  - aminoglutethimide
  - ortho-para-DDD (OPDDD) (mitotane)
  - ketoconazole
  - etomidate
  - rifampicin, phenytoin and phenobarbarbitone (see note below)

## Management

- IV N/saline or colloid (PPF or haemaccel) for hypotension
- IV 50% Dextrose (50ml) if hypoglycaemic
- Serum cortisol (save for routine assay later)
- Short synacthen test prior to starting hydrocortisone (omit if patient known to have Addison's disease) (see below)
- IM Hydrocortisone (100mg stat), then 100 mg x3 daily PO. If the patient has already taken an adequate dose of steroids, this single extra dose can do no harm and may be life saving. If the patient needs glucocorticoids urgently (and cannot wait an hour), use dexamethasone 2 mg IV which will not interfere with the cortisol assay.
- Fludrocortisone (100 mcg daily orally) is not required until the patient is on only replacement doses of hydrocortisone.
- Once the crisis is over, hydrocortisone replacement is usually 20 mg daily given as 10 mg (6am) + 5 mg (noon) + 5 mg (4pm) to try and mimic the physiological diurnal variation.

*Note 1:* **Rifampicin, phenytoin and phenobarbitone** accelerate the metabolism of cortisol and may precipitate Addisonian crisis in partially compromised individuals, or in those on a fixed replacement dose. Most adrenal crises precipitated by rifampicin occur within two weeks of initiating therapy.

*Note 2:* **Short synacthen test:** Take baseline blood sample and administer tetracosactrin (Synacthen) 250 mcg IM or IV. Take further blood samples at 30 and 60 minutes and send all blood samples to lab for cortisol assay (serum).

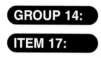

**GROUP 14:**

**ITEM 17:**

# Endocrinology and diabetes
# Patients on steroids for surgery

### CASE HISTORY 1

A 30-year-old lady who is known to have chronic asthma who has been on prednisolone between 10mg and 40 mg for at least the last 10 years is admitted for a routine cholecystectomy. Her asthma has been difficult to control and she finds that her asthma worsens whenever her dose of prednisolone is reduced to 10 mg. She is currently taking prednisolone 10 mg daily, aminophylline 225 mg twice daily, Salbutamol and Becloforte inhalers.

### How should the patient's steroids be continued following surgery?

Patients who have been on such doses of corticosteroids will have a completely suppressed pituitary adrenal axis (Fig 14.16.1), with adrenal atrophy. However the adrenal mineralocorticoid production will be normal so that the risks of an Addisonian crisis are small. This contrasts with patients who are on replacement steroids following adrenalectomy or if they have Addison's disease (see below). Nevertheless hydrocortisone 50 mg 12 hourly should be administered to replace the missing glucocorticoid at the time of surgery.

### CASE HISTORY 2

A 47-year-old lady is admitted for a cholecystectomy. She is known to have Addison's disease and is on replacement hydrocortisone, 15 mg in the morning and 5 mg at 4pm and fludrocortisone 50 mcg daily. In the past, she had an Addisonian crisis after she stopped her tablets for three days.

### Again you are asked for advice as to her steroid replacement perioperatively.

This patient is far more at risk of an Addisonian crisis if her steroids are not continued perioperatively. Intravenous boluses of hydrocortisone are rapidly cleared from the circulation and while such treatment is fine in patients who have their own adrenals, this patient will have undetectable plasma concentrations of hydrocortisone within three hours of intravenous hydrocortisone.

She should either be given 100 mg hydrocortisone IM (NOT IV) every six hours, until she can take steroids orally, or have an intravenous infusion of hydrocortisone, 100 mg over 24 hours (i.e. 4 mg per hour). The pharmacokinetics of hydrocortisone are such that such a continuous infusion will achieve a steady state plasma cortisol level of 1000 nmol/l, similar to normal individuals

## 𝑖

### Information

*Once daily* steroids are used in pharmacological doses to treat inflammatory conditions. Such treatment is not appropriate for hydrocortisone replacement in patients with Addison's disease, patients who have congenital adrenal hyperplasia (who may not be able to synthesise any adrenal steroids) or following adrenalectomy, where patients are at risk of true Addisonian crises.

having surgery. Hydrocortisone 100 mg every six hours when given IM will also achieve a similar concentration of cortisol. Oral hydrocortisone also has a much longer half life than intravenous hydrocortisone.

## Endocrinology and diabetes
## Incidental hypercalcaemia

### CASE HISTORY

A 56-year-old female patient has been admitted for a hysterectomy. She has treated hypertension but no other known illness, and no other symptomatology. A routine biochemical screen has revealed a corrected calcium of 2.75 mmol/l (NR 2.20-2.60 mmol/l). Ask the patient about specific symptoms and complications of this mild -moderate hypercalcaemia (see below).

### What is the appropriate management of this case with mild hypercalcaemia?

(Mild to moderate hypercalcaemia corrected calcium <3.0mmol/l)

• Ensure adequate hydration pre op
• Urea and electrolyte measurement essential
• Continue I.V. N/Saline (1L 8 hourly) post operatively until patient is drinking freely
• Follow-up with full investigation (see below)

### Symptoms of hypercalcaemia
• Malaise
• Thirst and polyuria
• Non-specific musculoskeletal symptoms
• Epigastric pain (abdominal groans)

### Complications
• Renal calculus (stones)
• Peptic ulceration
• Hypertension
• Increased incidence of ischaemic heart disease
• Osteoporosis ('bones')
• Confusion ('psychic moans')

### Information

An incidental finding of a raised serum calcium is now a common presentation of hypercalcaemia.

### Information

Primary hyperparathyroidism is the most common cause of mild-moderate hypercalcaemia. Malignancy is usually apparent with physical examination + CXR, breast examination should not be overlooked.

### Investigations

- Urea + electrolytes
- Serum PTH (modern assays are very reliable)
- ESR
- Serum electrophoresis
- Urine for Bence-Jones protein
- 24-hour urine collection for calcium * and creatinine clearance
- CXR  – TFTs – serum ACE levels (for sarcoidosis)

## Causes

- Primary hyperparathyroidism (also causes severe primary hypercalcaemia)
- Myeloma
- Solid tumours (also cause severe primary hypercalcaemia)
  - breast
  - bronchus
  - kidney
  - lymphoma
- Vitamin D excess (especially the 1 alpha analogues of vitamin D)
- Sarcoidosis
- Thyrotoxicosis
- Addison's disease

## Biochemical features of primary hyperparathyroidism

- "Normal" or elevated PTH. Any other cause of hypercalcaemia should suppress the PTH
- Low bicarbonate 15-20 mmol/l (PTH excess causes a mild secondary renal tubular acidosis [hyperchloraemic acidosis])
- High serum chloride (PTH excess causes a mild secondary renal tubular acidosis [hyperchloraemic acidosis])
- Moderately elevated ESR
- Normochromic anaemia

*FHH – Familial hypocalciuric hypercalcaemia is a benign familial autosomal dominant condition caused by a mutation of the calcium sensing receptor. It can be difficult to distinguish from asymptomatic primary hyperparathyroidism. A low urinary calcium suggests the diagnosis which is confirmed by examining family members.

## Treatment for primary hyperparathyroidism

Patients who are symptomatic or who have complications should all be referred for parathyroid surgery, whatever the serum calcium level.

Current thinking suggests that the majority of asymptomatic patients should also be treated surgically as they are at risk of developing complications, and should certainly be referred for specialist opinion.

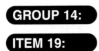

# Endocrinology and diabetes
# Severe hypercalcaemia

**GROUP 14:**

**ITEM 19:**

## CASE HISTORY

A 72-year-old woman was referred to a specialist unit with a diagnosis of "recurrent hyperparathyroidism". She had a past history of primary hyperparathyroidism treated surgically 10 years previously and had been maintained on a low dose of oral calcium.

Three months prior to admission she had become generally unwell, weak and lethargic. She reported weight loss of 5kg. The GP had performed blood tests which were as follows: corrected calcium 3.5 mmol/l, urea 16mmol/l, creatinine 150µmol/l. Renal function was previously normal. The patient arrived dehydrated and vomiting. She was found to have a fungating breast carcinoma which she had kept secret.

- Recurrence of hyperparathyroidism after surgical cure is unusual and suggests multiple endocrine neoplasia or an alternative cause
- Hypercalcaemia causes dehydration by creating a secondary type of nephrogenic diabetes insipidus. As calcium clearance is itself dependent on GFR, hypercalcaemia can rapidly decompensate in the presence of fluid depletion

### Management of severe hypercalcaemia

Defined as calcium > 3.5mmol/l or calcium > 3.0 with evidence of dehydration

### Correct fluid deficiency

- Aggressive rehydration with N/Saline
- Central venous pressure monitoring is usually necessary to prevent pulmonary oedema
- Patients frequently require four to eight litres of N/Saline over the first 24 hours
- This is usually sufficient to bring calcium down to 3.0 mmol/l

### Specific therapy

- Bisphosphonate treatment
  - 60mg I.V. pamidronate causes normalisation of serum calcium in 80% of patients after 48 to 72 hours. Bisphosphonates are most effective in malignant disease. The onset of action is delayed by at least 48 hours, so recurrent dosing at 24h is inadvisable, if late hypocalcaemia is to be avoided

• Forced diuresis
 – after normal saline rehydration, oral frusemide 20mg
 8 hourly with 4 – 6 L N/Saline per 24 hours. Very careful
 monitoring of fluid balance and electrolytes is required

**GROUP 14:**

**ITEM 20:**

# Endocrinology and diabetes
# Hypocalcaemia

### Clinical features
• General malaise
• Abnormal neurological sensations and neuro muscular
 excitability
• Numbness around the mouth and paraesthesia of the distal
 limbs
• Hyperreflexia
• Carpal and pedal spasms
• Tetany contractions (may include laryngospasm)
• Generalised seizures
• Hypotension,bradycardias, arrhythmias and congestive cardiac
 failure
• Prolonged QT interval on ECG
• Chvostek's sign is elicited by tapping the facial nerve just
 anterior to the ear, causing ipsilateral contraction of the facial
 muscles. (Positive in 10% of normals)
• Trousseau's sign is elicited by inflating a blood pressure cuff
 for three to five minutes at the level of systolic blood pressure.
 This causes mild ischaemia, unmasks latent neuromuscular
 hyperexcitability and carpal spasm is observed

### How do you assess severity?
Acute hypocalcaemia is much more life threatening than chronic
hypocalcaemia. The presence of symptoms and signs above are a
much better guide to prognosis than the absolute value of the
plasma calcium. In the presence of a low calcium (corrected
calcium less than 2.0 mmol/l) any of the above features should be
taken as evidence that urgent treatment is required.

Trousseau's sign can be graded as follows:

**Grade 1:** Carpal spasm occurs which the patient can overcome
herself

**Grade 2:** Carpal spasm occurs which the patient cannot
overcome but the examiner (you) can overcome

**Grade 3:** Carpal spasm occurs which neither of you can
overcome once the cuff has been inflated for 60 seconds

## Information
**Causes of TETANY**
• In the presence of alkalosis
 – hyperventilation
 – excess antacid therapy
 – persistent vomiting
 – hypochloraemic alkalosis
 e.g. 1° hyperaldosteronism
• In the presence of
 hypocalcaemia
 causes – see below

## Investigations
• Plasma calcium (and albumin)
 and phosphate
• Plasma magnesium
• "Routine" biochemistry
 including sodium, potassium
 and renal function
• Plasma PTH level
• SXR (intracranial calcification
 of chronic hypocalcaemia)

**Grade 4:** Carpal spasm occurs which neither of you can overcome before the cuff has been inflated for 60 seconds

## Causes of hypocalcaemia

- Hypoparathyroidism (primary, secondary or most commonly postsurgical)
- Renal failure (associated hyperphosphataemia)
- Vitamin D deficiency or abnormal vitamin D hydroxylation (giving rickets and osteomalacia).
- Pseudohypoparathyroidism
- Severe magnesium deficiency (causes both reduced PTH secretion and resistance to PTH action)
- Acute complexing or sequestration of calcium
- Acute pancreatitis
- Rhabdomyolysis
- Alkalosis (eg hyperventilation)

## How would you manage hypocalcaemia?

- The aim of acute management is not to return the calcium to normal but to ameliorate the acute manifestations of hypocalcaemia
- For frank tetany, 10 ml of 10% calcium gluconate (2.25 mmol) can be given by slow intravenous injection over five minutes. Intravenous calcium should never be given faster than this because of the risk of arrhythmia
- Depending on the symptomatology and clinical signs present, a constant infusion of calcium gluconate 0.05 mmol/kg/hour for 4 hours can be infused
- Post parathyroidectomy, mild hypocalcaemia normally ensues, requiring observation only in the absence of symptoms. A nadir occurs at five days after surgery. In patients who have parathyroid bone disease however, "hungry bones" may cause profound hypocalcaemia shortly after the parathyroids are removed. This may cause a severe and prolonged hypocalcaemia which requires prolonged (several days) treatment
- Chronic hypocalcaemia is best managed with oral calcium together with either vitamin D, or, if the cause is hypoparathyroidism or an abnormality in vitamin D metabolism, a form of activated (hydroxylated) vitamin D such as one-alpha cholecalciferol.

## CASE HISTORY

You are called to A&E to see a 30-year-old lady who complains of carpal spasm. She has had a total thyroidectomy for papillary thyroid carcinoma four weeks previously and was discharged on thyroxine 100mcg daily. Electrolytes had not been checked following surgery.

**i**

**Information**

Administration of alfacalcidol
(500 nanograms [= 0.5 mcg]
twice daily) together with oral
calcium gluconate which may
be needed chronically

### What are the most important steps in her management?

- The patient's parathyroid glands may have been inadvertently removed. Before the plasma calcium result is available, an urgent assessment of the patient must be made to determine the severity as above. This includes looking for carpal spasm when measuring blood pressure and an ECG looking for a prolonged QT interval. These will give an indication of the risk of cardiac arrhythmia or an epileptic fit
- Administer 10 ml calcium gluconate (10 ml of 10% calcium gluconate (2.25 mmol) before the plasma calcium result is back
- Long term aim of plasma calcium should be no higher than 2.30 mmol/l as one-alpha increases both calcium and phosphate, increasing the risk of nephrolithiasis. Natural PTH increases plasma calcium and reduces plasma phosphate

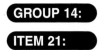

**GROUP 14:**

**ITEM 21:**

# Endocrinology and diabetes
# Phaeochromocytomas (Catecholamine crisis)

Phaeochromocytomas are rare catecholamine producing tumours derived from chromaffin cells, usually involving one or more adrenal glands. It is known as the 10% tumour (see box). Most are diagnosed during routine screening of hypertensive patients (they are found in only 0.1% of hypertensives). They usually secrete adrenaline (epinephrine) or noradrenaline (norepinephrine). A small proportion secrete dopamine, when hypotension may occur. Patients with pure adrenaline producing tumours may mimic septic shock due to adrenaline induced peripheral vasodilatation (due to β receptor stimulation)

**i**

**Information**

Phaeochromocytoma – the 10%
tumour
- 10% are bilateral
- 10% are extra-adrenal, usually
  around the sympathetic
  chain, when they are known
  as paragangliomas
- 10% are malignant

### How do they present?

Symptoms and signs of catecholamine excess include:
- Hypertension (mild to severe sustained uncontrolled hypertensive episodes)
- Paroxysmal hypertension
- Anxiety attacks
- Palpitations and tachycardia
- Cold extremities
- Sweating
- Tremor
- Pallor
- Cardiac arrhythmias including atrial and ventricular fibrillation

- Hypertensive crises may be precipitated by ß blockers, tricyclic antidepressants, metoclopramide, and naloxone
- Unexplained lactic acidosis
- Apparent Type 2 diabetes

### Associations

High risk groups are families of patients with the following autosomal dominant conditions:

- Von-Recklinghausen disease (Neurofibromata, café au lait spots, Lisch nodules, [iris hamartomas] and axillary freckling)
- Von-Hippel Lindau disease (cerebellar haemangioblastomas, retinal haemangiomas and other neoplasms including renal cell carcinoma)
- Multiple endocrine neoplasia Types 2a (hyperparathyroidism and medullary thyroid carcinoma) and 2b (medullary thyroid carcinoma, bowel ganglioneuromatosis and hypertrophied corneal nerves)

### How do you diagnose it?

There are no tests which will diagnose a phaeochromocytoma acutely. Hypertensive patients with hyperglycaemia and hypokalaemia may have a phaeochromocytoma, but these are both common features of treated hypertension (e.g. thiazides), or may indicate other endocrinopathies (e.g. Cushings, Conns, secretory adrenal carcinoma).

### Supportive tests include

- U&E (potassium often low, urea may be high if dehydrated)
- Glucose (hyperglycaemia)
- Urinary catecholamines (adrenaline, noradrenaline and dopamine) are now measured by most laboratories. Some laboratories measure urinary vanillyl mandelic acid (VMA)(a catecholamine metabolite) levels as a screen, but this test is prone to false positives because several dietary substances, including vanilla essence can give a false positive test result. Fifteen per cent of patients with essential hypertension have a false positive VMA

**Fig 14.21.1 The synthesis and metabolism of catecholamines**

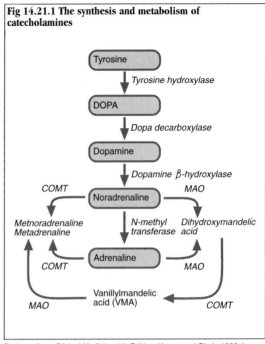

Redrawn from *Clinical Medicine*, 4th Edition, Kumar and Clark, 1998, by permission of the publisher WB Saunders

- Plasma (heparinised) catecholamines (adrenaline, noradenaline and dopamine)     – best investigation. The blood must be taken directly to the lab for centrifugation
- MRI scan of adrenals
- MIBG scan. MIBG ([131]I-metaiodobenzylguanidine) is taken up selectively by adrenal tissue. It is not used to diagnose a phaeochromocytoma, but is useful for *localisation* of tumour

**How would you manage a case?**

Patients are usually volume depleted at presentation, and should be rehydrated prior to initiation of α and ß blockade, with a litre of normal saline every eight hours, otherwise severe hypotension may occur. ß blockade alone may precipitate a hypertensive crisis and must never be given prior to adequate α blockade. Labetalol is predominantly a ß blocker and should not be used alone. Long acting non-competitive α blockers eg phenoxybenzamine should be used to prevent escape episodes.

- Adequate fluid replacement with CVP monitoring
- Initiate oral α blockade: phenoxybenzamine 10mg daily increasing gradually to 40 mg x3
- When the blood pressure is controlled with phenoxybenzamine, add propranolol 10-20 mg x3
- Surgery. Hypotension commonly occurs intra-operatively when the tumour is removed, and this should be managed with

blood, plasma expanders and inotropes as required. Inotropes should only be used when the patient is appropriately fluid replete. Expansion of intravascular volume 12 hours before surgery significantly reduces the frequency and severity of postoperative hypotension

- In emergency, (hypertensive crisis) intravenous phentolamine (1-5 mg) should be used, but great care should be taken to adequately rehydrate the patient in order to prevent severe hypotension

---

**GROUP 14:**

**ITEM 22:**

# Endocrinology and diabetes
# Hypopituitary coma and apoplexy

Hypopituitarism does not become evident until 75% of the adenohypophysis is destroyed, and at least 90% destruction is required for total loss of pituitary secretion. Complete loss of hormone secretion can rapidly become life-threatening and requires immediate therapy. In a mild or incomplete form, hypopituitarism can remain unsuspected for years and may only become apparent under the stress of surgery or infection.

### How do patients present?

- Patients may present at times of stress ( e.g. following a general anaesthetic) with hypoglycaemia and coma, due to the combination of a lack of GH, cortisol and thyroxine, all of which have a counter-regulatory effect on insulin
- Postpartum infarction of the gland is an important cause of hypopituitarism. This occurs following postpartum haemorrhage and vascular collapse during a difficult delivery. The pituitary is enlarged at the end of pregnancy, resulting in pituitary infarction with a relatively trivial fall in BP (Sheehan's syndrome)
- The first sign post-partum is failure of lactation, caused by a deficiency of prolactin (and occasionally oxytocin)
- Failure of menses then occurs due to a lack of gonadotrophins
- These signs are both often missed as patients are commonly commenced on an oral contraceptive pill
- Other features are non-specific and include tiredness, weakness, loss of body hair and loss of libido due to ACTH deficiency, hypothyroidism and gonadotrophin deficiency
- There is no postural drop as adrenal mineral corticoids (aldosterone) are unaffected

### Investigations

- Baseline blood samples must be taken for cortisol, ACTH, thyroid function, LH, FSH, prolactin and GH levels.
- A short synacthen test (see Group 14, Item 16) must be performed to test for adrenocortical reserve, and an LHRH and TRH test can be performed at the same time.
- It is best to defer an insulin induced hypoglycaemia test until the patient is stable.
- Imaging using CT with fine cuts through the pituitary or MRI is indicated to find any space occupying lesion

### Assessment of severity

The degree of hypopituitarism bears little relationship to the clinical state of the patient. In the absence of stress, patients with severe hypopituitarism may show few signs. Patients with mild hypopituitarism may become profoundly unwell at times of stress such as during an intercurrent infection.

### Causes

- Ischaemic necrosis (postpartum haemorrhage, eclampsia, temporal arteritis, arteriosclerosis)
- Destruction of the pituitary gland by primary or metastatic tumour
- Pituitary apoplexy
- Post pituitary surgery or radiotherapy
- Primary empty sella syndrome

### Management

- Hydrocortisone 100 mg IV should be administered if the diagnosis is suspected.
- Administer normal saline (1 litre over one hour then reassess) if the patient is in shock
- Administer glucose (50 ml of 50% dextrose) if the patient is hypoglycaemic.
- Investigate and treat any precipitating intercurrent infection.

## PITUITARY APOPLEXY

Is a rare syndrome caused by haemorrhage or infarction of the pituitary gland, usually occurring in patients with a pituitary adenoma, which may mimic a subarachnoid haemorrhage. The apoplectic episode may be the presenting symptom of the pituitary tumour.

### How would this present?

Pituitary infarction may be silent. Apoplexy implies the presence of symptoms:

- Headache occurs in 75% of cases (may be sudden onset, very severe, or mild)
- Visual disturbance (compression of optic tract, usually causing bitemporal hemianopia)
- Ocular palsy present in 40% of cases. Unilateral or bilateral
- Nausea/vomiting
- Meningism
- Hemiparesis
- Fever, anosmia, CSF rhinorrhoea, hypothalamic dysfunction (disturbed sympathetic autoregulation with abnormalities in BP control, respiration and cardiac rhythm) have all been described, but are rare

- Clinically, pituitary apoplexy may be very difficult to distinguish from subarachnoid haemorrhage, bacterial meningitis, midbrain infarction (basilar artery occlusion) and cavernous sinus thrombosis.

### How do you investigate?

A CT brain scan with fine cuts through the pituitary will reveal a tumour mass and will often reveal the haemorrhage within 24-48 hours with administration of intravenous contrast. MRI will not replace CT scanning in the acute setting due to its inability to detect fresh bleeding, although it is especially useful in the subacute setting (four days to one month). A single clotted blood sample should be taken to measure cortisol, thyroid function, prolactin, growth hormone and the gonadotropic hormones.

### Assessment of severity

The course of pituitary apoplexy is variable. Headache and mild visual disturbance may develop slowly and persist for several weeks. In its most fulminant form, apoplexy may cause blindness, haemodynamic instability, coma and death. Residual endocrine disturbance invariably occurs. Panhypopituitarism is the usual result.

### Causes

- Spontaneous haemorrhage of a pituitary tumour without antecedent events is the commonest cause of pituitary apoplexy. Apoplexy is known to occur in patients with pituitary tumours with the following antecedent events:
- Anticoagulant therapy
- Head trauma
- Radiation therapy
- Drugs, including bromocriptine and oestrogen
- Following tests of pituitary function

### How would you manage this patient?

- Hydrocortisone 100 mg IV should be given if the diagnosis is suspected after the blood samples above have been collected
- Monitor U&E and urine output for evidence of diabetes insipidus
- Urgent neurosurgical opinion (*see note a*)
- Pituitary function once the acute apoplexy has resolved and treat as necessary (*note b*).

*Note a*
Neurosurgical decompression via a trans-sphenoidal route is the definitive treatment for pituitary apoplexy. Obtundation, and visual deterioration are absolute indications for neurosurgery. Patients without confusion or visual disturbance generally do well without surgery.

*Note b*
A TSH in the normal range may be inappropriate if the T4 is low in pituitary disease, but this may occur in the sick euthyroid state characteristic of many patients seriously ill.

*Note c*
Pituitary apoplexy has been associated with resolution of hypersecretory states

**GROUP 14:**

**ITEM 23:**

# Endocrinology and diabetes
# Diabetes insipidus

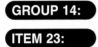

### Investigations
- Na 146   K4.0   U4.7   Cr90
- Urine SG (dipstick):  1.001
- This patient probably has transient diabetes insipidus.

Transient diabetes insipidus often occurs following pituitary surgery because of vasopressin deficiency. You may be called to see a patient with polyuria and polydipsia for assessment. Following transphenoidal surgery, patients have their noses packed and therefore breathe thorough the mouth. For this reason, there is often superadded polydipsia, with associated polyuria.

## CASE HISTORY

You are called to see a patient who had a transphenoidal hypophysectomy the day before for a macroprolactinoma. He made a good recovery from surgery but now complains of extreme thirst.

### How would yo manage this patient?
- Continue IV Dextrose/saline 2 L/24 hours.
- Make sure an accurate fluid balance chart is being maintained
- Diabetes Insipidus (DI) is usually self-limiting in this situation. Allow free fluids orally.
- If urine output>1L per 4 hours consider desmopressin (adult dose 0.5-1.0 mcg sc six-hourly is required). Prior to administration check plasma and urine osmolality
- DI is confirmed by the presence of a high plasma osmolality (>295) in the presence of an inappropriately low urine osmolality (U:P ratio <2:1). If the plasma osmolality is low the patient may be over-drinking due to a dry mouth, and a low urine osmolality is appropriate. In this circumstance, administration of desmopressin will cause a further fall in plasma osmolality and can be dangerous.

### Other causes of diabetes insipidus

Diabetes insipidus is either cranial (CDI) or nephrogenic (NDI) (due to the inability of ADH to act on the kidney).

| CDI | NDI |
|---|---|
| Pituitary or brain tumour | Drugs |
| Basal skull fracture | – diuretics |
| Neurosarcoidosis | – lithium |
| (affects hypothalamus) | Hypercalcaemia |
| | Hypokalaemia |

## GROUP 14:     Endocrinology and diabetes

## ITEM 24:     The syndrome of inappropriate ADH (SIADH)

This is a popular condition for examiners in vivas and written exams, but often overdiagnosed in patients.

### How would it present?

Most commonly, patients present with incidentally discovered hyponatraemia. (see Group 9, Item 2). Alternatively, they may present with a fit or episodes of confusion.

### Causes

Small cell lung carcinoma is well recognised but other pathologies also cause SIADH.

• Drugs
• Pneumonia
• Tuberculosis
• Hypotension following bleeding
• Intracranial pathology

### What other causes should you think of?

It is essential that other causes of hyponatraemia (in particular diuretics) are excluded. The diagnosis of SIADH cannot be made in a patient who is on diuretics, although of course a patient may have SIADH and also be on diuretics. The differential diagnosis (especially for exam purposes) is psychogenic polydipsia, where a patient may drink 6 litres of water within an hour and present with a fit and hyponatraemia. These patients usually have a

## Investigations

- Take a careful drug history, and ensure the patient is not on any drugs e.g.diuretics, lithium or carbamazipine.
- U&E and plasma osmolality (hyponatraemia will be seen)
- Urinary electrolytes and osmolality
- The patient will have a low plasma osmolality (< 276) and an inappropriately concentrated urine (>300).
- Free T4 and TSH to exclude hypothyroidism
- Cortisol and short synacthen test to exclude Addison's disease
- Both of these reduce the patients ability to clear free water.
- CXR (TB, carcinoma)
- AXR (adrenal calcification)
- SXR, CT / MRI brain and pituitary (exclude intracranial pathology)

## Information

Syndrome of inappropriate antidiuretic hormone (SIADH)

- Dilutional hyponatraemia due to excessive water retention
- Low plasma osmolality with higher "inappropriate" urine osmolality
- Continued urinary sodium excretion> 30 mmol/l
- Absence of hypokalaemia (or hypotension)
- Normal renal, adrenal and thyroid function

psychiatric history, and their polydipsia may be part of a behavioural disorder. In these patients, urinary osmolality is usually low and a diuresis occurs. With fluid restriction, electrolytes should normalise within 6 hours, as the patients pass the six litres excess water! If a patient is on diuretics, the urinary sodium and hence osmolality will be artificially raised, causing confusion.

Following a rapid loss of blood (10% of ones blood volume), the pituitary also appropriately secretes ADH to maintain circulating volume. Following surgery, this backup emergency system may be activated if a patient has bled perioperatively. If the patient is also given dextrose postoperatively, the patient may be found to be hyponatraemic the next day, with an apparently inappropriate secretion of ADH (concentrated urine). The patient must be reassessed following adequate rehydration, and the surgeons can be reassured that the patients ADH secretion was appropriate at the time!

## CASE HISTORY

A 65-year-old smoker complained of a chronic cough and haemoptysis. A chest X-ray revealed a hilar mass. He was referred to the chest clinic for further investigation.

Electrolytes: Na 118, K 4.4, U 3.3, Cr 100, Glucose 4.9

Measured plasma osmolality: 255

In view of the low plasma osmolality, a spot urine was also sent to the biochemistry department:

Urinary sodium: 30mmol/l Urinary osmolality 350 mosm/kg.

This patient's urinary osmolality is high for his current plasma osmolality. Normally the kidney can make urine as dilute as 100 mosm/kg (urine SG=1.0001) (40 mosm/kg in young fit people), and as concentrated as 1300 in a patient who is dehydrated (urine SG=1.4000). The appropriateness of the current urinary osmolality has to be interpreted with the knowledge of the current plasma osmolality.

This patient does indeed have inappropriate ADH. He was put on a one litre fluid restriction daily and commenced on deme-clocyline.

## Treatment

Fluid restriction
Demeclocycline

# Notes

**GROUP 15:**

**ITEM 1:**

# Neurology
## Diplopia

### Information

A painless III<sup>rd</sup> nerve palsy with preserved pupil reactions commonly occurs in the setting of diabetes. If there is headache, especially of sudden onset, one must also consider a posterior communicating artery aneurysm compressing the IIIrd nerve in front of the midbrain. Such a lesion also commonly involves the parasympathetic pupillary constricting fibres. Depending upon the strength of suspicion, MR angiography or formal intra-arterial angiography is indicated.

### CASE HISTORY 1

A 78-year-old woman with diabetes presents with double vision of acute onset. There is ptosis in the left eye and the eye is deviated downward and laterally on primary gaze and fails to elevate or move medially. The pupils both react normally. She is otherwise well. Her blood glucose is found to be 11.5 mmol/l.

### What immediate action would you take?

• Achieve diabetic control
• Patch over eye
• Reassure that recovery likely (but not definite) over weeks
• The diagnosis is **mononeuritis multiplex**, a complication of diabetes mellitus

If no recovery, refer to a neurologist for MRI scan and investigation of other causes of mononeuritis multiplex (see Group 15, Item 3)

### CASE HISTORY 2

A 35-year-old woman presents with three months of intermittent double vision. Examination reveals mild restriction of upgaze and lateral gaze of the left eye and mild restriction of upgaze of the right eye. There is mild bilateral ptosis. Further examination reveals fatiguability of the ptosis and of the eye movements.

### What action would you take?

Confirm diagnosis of myasthenia by:
• Serum acetyl choline receptor antibodies (90% of cases with 100% specificity)
• Tensilon test (see Kumar & Clark 4th Ed. p 1102)
• EMG studies, including the extraocular muscles

This patient was diagnosed as having **Myasthenia Gravis** and will need urgent referral to a neurologist. Myasthenia Gravis is sometimes restricted to the ocular system and can present as a variable gaze palsy difficult to interpret in terms of individual muscles or cranial nerves. There is not always a history of fatiguability. Some of the many causes of diplopia are listed in Table 15.1.1.

> **Table 15.1.1. Causes of diplopia**
>
> | | |
> |---|---|
> | Muscle / obstructive | thyroid eye disease |
> | | orbital masses |
> | | orbital pseudotumour (ocular myositis) |
> | | myasthenia |
> | | breakdown of latent squint |
> | | |
> | Cranial nerves | mass lesion in path of III, IV or VI nerves |
> | | mononeuritis multiplex |
> | | false localizing due to raised intracranial pressure |
> | | |
> | Central | brainstem inflammation, demyelination |
> | | brainstem mass lesion, infarction, haemorrhage |

Treatment of Myasthenia Gravis includes pyridostigmine, gradually increased steroids, immunosuppression, and plasmapheresis. Restricted ocular myasthenia carries an improved prognosis, as swallowing and the respiratory muscles may be permanently spared.

MRI of the chest and consideration of thymectomy is necessary.

## CASE HISTORY 3

A 30-year-old, 27-weeks-pregnant woman complains of four weeks of headache, nausea, brief one-second episodes of visual obscuration and horizontal double vision worse on distance gaze. She is found to have bilateral papilloedema and bilateral restriction of lateral gaze consistent with VI[th] nerve palsies.

### What action would you take?

- MR scan of head (if available) or CT. In this case the ventricles were normal and therefore it was safe to proceed to:
- a lumbar puncture and record the opening pressure
- if pressure >25 cm, remove a volume of CSF, usually around 20 ml, such as approximately to halve the opening pressure

This lady has **clinical idiopathic intracranial hypertension (IIH).** It is most common in overweight females and rare in males.

### Precipitating factors are

- Pregnancy
- Weight gain
- Polycystic ovaries
- Tetracyclines
- Vitamin A excess
- Steroids

**Remember**

There are a number of secondary causes of raised intracranial pressure without dilated ventricles or other space occupying lesion, the most important of which in these circumstances being venous sinus thrombosis and meningeal disease. MRI/MR venography and examination of CSF constituents is therefore mandatory.

## Management

Repeated lumbar puncture and removal of CSF e.g. every one to two weeks has been used but is probably not helpful. Drugs such as acetazolamide can be helpful. Treatment is directed primarily at preventing visual loss due to uncorrected papilloedema and secondarily at relief of headache/diplopia. The visual fields must be checked formally at intervals by Goldman-Bjerrum screen perimetry to monitor any enlargement of the blind spots. If repeat puncture is unsuccessful in this usually self-limiting condition, then lumboperitoneal shunting, optic nerve fenestration or even ventriculoperitoneal shunting may be necessary.

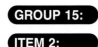

# Neurology

# Visual impairment or failure (acute/subacute)

## CASE HISTORY

A 64-year-old man presents in the A&E with three hours of visual loss in the right eye. There was a previous episode several months earlier. He describes the loss as a horizontal screen descending over his vision. You are called by the A&E officer to give an opinion. When you arrive the visual loss has recovered.

### What is the most likely diagnosis?

Temporary monocular visual loss with a horizontal defect in this age group is very likely to be **amaurosis fugax**; this is an ophthalmic artery TIA. It is often the first clinical evidence of an internal carotid artery stenosis.

### Investigation and management

See Group 7, Item 8 and Group 15, Item 5.

### What is the differential diagnosis?

TIAs are usually diagnosed clinically. Other causes are shown in Table 15.2.1.

Remember giant cell arteritis which causes acute visual loss. It responds to steroids see Group 8, Item 7.

Abrupt and progressive visual loss over days is also seen in the elderly hypertensive. There is often disc swelling and later disc pallor. This is due to an arteriopathy of the posterior ciliary artery resulting in ischaemia of the optic disc causing an anterior ischaemic optic neuropathy. Urgent management by a specialist with heparin infusion and mannitol.

**Table 15.2.1. Causes of relatively acute or transient visual disturbance**

| Ophthalmological: | Neurological: |
|---|---|
| – glaucoma | – optic neuritis/demyelination |
| – amaurosis fugax | – compressive lesion of the optic nerve, chiasm, tract |
| – giant cell (temporal) arteritis | – TIA/stroke of posterior cerebral circulation |
| – anterior ischaemic optic neuropathy | – migraine |
| – central retinal vessel occlusion | – occipital, temporal, parietal haemorrhage |
| – vitreous haemorrhage | – occipital, temporal, parietal space occupying lesion |
| – retinal detachment | – epileptiform phenomena |
| – uveitis, keratitis | – obscurations of raised intracranial pressure |

## CASE HISTORY 2

A 24-year-old woman complains of several attacks of an hour's duration of loss of vision in the right eye accompanied by a left sided pounding headache. Closer questioning reveals that the defect is in fact in the right visual field of both eyes.

Visual hemifield disturbance, sometimes with shimmering or jagged line scotomata, is a relatively common aura experienced by patients with migraine. Occasionally there is no headache.

If the symptoms are dramatic or atypical or especially if there are any fixed symptoms or signs, an **MRI** scan should be performed to check for an underlying vascular lesion such as an arteriovenous malformation or underlying epileptogenic lesion, including occipital tumour.

(see Group 15, Item 8)

**GROUP 15:**

**ITEM 3:**

# Neurology
# Bell's Palsy

## CASE HISTORY 1

You are called to see a 45-year-old man who woke up this morning with a 'numb' left face, a droopy left eyelid and drooling from the left side of his mouth. On examination, it is apparent that his 'numbness' in fact represents left facial weakness in the upper and lower distributions. There is no sensory loss and no lesions of the skin around or inside the ear.

**An acute VII nerve lesion, Bell's Palsy,** is usually idiopathic and the correct management is reassurance, combined with protection of the cornea if left exposed. Steroids (e.g. 60 mg prednisolone for a week and tailing down over the subsequent one to two weeks) may be given if diagnosed early, but the evidence for benefit is unclear. There should be no sensory loss or any other cranial nerve abnormality. Sometimes recovery is incomplete and there may be faulty reinnervation of the facial muscles or of the lacrimal gland. Relapses may occur.

Bilateral or recurrent Bell's Palsy, or one that shows no recovery after several weeks, should be investigated with an MRI scan, possibly CSF analysis, and investigations for causes of mononeuritis multiplex (see box).

Note: One should suspect sarcoidosis in cases of bilateral Bell's Palsy. A rare condition causing bilateral Bell's Palsy and tongue swelling with other features is Melkersson-Rosenthal syndrome. Progressive multiple cranial nerve palsies should lead to suspicion of malignant meningitis, or lymphomatous or carcinomatous infiltration.

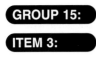

### Investigations

Mononeuritis multplex
- FBC
- U&Es
- Glucose
- Autoantibodies
- Anticardiolipin antibodies
- ANCA
- Treponemal serology
- Borrelia serology
- CXR
- Serum and CSF ACE
- Serum electrophoresis and Bence Jones protein

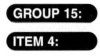

## GROUP 15:
## ITEM 4:

# Neurology
# Vertigo

## CASE HISTORY 1

An 85-year-old lady presented to A&E with a history of severe nausea, vomiting and dizziness which started on waking one morning two weeks ago. She was confused and dehydrated. On rehydration she was able to give a clear history of true vertigo, (the sensation of the environment spinning or rotating about her). The symptoms are precipitated by head movement, especially when she turns her head in bed. On examination, she has normal eye movements but rotational nystagmus in both eyes is brought on by sudden head movements (Hallpike's manoeuvre).

## What is the likely diagnosis?

This history is typical of **vestibular neuronitis** (or so-called viral labyrinthitis, although the aetiology is uncertain). It occurs at any age. Recovery generally takes place to a large extent over two to three weeks, although complete recovery may take several months. Cinnarizine and other vestibular suppressants give symptomatic relief but are best avoided in the long term.

Peripheral vestibular lesions are characterised by positional vertigo ie influenced, often in a stereotyped way, by head movement. This is manifest in the Hallpike's test, which characteristically reveals a torsional nystagmus.

A central vestibular lesion is sometimes also positional but generally fails to habituate; (i.e. on Hallpike's testing, continued repetition of the same movement results in no reduction in the unpleasantness or in the nystagmus).

The definitive investigation to differentiate the two sites and to lateralize the lesion is by caloric tests.

## Main causes of vertigo

- Peripheral:
  - viral labyrinthitis
  - benign positional vertigo
  - Ménière's syndrome
  - lesion of the VIII nerve e.g. Schwannoma
  - inner ear infections, infiltrations
- Central:
  - brainstem infarction, inflammation or demyelination
  - brainstem space occupying lesion
  - posterior territory TIA
  - migraine
  - complex partial seizures

**Remember**

If there is a suspicion of a central lesion, an MRI scan should be performed.

One should always check for associated deafness, tinnitus, cranial nerve lesions or cerebellar disturbance because of the importance of early identification of a cerebellopontine angle lesion, most commonly an VIII nerve Schwannoma ('acoustic neuroma').

## CASE HISTORY 2

A rather anxious lady presented to A&E with occasional very brief blackouts and a long history of dizziness in crowds or when walking past fast moving traffic. She prefers to avoid any sudden head movements, especially in certain directions and when turning in bed. Hallpike's test is positive.

### What is the likely diagnosis?

**Benign positional vertigo.** This is a relatively common disorder presenting with true vertigo particularly on head movement. There are often vague 'vestibular hypersensitivity' symptoms, especially precipitated when there are conflicting visual inputs such as being stationary in a fast-moving visual field. Occasionally, the vertigo may be so sudden and dramatic as to present as a blackout.

### Diagnosis

Largely clinical, although caloric testing may reveal mild dysfunction and MRI helps to exclude other conditions.

### Management

With vestibular physiotherapy in the form of Cawthorne-Cooksey exercises and vestibular suppressants. At least in some cases the cause is said to relate to fragments of calcification in the semicircular canals; some specialists perform the Eppley manoeuvre in an attempt to dislodge these fragments away from the receptors. Some severe cases may be successfully treated by surgical section of the nerve to the ampulla of the posterior semicircular canal.

## CASE HISTORY 3

A 70-year-old man presents with sudden onset of vertigo, vomiting, gait unsteadiness and left facial numbness. On examination there is coarse unidirectional nystagmus, reduced left corneal reflex, left Horner's syndrome, mild dysphagia and palatal deviation to the right, left sided ataxia, and impaired pinprick on the right arm and leg.

This is a **partial left lateral medullary syndrome** due to a stroke in the territory of branches of the posterior or anterior inferior cerebellar arteries. The vertigo is usually not positional. Nystagmus of brainstem origin is often coarse, may be in any direction, often unidirectional and sometimes monocular.

### Management

As for a stroke – Group 15, Item 5.

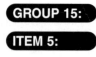

## Neurology
## Stroke and TIAs

### CASE HISTORY 1

A 70-year-old man presents with a four-hour history of right sided arm, leg and face weakness and loss of speech. He has no headache and is mildly confused. He has a history of ischaemic heart disease. Examination reveals a global dysphasia, full visual fields, UMN distribution right facial weakness and dense weakness (upper motor neurone distribution) of the right side with absent reflexes and an upgoing plantar response on that side.

A clinical diagnosis of left middle cerebral artery ischaemic stroke is made.

### What immediate action would you take?

- Give oxygen by mask
- Do blood tests (Hb, WCC, U&Es, glucose, ESR)
- CT scan – to check if haemorrhagic

### How would you manage a case with the following CT diagnoses?

- If haemorrhagic stroke (particularly in the posterior fossa)
  - refer to neurosurgeons for emergency clot evacuation
- If stuttering stroke in evolution and CT indicates that it is not haemorrhagic
  - give IV heparin
- If evidence of cerebral oedema and risk of coning
  - give mannitol
- If not haemorrhagic stroke after a delay of two weeks
  - start aspirin 75 mg and dipyridamole slow release. Start anticoagulants if atrial fibrillation
- Pravistatin (or other statin ) if fasting cholesterol > 5.4 mmol/l
- For all
  - supportive care
  - treatment of any concurrent infection, other illness, electrolyte disturbance
  - do not overcorrect systemic hypertension in the acute phase
  - keep nil by mouth with iv fluid replacement in any major stroke until swallowing is assessed properly, preferably by speech therapists. Asymptomatic aspiration is common
  - early referral to physiotherapy and other support services

An early CT scan is very useful in stroke to check for subarachnoid or intracerebral haemorrhage and to help exclude other conditions that may masquerade as stroke, such as tumour,

**Remember**

Present UK guidelines do NOT indicate thrombolysis – even if a stroke is diagnosed within four hours with a normal CT (ie not a haemorrhagic stroke)

cerebral abscess and cerebral venous sinus thrombosis. The last of these may present with bilateral or even unilateral hemispheric, sometimes haemorrhagic, infarction; the 'delta' sign may be seen on CT or MRI. This condition is treated with intravenous heparin followed by warfarin.

One should attempt as far as possible to localise and determine the nature of the stroke. There are a number of common causes (see below). This will guide management to prevent recurrence. Most investigations are directed to this goal. In addition, identification of hypertension is important. This is particularly associated with lacunar strokes and with amyloid angiopathy, the most common cause of hemispheric haemorrhage.

### Common types of stroke
- Thrombotic – often in the middle cerebral artery distribution
- Embolic from neck vessels
- Embolic from cardiac structural abnormality or arrhythmia
- Lacunar – deep (often capsular or thalamic) infarct or haemorrhage
- Intracerebral haemorrhage. Amyloid angiopathy
- Watershed infarction eg from episode of loss of cardiac output or anoxia.

### CASE HISTORY 2

A 56-year-old man presents with weakness of the left hand and face lasting three hours and resolving gradually. He had a similar episode three months earlier with complete recovery. He is a Type 2 diabetic and a smoker. A Doppler U/S reveals that he has a 90% stenosis at the origin of the right internal carotid artery.

### What are the options for treatment?
- Carotid endarterectomy is indicated when there is symptomatic carotid stenosis greater that 70%. Most surgeons require subsequent formal angiography to confirm the degree of stenosis and to check the anatomy of the stenosis and the other vessels. To be symptomatic, the TIA symptoms must correspond to the stenosed vessel. Some surgeons advocate endarterectomy for asymptomatic stenoses, but this is not standard practice at this time. It is not appropriate to operate on a stenosed vessel when the area supplied is already completely infarcted. A 100% blockage does not require surgery because in this situation there is not the same risk of embolus. Angioplasty of the carotid vessels and surgery or angioplasty for posterior circulation stenoses are currently not routinely performed.
- As well as offering surgery, one should also address remediable risk factors such as smoking, hypertension and hypercholesterolaemia and optimize control in diabetics. Lifelong aspirin and dipyridamole are indicated.
- Warfarin is given when there is a structural cardiac lesion or

### Investigations
Guidelines for investigation of older age group stroke/TIA
- CT head
- Hb/PCV
- WCC
- U&Es
- Glucose
- ESR
- TFTs
- Fasting cholesterol (after acute phase)
- CXR
- ECG and cardiac enzymes
- Vit B12
- Treponemal serology
- Doppler U/S carotids ± vertebrals or MR angiogram neck vessels
- If a cardiac lesion is suspected – consider echocardiogram, 24-hour ECG

cardiac arrhythmia (particularly atrial fibrillation) that would lead to a risk of cardiac thrombosis and subsequent embolus.It is not indicated for carotid disease.

## CASE HISTORY 3

A 40-year-old man presents with a one-week history of headache followed by loss of speech and a right hemiparesis. His weakness worsens over the next 24 hours and he becomes confused. A CT scan is normal at this time. A subsequent MRI scan reveals an infarct in the left frontal lobe with small petechial haemorrhages here and elsewhere in the hemispheres. His ESR and autoantibodies are normal. CSF analysis reveals 35 lymphocytes /mm$^3$ but is otherwise normal. A right frontal brain biopsy reveals primary **cerebral granulomatous angiitis**. He is treated with high dose steroids and cyclophosphamide.

### What are the causes of strokes in this young age group?

In the younger age group, one must consider other causes of stroke, such as vasculitis or structural cardiac lesions. In many of these conditions, specific treatment is indicated. Cerebral vasculitis is difficult to diagnose, since systemic inflammatory markers may be normal. The CSF and intra-arterial angiography are sometimes also normal. Even a cerebral/ meningeal biopsy may miss involved vessels since the condition is often patchy.

### Investigations

Additional investigations in the younger age group
- MRI head
- Autoantibodies inc. anticardiolipin, ANCA
- Lupus anticoagulant
- Urine for protein and casts
- Serum electrophoresis
- Serum lactate/pyruvate
- Urine homocysteine
- Echocardiogram
- 24-hour ECG
- Consider CSF analysis

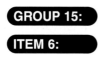

**GROUP 15:**

**ITEM 6:**

# Neurology
## Subdural haemorrhage

### CASE HISTORY 1

A 77-year-old woman was admitted two weeks ago with failure to manage at home alone. There had been a two-year history of cognitive decline that seemed to have accelerated to precipitate the admission. On examination, she was confused, unable to repeat a five digit number, disorientated and had an upgoing left plantar. After several days on the ward, a CT scan was requested and revealed **bilateral subdural haematomas**.

Subdural haemorrhage may present rather acutely following a fall and occasionally presents spontaneously with sudden onset of headache and obtundation or other features. The diagnostic challenge lies in identifying other cases that present vaguely without focal signs and with no history of trauma. A number of factors are associated with increased risk of subdural haemorrhage.

• Old age
• Cerebral atrophy, dementia
• Alcoholism, general debility
• Bleeding diathesis
• Intracranial lesion such as tumour
• Brain surgery, especially ventricular shunt insertion for normal pressure hydrocephalus

### Management

Subdural haematomas depends on their size and the severity of symptoms. Small ones may simply be managed conservatively with follow up CT scanning. Larger or more acutely symptomatic subdurals should be surgically evacuated.

**GROUP 15:**

**ITEM 7:**

# Neurology
# L-DOPA therapy

## CASE HISTORY 1

A 75-year-old man with **Parkinson's disease** presents with uncontrollable gyrating movements of his arms and legs. On obtaining a detailed history it transpires that he is on levodopa therapy and it was recently increased to Sinemet CR three tablets four times a day.

### What is the problem?

This patient has dyskinesia – a common late side-effect of levodopa therapy for parkinsonism. About 10% of patients per year of therapy will develop such dyskinesias, involving uncontrollable choreoathetoid movements and dystonic posturing. At this stage in the illness, the severity of dyskinesia is dose dependent and so a balance has to be struck between 'off' symptoms of bradykinesia and rigidity and 'on' dyskinetic symptoms. In the above case, the sinemet was prescribed inappropriately.

When commencing levodopa therapy, patients are generally started on 1 Sinemet-Plus or 1 Madopar (100mg/25mg tablets) three times a day. These drugs consist of a combination of levodopa and a peripheral DOPA decarboxylase inhibitor to prevent inappropriate peripheral activation to dopamine. The dose of these drugs can be gradually increased in amount and frequency as the underlying disease worsens.

Alternatively, patients may receive a controlled release preparation; Sinemet CR has nearly twice the bioavailable strength of straight Sinemet but the Madopar CR preparation is a more equivalent dose. The controlled release preparations may be given once at night to help with nocturnal or early morning 'off' symptoms, or may be given two to three times a day alone or in combination with straight levodopa in an effort to smoothen fluctuating symptoms.

Occasionally dyskinesias occur in relation to dramatic fluctuations in levodopa levels rather than to high peak level; the solution in this situation is to place the patient on a higher dose of longer acting medication.

*i*

**Information**

Some physicians start off with controlled release preparations. This is to minimize dose fluctuations that may result in dyskinesias later in the course of the disease, but there is no clear evidence for this protective effect.

**GROUP 15:**

**ITEM 8:**

# Neurology
# Multiple sclerosis

### CASE HISTORY 1

A 28-year-old man presents with several days of pain and progressive loss of vision in one eye. Examination reveals loss of colour vision, acuity of 6/36 and disc swelling. It comes to light that he previously had an episode of gait and bladder disturbance that recovered fully after several weeks.

### What is the diagnosis of his eye problem?

**Optic neuritis.** This is a common first presentation of **multiple sclerosis (MS)**; the previous history suggesting an episode of transverse myelitis indicates dissociation in space and time, providing strong clinical support for the diagnosis of multiple sclerosis.

### What action would you take?

• Recovery after an episode of optic neuritis is aided by intravenous methylprednisolone e.g. 1g/day for three days.

• An MRI should be performed to look for demyelinating lesions of MS and to check for MS-mimicking conditions such as sarcoidosis. In the latter condition, meningeal enhancement may occur.

• CSF analysis for oligoclonal bands may be performed further to corroborate the diagnosis.

• Visual evoked potentials are likely to be delayed in the affected eye but may also reveal subclinical involvement of the other eye, providing evidence for dissociation in space.

### CASE HISTORY 2

A previously well 25-year-old woman develops double vision, vertigo, unsteadiness and speech and swallowing problems over two days. She is admitted to hospital where she rapidly deteriorates, becoming confused and hypoxic. She requires ventilatory support. An MRI scan reveals a number of small bilateral periventricular white matter lesions and lesions in the brainstem and cerebellar peduncles. CSF examination reveals oligoclonal bands. She is given intravenous methylprednisolone and recovers well over the next two weeks apart from residual mild vertigo and intermittent diplopia.

**Remember**

Multiple sclerosis may sometimes present dramatically as a brainstem syndrome with central respiratory problems and rapid severe bulbar failure. Early supportive management is essential in such cases. There may be excellent recovery following the relapse. Patients with known MS who suffer a relapse involving bulbar function or dysarthria should similarly be carefully observed.

## CASE HISTORY 3

A patient with **known multiple sclerosis** with frequent severe relapses, bladder instability and incontinence and painful leg spasms wonders if anything can be done for her incurable condition.

### What would you suggest?

There are a number of aspects of management of MS:

- **Intravenous methylprednisolone** or a short course of high dose oral prednisolone have clear benefit in speeding recovery after a relapse but have no effect on the underlying disease. There is no role for maintenance steroids. If a patient exhibits steroid dependence (tending to deteriorate whenever steroids are withdrawn) they probably do not have multiple sclerosis but some other inflammatory condition such as sarcoidosis, Behcets, SLE or vasculitis.

- **Beta interferon** is now available for management of relapsing-remitting multiple sclerosis. The indications for treatment, in a committed patient willing to embark on long-term intramuscular or subcutaneous self administration and for whom funding is available, are:
  - At least three significant relapses in the past 18 months
  - Sufficiently good between relapses to walk 50 m

The benefit is a reduction in number of relapses by one third and a possible modest benefit in underlying disability. The side-effects include "flu" like symptoms and injection site problems.

- **Bladder problems and sexual dysfunction** are common in MS. It may be appropiate to refer to a specialist. Hyperirritability symptoms can be treated with an anticholinergic such as oxybutynin. However, if the residual urine after micturition is greater than 100-200 ml as measured by U.S, then the risk of urinary infection and possible pyelonephritis is significantly increased; it is best in this situation to combine anticholinergics with intermittent catheterization which the patient can sometimes be taught to perform. When incontinence is severe, a permanent catheter, preferably suprapubic, may be the best solution.

- **Tonic and clonic spasms** are also a common problem that can be successfully managed. These spasms can be extremely painful and may limit patents' mobility and posture maintenance more than does their weakness. Since most treatments result in some voluntary weakness, in ambulatory and transferring patients a balance must be struck between weakness and spasticity. In some, spasticity is actually beneficial in enabling the legs to be rigid for standing. Treatments include baclofen (oral or intrathecal pump), tizanidine, diazepam, dantrolene and injections of baclofen or application of nerve blocks.

### Information

Sometimes hyperreflexia is so bad, despite permanent catheterization, that bladder contraction is deliberately weakened by a treatment with intravesical capsaicin or phenol.

• MS patients experience severe **neuropathic** pain. Carbamazepine and amitriptyline may be very helpful in some cases as may specialist procedures for pain management.

**GROUP 15:**

**ITEM 9:**

# Neurology
# Encephalitis

### CASE HISTORY 1

A 45-year-old man presents with a week's history of malaise, followed by increasing confusion, headache, meningism and a seizure. On examination he has fever, neck stiffness and hyperreflexia of the left arm and leg.

### What action would you take?

• Supportive care, including respiratory support if necessary
• Treatment of any seizures. Ictal and post-ictal states are an important reversible element of obtundation
• CT scan followed by lumbar puncture, looking for lymphocytosis, Serology and PCR for likely aetiological agents (see below)
• Commence aciclovir. Recommendations are now for at least two weeks of treatment in cases strongly suspected to have herpes simplex encephalitis (HSE). Patients have been known to relapse and respond to further treatment even after this period. In suspected herpes zoster infection, especially if there is outer retinal necrosis in the immunocompromized, foscarnet may be added

If the patient survives, there is often significant residual deficit and attention should be directed to ongoing rehabilitation. Memory problems are particularly common following HSE.

### Causes of Encephalitis/Meningoencephalitis

• Viral include
  – herpes simplex
  – measles
  – rubella
  – EBV
  – VZV
  – ECHO
  – coxsackie

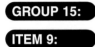

**Other investigations**

• An MRI scan is very useful (see case 2)
• An EEG to exclude generalized or complex partial status epilepticus.
• The possibility of immunosuppression (as a result of AIDS, lymphoproliferative disorders or iatrogenic) should be investigated

- CMV
- HIV
- Japanese B (commonest worldwide)
- post-viral  – acute disseminated encephalomyelitis (ADEM)
• Bacterial include
  - Legionnaire's
  - mycoplasma
  - listeria
  - tuberculosis
• In immunocompromised people think of unusual organisms eg fungal

The term 'encephalitis' effectively encompasses any acute febrile illness, perhaps with some meningeal involvement, that is accompanied by acute generalized or focal cerebral disturbance. Thus there is considerable overlap with meningitis. In addition, for practical purposes, the differential should often include other causes of acute obtundation, since one cannot rely on finding fever and meningism to distinguish an infective encephalitis from other acute or subacute encephalopathies.

⚠️

**Remember**

All cases of encephalitis should be given Aciclovir; HSV is treatable. Most other causes are not.

## CASE HISTORY 2

A 30-year-old woman is admitted with a three-week history of progressive confusion, double vision, swallowing problems and walking difficulty. Blood and CSF culture reveal Listeria. An MRI scan showed brainstem lesions. Treatment is commenced with intravenous ampicillin and tobramycin and the patient makes a full recovery.

Encephalitis often has characteristic features that lead one to suspect certain aetiological agents:

• Listerial encephalitis may be rather focal, particularly affecting the brainstem and may result in multiple abscesses, as may pseudomonas, E. coli and fungi. Legionnaires' encephalitis may also affect the brainstem
• Herpes simplex virus typically has a predilection for the temporal lobes that may be seen on MRI scanning and may result in memory problems as a prominent feature
• Measles and mycoplasma may produce an acute haemorrhagic leukoencephalitis. An immune reaction to measles may result in subacute sclerosing panencephalitis, a more insidious disorder
• Varicella zoster initial infection may cause an acute cerebellitis in children that is normally self-limiting

## CASE HISTORY 3

A 25-year-old woman has an upper respiratory tract infection. Following recovery she becomes obtunded over a period of 48 hours. On examination, she is apyrexial, gaze is incomitant and there is gaze evoked nystagmus. She requires intubation to protect the airway. In the limbs there is marked spasticity. CT shows effacement of cerebral sulci but it is safe to do a lumbar puncture. Lumbar puncture reveals 40 lymphocytes/mm$^3$. She is treated with aciclovir. A subsequent MRI scan reveals diffuse and confluent T2 hyperintensities in the periventricular white matter, in the brainstem and also within cerebral grey matter. She is treated with intravenous methylprednisolone followed by a course of oral steroids and makes a good recovery after several weeks, with some residual pyramidal gait difficulty.

### What has this patient got?

**Acute disseminated encephalomyelitis (ADEM).** This is considered to be a post-viral (sometimes post-mycoplasma), mainly white matter inflammatory condition, although the distinction from a direct viral encephalitis may be blurred. At the other end of the scale, the distinction from a severe initial attack of multiple sclerosis may be unclear; the latter attack is usually milder, more likely to be associated with CSF oligoclonal bands, and of course is characterized in retrospect with repeated attacks. However, treatment of both ADEM and multiple sclerosis attacks is similar, namely with high doses of steroids. Because of the nature of presentation of ADEM, antivirals are usually also given.

**GROUP 15:**

**ITEM 10:**

# Neurology
# Falls

### Information
- Steele-Richardson Syndrome
- Axial rigidity
- Dementia
- Defective up-and-lateral gaze and Parkinson's

## CASE HISTORY 1

A 70-year-old man presents with recurrent falls. On examination he has a rigid increase in tone worse in the trunk than the limbs, marked bradykinesia and extreme mental slowness. He walks with a rather upright gait. He is thought to have Parkinson's disease but has a poor response to levodopa.

### What is the diagnosis?

This man has **progressive supranuclear palsy (PSP – Steele-Richardson syndrome)**. Parkinson's disease usually results in falls late on in the disease. Early falls should lead to suspicion of PSP or multisystem atrophy (which does not cause early cognitive problems).

Some common causes of falls are listed below. Some simply relate to stance or gait difficulties.

### Causes of falls

- Preserved consciousness:
  - leg weakness
  - spasticity
  - extrapyramidal syndromes
  - ataxia, periodic ataxia
  - vertigo
  - drop attacks
  - cataplexy
  - epilepsy, myoclonus

- Loss of consciousness:
  - epilepsy
  - faint
  - syncope (cardiac or vascular insufficiency)
  - vertebrobasilar TIA, migraine
  - intermittent hydrocephalus
  - metabolic e.g. hypoglycaemia
  - toxic encephalopathy
  - other encephalopathies

## CASE HISTORY 2

A 40-year-old woman is worried she has epilepsy. She suffers repeated falls on walking outside. There is no warning before falling, she grazes her knees and hands and recovers immediately in a state of embarrassment. If she loses consciousness at all, it could only be for a split second because she is certainly aware when she hits the ground.

### What is the diagnosis?

The diagnosis is of drop attacks; these are benign episodes of uncertain aetiology that commonly occur in middle-aged to elderly women. There is no loss of consciousness and they are not considered epileptic (see Group 15, Item 13)

**GROUP 15:**

**ITEM 11:**

# Neurology
# Head injuries

### CASE HISTORY 1

A 25-year-old man is knocked unconscious by a blow from a sledgehammer. He regains consciousness after a few minutes and attends casualty. He is nauseated and in pain but reasonably alert with a Glasgow coma scale (GCS) of 14. A skull X-ray shows no skull fracture. After being reasonably well for many hours his conscious level rapidly deteriorates to a GCS of 5. A subsequent CT scan reveals a large extradural blood collection that requires emergency drainage by craniotomy.

**Extradural haemorrhage** is an important secondary effect of head injury. These bleeds occur into a tight space resulting in a rather long lucid interval as the blood slowly accumulates. CT reveals a convex hyperdense collection in the acute phase. In contrast, subdural haemorrhages bleed more freely into a more easily opened space so the shape is concave on CT and there is little lucid interval.

### Effects and complications of head injury

- Primary effects:
  - diffuse axonal injury
  - contusion
  - laceration
  - vascular lesions
- Secondary effects:
  - extradural haemorrhage
  - subdural haemorrhage
  - CSF leak, infection
  - hydrocephalus

**Remember**

- Always carefully monitor head injuries and record changes in GCS rather than simply considering one value in isolation.
- The result of secondary swelling by haemorrhage or oedema (latter common in children) is raised intracranial pressure (ICP) leading to reduced perfusion pressure and coning.

– compromised airway, respiration
– hypotension
• Late sequelae:
  – chronic daily headache
  – post traumatic stress disorder – rare
  – vertigo
  – cognitive impairment

**Table 15.11.1 Glasgow coma scale**

| | Score |
|---|---|
| **Eye opening (E)** | |
| Spontaneous | 4 |
| To speech | 3 |
| To pain | 2 |
| No response | 1 |
| **Motor response (M)** | |
| Obeys | 6 |
| Localises | 5 |
| Withdraws | 4 |
| Flexion | 3 |
| Extension | 2 |
| No response | 1 |
| **Verbal response (V)** | |
| Orientated | 5 |
| Confused conversation | 4 |
| Inappropriate words | 3 |
| Incomprehensible sounds | 2 |
| No response | 1 |

Glasgow Coma Scale = E+M+V
(GCS minimum = 3; maximum = 15)

**Information**

**Post-traumatic amnesia**
of over 24 hours indicates
severe brain injury

### What action would you take in a patient with a head injury?

• Attend first to any secondary or concomitant general problems ie resuscitation, correct hypovolaemic shock, hypotension or compromised airway
• Assess severity, using circumstances of injury and period of amnesia as a guide.
• Establish whether there is anterograde amnesia, the inability to form memories from the time of injury to the time of continuous normal memory, is the most accurate guide.
• Brainstem damage in head injury can affect central respiratory drive, bulbar function and pressor responses
• Regular GCS measurements; below 5 at 24 hours implies severe injury and 50% of such patients die
• Do CT scan

## How would you manage the following problems?

- If the patient is deteriorating, or has evidence of raised ICP. Consider insertion of a bolt which is simply a tube into the ventricle through which one can record ICP.
- If ICP >20mmHg, need to treat. Give enough mannitol iv to raise the plasma osmolality to 300. Mannitol also has poorly understood neuroprotective effects. Hyperventilation with IPPV will also lower the ICP.
- If the patient has haemorrhages. The definitive procedure is a craniotomy which, since the advent of CT making localization easy, is preferred to burr holes.

### Follow up

Check for continued improvement in the weeks subsequent to the head injury. At two to three weeks post injury, the development of hydrocephalus is an important complication.

## CASE HISTORY 2

A 30-year-old man falls from a second storey building and is immediately unconscious. He is admitted comatose, although he is breathing spontaneously. There are no external injuries and CT scan of the head is normal. He does not regain consciousness.

Diffuse axonal injury is the most important primary effect of head injury and a common cause of vegetative state. There is usually immediate LOC followed by prolonged coma.

Milder versions are reversible (called traumatic brain injury) and may be the basis of concussion. The injuries occur with brain accelerations or decelerations such as hitting the floor or wall rather than by a direct blow to the head. Certain areas are particularly vulnerable, such as the parasagittal white matter, internal capsule, cerebellar peduncles, posterior corpus callosum and dorsolateral midbrain. The mechanism of damage relates to stretch of axons causing $Ca^{++}$ entry and neurofilament damage, interrupting axonal transport over the next 12 hours. The changes are theoretically reversible in this period.

# Neurology
# Meningitis

## CASE HISTORY 1

A 55-year-old alcoholic is brought to A&E with headache, confusion and a high fever. He is found to be photophobic and have neck stiffness. He is thought by the casualty staff to have meningitis and is immediately given IV benzyl penicillin as they were unclear about the most likely organism.

You are called urgently to A&E.

**Remember**

CMO advice: give immediate penicillin if meningococcal meningitis suspected.

### What would you do?

You quickly check the neurological signs and agree this is meningitis. You also note that there is no purpuric rash of meningococcal septicaemia. You try and see his fundi but are unsure that papilloedema is present. You are worried about doing a lumbar puncture as he is semi-conscious and you are concerned about the possibility of 'coning'. You arrange an immediate CT scan which is normal. You proceed with a lumbar puncture and the CSF which is turbid is sent urgently to the microbiologists.

### What do you do next?

This man has meningitis , presumably bacterial. You re-check for purpuric spots of meningococcal meningitis.

The CSF results phoned through are:

- Protein 2g/l
- Glucose 1.5 mmol/l
- Leucocytes 500/mm$^3$
- Pneumococcus seen on Gram stain

**Other investigations**

- Blood culture
- CXR

Diagnosis:

**Pneumococcal meningitis**

You immediately start treatment with Cefotaxime as there is a high incidence of penicillin resistant pneumococcus. If there is raised intracranial pressure, mannitol and steroids are given. Get neurosurgical advice as ventricular pressure monitoring or shunting may be indicated. For other causes of meningitis – see below.

### Causes of Meningitis

- Bacterial:
  - meningococcus
  - pneumococcus
  - listeria
  - staphylococcus aureus
  - E.coli
  - pseudomonas
- Viral:
  - enteroviruses
  - mumps (meningoencephalitides)
- Atypical:
  - tuberculosis
  - cyptococcus
  - leptospirosis
- Non-infective:
  - subarachnoid haemorrhage
  - chemical meningitis
- Recurrent:
  - nasal sinus fistula
  - traumatic CSF leak
  - Epstein Barr virus
  - sarcoidosis, Behcet's
  - Mollaret's meningitis (?HSV type VI)
  - Vogt-Koyanagi-Harada syndrome

- **Pneumococcal meningitis** most commonly occurs in the debilitated or in those with a chest or sinus infection, valvular disease, splenectomy or a fistula from the paranasal air sinuses to the brain.
- **Meningococcal meningitis** (see also Group 1 Item 3) occurs in epidemics and is associated with a petechial or purpuric rash and very rapid evolution. It is seen in young adults. Nasopharyngeal swab culture is useful for typing meningococcus and haemophilus.
- **Staphylococcus aureus meningitis** generally occurs in the context of systemic infection, abscesses or neurosurgical procedures.
- **Pseudomonas** and other gram negative Enterobacillae are usually a consequence of surgical access to the CSF.
- **Listeria meningitis** is now quite common. It should be treated with ampicillin and gentamicin. It is also associated with an encephalitis.
- **Haemophilus Influenza** type B used to be extremely common but has been virually eliminated in the UK by immunisation (Hib vaccine) in children.

**Table 15.12.1 Treatment regimens**

**Antibiotics and Acute Bacterial Meningitis**

| Organism | 1st Choice | Alternative |
|---|---|---|
| Unknown | Cefotaxime | Benzylpenicillin and cefotaxime |
| Meningococcus | Benzylpenicillin | Cefotaxime |
| Pneumococcus | Cefotaxime | Penicillin if organism sensitive |
| Haemophilus | Cefotaxime | Chloramphenicol |
| Listeria | Amoxicillin + Gentamicin | |

This table shows the value of Cefotaxime in practice.

## CASE HISTORY 2

A 22-year-old Asian man is admitted from A&E with an insidious two-week history of malaise, headaches and marked confusion. On examination, he is pyrexial, drowsy, has neck stiffness and has upgoing plantar responses. A presumptive diagnosis of **tuberculous meningitis** is made.

### What action would you take?

- Routine blood tests
- CXR – important – may show evidence of TB
- CT scan – an immediate scan is done because with his confusion and possible raised intracranial pressure coning is a possibility following lumbar puncture
- Lumbar puncture

The CSF results phoned back to your house officer are:

- Glucose 1.8 mmol/l (blood level 6.5 ie low glucose)
- Protein 2.3 g/l (very high protein)
- 250 white cells (70% lymphocytes)

**Table 15.12.2 Typical changes in the CSF in meningitis**

| | Normal | Viral | Pyogenic | Tuberculosis |
|---|---|---|---|---|
| Appearance | Crystal-clear | Clear/turbid | Turbid/purulent | Turbid/viscous |
| Mononuclear cells | <5 mm$^3$ | 10-100 mm$^3$ | <50 mm$^3$ | 100-300mm$^3$ |
| Polymorph cells | Nil | Nil[a] | 200-300/mm$^3$ | 0-200/mm$^3$ |
| Protein | 0.2-0.4 g/l | 0.4-0.8 g/l | 0.5-2.0 g/l | 0.5-3.0 g/l |
| Glucose | 2/3 to 1/2 blood glucose | >1/2 blood glucose | <1/2 blood glucose | <1/3 blood glucose |

[a]Some polymorph cells may be seen in the early stages of viral meningitis and encephalitis

Reprinted from *Clinical Medicine*, 4th Edition, Kumar and Clark, 1998, by permission of the publisher WB Saunders

Note: the CSF protein can be so high as to cause the formation of a fine clot ('spider web')

Note: Tubercle bacilli are only occasionally seen in the CSF and the CSF must be sent for culture – which takes six weeks.

### How would you manage this case?

Start anti-TB chemotherapy in this case which strongly suggests tuberculous meningitis on the basis of the clinical picture and high protein in the CSF. Don't wait for the culture! Start quadruple therapy (rifampicin, isoniazid and pyrazinamide with pyridoxine cover together with ethambutol – see Group 11 item 11) for six weeks when culture and sensitivities are back: Four drugs should be given for three months followed by rifampicin and isoniazid for nine months. Specialist advice should be sought for treatment, notification and contact tracing.

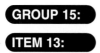

**GROUP 15:**
**ITEM 13:**

# Neurology
# Fits and faints

### CASE HISTORY 1

A 16-year-old girl is referred with a suspected seizure. Earlier that day in her office she had felt unwell for about an hour. On getting up from her chair she suddenly lost consciousness without warning. She was incontinent of urine. She woke some minutes later, but had nausea and malaise for the rest of the day. Witnesses said that when unconscious, she was flaccid, twitching her mouth, hands and feet and was pale.

### Is this a fit or a faint?

The patient has **suffered a faint**. Some factors are good at distinguishing fit from faint while others are unreliable. In the above case, it is noted that faints, other than cardiac syncope, only occur on standing; the preceding symptoms are prolonged or ill defined. Twitching is not usually as violent as in a clonic seizure and the underlying muscle tone is not increased.

**Table 15.13.1 Features of fits and faints**

| | Fit | Faint |
|---|---|---|
| Prodrome | none or characteristic brief aura | Short or prolonged. Blood draining, visual darkening, rushing noise. Cardiac syncope may have no prodrome |
| Posture at onset | Any | Standing unless cardiac |
| Injury | Common | Rarer. Protective reflexes may act. |
| Incontinence | Sometimes | Sometimes |
| Skin colour | Normal, flushed or pale | Pale |
| Recovery | Slow return of consciousness | Rapid, more physical weakness with clear sensorium |
| Frequency | Rare to many a day | Not repeated attacks each day |
| EEG | May be abnormal | Normal |

Vasovagal faints are generally idiopathic but there are often precipitating or predisposing factors.

### Associations with faints

• Adolescent, young adult female
• Low blood pressure
• Postural hypotension
• Heavy periods
• Micturition with prostatic problems
• Hot, stuffy surroundings
• Fasting, hypoglycaemia
• Dehydration
• Vagal stimuli such as distress or nausea

### Investigations

in suspected cardiac syncope include :
• ECG
• 24-hour ambulatory monitoring
• perhaps echocardiogram.

One must distinguish vasovagal attacks from cardiac syncope (Group 10 Item 1). In the latter there is often no warning, there may be breathlessness and engorged jugular veins and the heart rate may be faster than 140 or slower than 40.

### CASE HISTORY 2

A 16-year-old boy presents with repeated brief falls. He does not seem to lose consciousness but has been admitted to casualty several times with severe head and facial injuries resulting from these episodes. Recovery, apart from associated injury, is immediate.

### What is the diagnosis?

This history is suggestive of **atonic seizures**. This seizure disorder usually presents in childhood, often as one aspect of a complex epileptic syndrome. It is important to remember that not all seizures resulting in falls are generalized tonic-clonic in nature.

The loss of tone is immediate and absolute so that no protective reflexes occur and injury can be severe. Some sufferers need to wear crash helmets.

## Epilepsy

An epileptic seizure is a convulsion or transient abnormal event experienced by the subject as a result of a paroxysmal discharge of cerebral neurones. Epilepsy, by definition, is the continuing tendency to have such seizures. Recurrent seizures can be prevented in most cases by anteconvulsant drugs.

## CASE HISTORY 3

A 28 year old is brought to A&E as he was found to be unconscious and shaking in the High Street. You called to see him urgently as he has had a further tonic/clonic generalised seizure.

How would you manage this situation?

**Remember**

Status epilepticus exists when seizures follow each other without recovery of consciousness

### General measures

• Secure the airway; remove any false teeth and insert oropharyngeal tube
• Administer 60% oxygen
• Secure venous access: many anticonvulsants cause phlebitis, so choose a large vein
• Glucose, 50 ml of 20% i.v. if hypoglycaemia is a possibility (Group 14 Item 4)
• Thiamine, 250 mg by slow i.v. injection if patient is a chronic alcohol abuser.

### Control seizures

• Lorazepam 0.1 mg/kg by slow (2 mg/min) intravenous injection. Give rectal diazepam (10-20 mg) or intramuscular midazolm (0.2 mg/kg) if intravenous access difficult
• If seizures continue give i.v. phenytoin;
*Phenytoin* Loading dose of 15 mg/kg at a rate not exceeding 50 mg/min. Give a further bolus up to total loading dose of 30 mg/kg if seizures persist. Continue with a maintenence dose of 100 mg i.v. at intervals of 6–8 hours; if seizures continue (despite phenytoin)

**Remember**

Full ventilatory support must be avaiable when treating status epilepticus

use:
*Phenobarbitone* 15 mg/kg at a rate not exceeding 100 mg/min and repeated at intervals of 6–8 hours if necessary.
*Chlormethiazole* (o.8%) 40–120 mg/min (15–15 ml) up to a maximum total dose of 320–800 mg to control seizures, followed by a continuous infusion at the lowest dose required to control seizures, usually 4–8 mg/min, is occasionally used
• If seizures continue despite these measures the patient is given a general anaesthetic, such as thiopentone or propofol, and management is continued with full anaesthetic support.

### Investigations

Serum anticonvulsant levels, blood glucose, serum electrolytes including calcium and magnesium. Consider brain CT scan, lumbar puncture and blood cultures, depending on clinical circumstances.

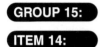

## GROUP 15:
## ITEM 14:

# Neurology
# Difficulty in walking

### CASE HISTORY 1

A 75-year-old man is referred with progressive difficulty with his walking over one year. He is hypertensive. On examination, he has cognitive deficit of frontal type, primitive grasp and snout reflexes and rather stiff, awkward legs when tested on the couch. His gait is upright, with difficulty getting started and short and high steps.

**An apraxic gait** is typical of frontal lobe pathology and can be regarded as a problem with high level programming and execution of gait. It is often related to cerebrovascular disease but one should always image these patients to exclude a frontal meningioma or other lesion. The only treatment is that for underlying cerebrovascular disease.

### CASE HISTORY 2

A 70-year-old woman has a three-week history of progressive difficulty walking and loss of bladder function. This is set against a background of milder problems with a stiff gait, numbness in the feet and pains down the left arm. On examination she has wasting and weakness of the hands and brisk triceps reflexes. In the legs there is a pyramidal distribution weakness, brisk reflexes, upgoing plantars and patchy sensory loss. She cannot walk at all.

### What is the diagnosis?

**Cervical myelopathy**, most commonly at this age due to spondylosis. She requires urgent imaging (MRI) of her cervical spine with a view to early decompression because relatively acute deficits are more potentially reversible. Sometimes steroids are given in the acute stage to reduce cord oedema.

Walking difficulties with upper motor signs in the legs should always be investigated by cervical imaging. Thoracic compression is relatively much less common in the elderly age group.

Other causes of difficulty in walking are listed below. (See also Group 15 Item 17)

> ⚠️
> **Remember**
> Lumbar spine imaging is inappropriate because the spinal cord ends at T12 and root disease gives lower motor neurone signs.

### Common causes of gait difficulty

**Neurological:**
- Myopathy – proximal, Trendelenburg positive, worse on stairs
- neuropathy – foot drop
- extrapyramidal – e.g. shuffling, stooped
- spasticity – stiff, circumducting hip
- apraxic – upright, high stepping
- ataxic – wide based

**Rheumatological/orthopaedic**
- ischaemic
- hysterical

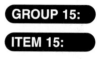

# Neurology
# Headaches

### CASE HISTORY 1

A 35-year-old woman is admitted with very severe headache of explosive onset. She is slightly drowsy and has photophobia and meningism. A CT scan is normal. Lumbar puncture is then performed and this shows no red cells in the CSF. An MR angiogram is then performed and this shows a saccular berry aneurysm in the right middle cerebral artery.

**Subarachnoid haemorrhage** presents with extremely sudden onset headache. CT scan and lumbar puncture do not have perfect sensitivity so a suspicious history alone may be grounds for going on to MR angiography, a risk-free investigation. A bloody tap may be more easily distinguished from subarachnoid haemorrhage if the CSF is taken more than 12 hours after onset of headache because beyond this time subarachnoid haemorrhage will have often resulted in xanthochromia. A bloody tap may also result in RBC-containing CSF on a subsequent collection.

### Action

- Formal intraarterial angiography is generally required preoperatively. Occasionally vasospasm may hide the aneurysm so the angiogram may be repeated after several days if negative, especially if the site of bleeding on CT scanning is suggestive of an aneurysm of the anterior circulation
- Careful monitoring for deterioration in conscious level, evidence of coning, focal deficits

- ECG monitoring may be indicated because of the increased risk of cardiac arrhythmias
- One may give an antispasmodic agent, but at the same time adequate perfusion must be maintained. (Raised blood pressure is a physiological response to maintain perfusion to the brain.) Nimodipine is recommended but low blood pressure should be avoided
- If sudden deterioration, hyperventilation, oxygen and mannitol may be appropriate while surgery is arranged urgently
- Some neurosurgeons prefer to operate (clipping the aneurysm) early while others delay by several days if the patient is stable because early surgery may lead to increased risk of cerebral ischaemia from vasospasm
- Postoperatively, particular attention is directed toward maintaining blood pressure and perfusion.

**Remember**

If a close family member has also had subarachnoid haemorrhage, then the rest of the family should be screened by MR angiography

Conditions which can mimic subarachnoid haemorrhage include sudden onset of meningitis or viral meningism, migraine, spontaneous subdural haemorrhage and coital headache. The last of these is a headache of very sudden onset but is a benign self-limiting condition, perhaps a variant of migraine. With the availability of MR angiography, patients are now often scanned to exclude aneurysms. Finally low pressure headache may be of sudden onset. This is a poorly understood condition where headache may occur suddenly on standing and generally settles when lying down. There is meningeal enhancement on MRI and a low CSF pressure. The condition is again self-limiting. At least some cases relate to CSF leaks, sometimes from lumbar puncture (post-lumbar puncture headache), occasionally from Valsalva manoeuvres.

## CASE HISTORY 2

A 35-year-old man complains of continuous headache day and night. He used to have a different headache that was episodic. This previous headache was unilateral, throbbing, and would last a few hours and was also associated with photophobia, visual scotomata and nausea. The new headache has no such features. He has to take about eight coproxamol tablets a day to control the pain.

### What is this new headache due to?

**Migraine headache**, which is clearly the nature of this man's original headache, sometimes becomes transformed into a more chronic headache punctuated by migraine-like exacerbations. Often the patient is given regular analgesia which has a well-known effect of actually perpetuating headache.

## What action should you take?

A brain scan is not often necessary in a clearly chronic headache with no signs, although the patient often seems to expect one. It is far more important to take a proper history and institute the correct management.

The patient can be reassured that he does not have malignant disease.

Chronic analgesia abuse should be stopped. This is best done gradually over a month and the patient can expect to be worse over this period. A migraine prophylactic agent should be given, such as amitriptyline, pizotifen, propranolol, gabapentin or sodium valproate.

## Management

Broadly similar for episodic migraine, i.e. sumatriptan prophylactics are given if the sufferer has more than about two migraines a month or finds then very debilitating.

## CASE HISTORY 3

A 40-year-old man comes to A&E with severe headache which then settles on arrival. This has happened before and he has always been immediately discharged. On taking a history, it transpires that he gets an excruciating headache coming on gradually at about the same time every day. The headache is unilateral, pounding, involves the side of the face and is associated with a watering eye and nose. He jumps up and down in agitation with the pain. The symptoms generally only last about an hour.

## What is the cause of this headache?

This description is typical for **cluster headache**. Each cluster may last a few weeks with several months of relief in between. Treatment is similar to that for migraine, but is generally less effective. Verapamil is said to be relatively more effective. Sometimes lithium or a course of high dose steroids may be tried for a severe cluster. For individual attacks, as well as triptans, breathing of 100% oxygen may be helpful and intramuscular opiates may be indicated in desperately severe attacks.

## CASE HISTORY 4

A 30-year-old woman has a long history of short but severe headaches on the side of the face lasting only a few minutes but occurring several times a day. There is considerable flushing and rhinorrhoea on the same side during each attack. There is no trigger to the attacks.

***

*i*

**Information**

For migrainous exacerbations, the patient can have a supply of a triptan drug, perhaps with an antiemetic.

### What is the cause of this headache?

The patient has **paroxysmal hemicrania**; the attacks are longer in duration than in trigeminal neuralgia but shorter than in cluster headaches or migraine. There is generally some associated autonomic disturbance. The important aspect of the condition is that there is a specific and often extremely rewarding response to indomethacin.

Some causes of acute, episodic and chronic and headache are listed below.

### Common causes of headache

• Acute:
  – subarachnoid haemorrhage
  – subdural haemorrhage
  – meningitis, encephalitis
  – inflammatory meningoencephalitis e.g. SLE
  – cerebral abscess
  – first migraine attack
  – coital headache
  – raised intracranial pressure
  – low pressure headache

• Episodic:
  – tension headache
  – migraine
  – paroxysmal hemicrania
  – cluster headache
  – trigeminal/occipital neuralgia

• Chronic:
  – tension headache
  – analgesia abuse
  – chronic hemicrania
  – chronic cluster headache
  – cervicogenic headache
  – Space occupying lesions
  – Raised intracranial pressure
  – Ongoing after many acute headaches
  – Psychiatric

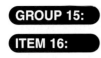

| GROUP 15: | **Neurology** |
|---|---|
| ITEM 16: | **Severe brain injury** |

### CASE HISTORY 1

Your patient has had a severe anoxic cerebral insult and is currently stable but comatose requiring ventilatory support on ITU. The ITU staff and the patient's relatives want an indication as to the likelihood of useful recovery.

### What action would you take?

It is most important to check for a remediable cause of coma or any confounding factors worsening the patient's responsiveness (see box). For example:

- Brain imaging may reveal a potentially treatable but unsuspected condition, possibly additional to the primary pathology, such as subdural or intracerebral haemorrhage, hydrocephalus or cerebral abscess
- An EEG may show abnormalities indicative of a unsuspected metabolic encephalopathy or subclinical seizure activity
- The patient may still be under the influence of long-acting anaesthetic agents or other sedative drugs

### Investigations

- Brain imaging
- EEG
- Recent drug history
- Check not still anaesthetized
- Electrolyte imbalance
- Sepsis
- Ongoing low cardiac output

### Aspects of examination to assess routinely

- Response to command, sound
- Response to visual menace
- Eye movements:
  - following, roving conjugate
  - optokinetic nystagmus (following a moving grid pattern)
  - vertical and horizontal Doll's head
  - any eye opening
- Pupils
- Corneal reflexes
- Bulbar function – ?tolerating the ET tube
- Respiratory function – level of ventilator support
- Spontaneous limb movements
- Limb movements to pain (localizing, withdrawal, extensor)
- Tone and reflexes
- General examination eg chest, infected pressure sores, abdominal guarding

### What are your prognostic indicators?

There are some clear prognostic values, depending on the time after the initial cerebral insult

**Table 15.16.1 Prognostic indicators for recovery at one year after hypoxic-ischaemic brain injury (Levy et al. (1985). JAMA 253, 1420)**

|  | Chance of moderate/good recovery |
|---|---|
| **On initial examination:** | |
| Absent pupil reflexes | 0% (0-7) |
| Pupils react but no motor response | 6% (2-16) |
| **At one day:** | |
| No withdrawal motor response nor spontaneous roving conjugate eye movements | 1% (0-6) |
| No withdrawal motor response but makes roving conjugate eye movements (or better) | 9% (1-29) |
| **At three days:** | |
| No withdrawal motor response | 0% (0-5) |
| **At one week:** | |
| Cannot obey commands nor make roving eye movements | 0% (0-26) |
| **At two weeks:** | |
| Defective dollís eye movements, but can obey commands or open eyes spontaneously or good improvement in eye opening | 22% (6-48) |
| If none of the above | 0% (0-20) |
| If normal doll's eye movements | 81% (61-93) |

Bracketed figures indicate 95% confidence intervals

Redrawn from *Clinical Medicine*, 4th Edition, Kumar and Clark, 1998, by permission of the publisher WB Saunders

In general, every case must be assessed on its merits, especially with regard to the nature of the original insult and whether it was a discrete event or likely to be resulting in ongoing brain injury.

Note: Relatives should not be given conflicting or inaccurate information.

**Beware:**

Determination of brain death is made only by the appropriate consultant specialists who assess on separate occasions various brainstem reflexes and responses listed under 'Aspects of examination'. The nature of the insult must be clear and remediable causes must be excluded. Since the criteria for brain death are heavily weighted towards brainstem function and, in the UK, EEG corroboration is not required, it is important to exclude locked-in syndrome. In this state, a severe pontine lesion prevents access to or from the outside world. The only signs of relatively spared higher level function may be preserved vertical optokinetic nystagmus or eye following and preserved vertical doll's eye reflexes. *(See also Kumar & Clark 4th Edition p858.)*

**Table 15.16.2 Differentiation of persistent vegetative state from other forms of unresponsiveness**

*(Modified from Journal of the Royal College of Physicians of London 30: 119-121 (1996))*

| Condition | Vegetative state | Locked-in syndrome | Coma | Brainstem death |
|---|---|---|---|---|
| Self-awareness | Absent | Present | Absent | Absent |
| Cyclical eye opening | Present | Present | Absent | Absent |
| Glasgow coma Scale | E4, M1-4, V1 | E4, M1, V1 | E1-2, M1-4, V1-2 | E1, M1-2, V1 |
| Motor function | No purposeful movement | Eye movement preserved in the vertical plane and able to blink volitionally | No purposeful movement | None or only reflex spinal movement |
| Perception of pain | No | Yes | No | No |
| Respiratory function | Normal | Normal | Depressed or varied | Absent |
| EEG activity | Polymorphic delta or theta: sometimes slow alpha waves | Normal or minimally abnormal | Polymorphic delta or theta waves; though sometimes silent | Electrocerebral silence or theta waves |
| Cerebral metabolism | Reduced by 50% or more | Minimally or moderately reduced | Reduced by 50% or more | Absent or greatly reduced |
| Prognosis | Depends on cause and length | Depends on cause though recovery unlikely | Recovery, vegetative state, or death within two to four weeks | No recovery |

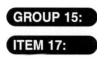

# Neurology
# Movement disorders

### CASE HISTORY 1

A 22-year-old woman develops an acute gastrointestinal illness with abdominal pain, vomiting and diarrhoea. After two days she becomes generally stiff and has prolonged episodes of painful spasm of the axial muscles with opisthotonic posturing. Her eyes periodically roll upwards involuntarily. She had been given metoclopramide for the vomiting symptoms.

**Oculogyric crises and acute dystonic reactions** can occasionally occur in sensitive individuals after relatively modest doses of drugs with central antidopaminergic action, such as neuroleptics or certain antiemetics e.g. metoclopramide. Neuroleptic malignant syndrome can also occur.

Treatment of oculogyric crisis involves identification of and stopping the responsible agent and, in serious cases, intravenous centrally acting anticholinergics may be given, e.g. procyclidine 5 – 10 mg.

Antipsychotic drugs with relatively few antidopaminergic side effects include sulpiride, olanzepine, sertindole. Suitable antiemetics in similar situations include domperidone and ondansetron or granesetron.

### Hypokinetic movement disorders

• Parkinson's disease
• Multisystem atrophy
• Progressive supranuclear palsy
• Dementia with Lewy bodies
• Corticobasal degeneration
• Some frontal dementias, mass lesions
• Tardive dyskinesia (+hyperkinetic)
• Psychomotor retardation

### Hyperkinetic movement disorder

• Choreoathetosis
• Ballismus
• Dystonia
• Myoclonus
• Tics
• Tremor
• Psychogenic

## CASE HISTORY 2

A 40-year-old man has a one-year history of involuntary facial movements and a shuffling gait. There is a past history of schizophrenia for which he was given haloperidol. On examination, he has intermittent involuntary protrusion of his tongue, grimacing and blepharospasm. He has some writhing movements of his left arm and repetitive rubbing of the soles of his feet on the floor when sitting. Voluntary arm movements are slow. He walks slowly with a shuffling gait and stooped posture.

**Tardive dyskinesia** may develop in patients previously, as well as currently, on antipsychotic medication. The movement disorder may be a complex mixture of hyperkinetic restlessness (akathisia), dystonia and choreoathetosis, and hypokinetic bradykinesia. They are late and difficult to reverse. The effects of antidopaminergics are thought to be due to long-term dysregulation of dopaminergic pathways. The immediate effects that sometimes also occur are more reversible (case 1). Sometimes, in the short term, increases in antipsychotic drug doses actually temporarily improve the hyperkinetic aspects (direct antidopaminergic action), but this is likely to lead to worsened long term problems. The drugs that are good for avoiding acute extrapyramidal side effects (case 1) are also good for minimizing long-term side-effects.

# Notes

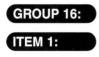

**GROUP 16:**   Psychiatry

**ITEM 1:**   Delirium

Delirium is the most commonly misdiagnosed psychiatric disorder in the general hospital. Yet it is the commonest psychosis met in this setting. Ten to 20% of surgical and medical inpatients have delirium during their admission. It is the best indication that the higher centres of the brain are failing.

### How would you recognise delirium?

The primary feature is disorientation in time and place (very rarely person). A well patient should know the day of the week, month and year (people who are well can occasionally get the date and time wrong). They should know the ward name and that they are in a hospital and its name and place. Other psychoses do not affect orientation.

- **'Clouding of consciousness'**
  Refers to the variable level of attention seen in delirium, so that the patient cannot learn information and therefore cannot recall it.

- **Visual hallucinations or illusions**
  Are commonly present, so the patient may mistake a curtain movement in a dimly lit ward as a threatening person causing extreme fear and agitation, especially at night.

- **Persecutory delusions**
  Are most common, which may make the patient refuse food, drink and medicines because they believe that they are being poisoned. Alternatively, these delusions may cause aggression as the patient defends themselves against a perceived threat.

**Remember**

The mental picture will change throughout the day. Commonly patients will be sleepy by day and awake all night.

### What are the predisposing factors?

Delirium occurs most commonly in a person with a developing or deteriorating brain, with predisposing factors such as:

- Extremes of age (the young and old)
- Damaged brain
- Any dementia (most common)
- Previous head injury
- Previous cerebro-vascular accident
- Alcoholic brain damage
- Dislocation to an unfamiliar environment (such as admission to hospital)
- Sleep deprivation
- Sensory extremes (overload or deprivation)
- Immobilisation

**Aetiology**

Primary brain diseases

Systemic diseases affecting the brain

Intoxication (drugs and poisons)

Drug withdrawal

Metabolic

## Dividing these causes into pathological entities:

- Drugs and poisons (see Group 16, Item 2)
- Withdrawal from drugs (e.g. alcohol and sedatives; see Group 16, Items 2, 4 & 5)
- Infections (intracranial and systemic)
- Metabolic encephalopathies (e.g. hypoglycaemia, hypoxia, hyponatraemia)
- Brain trauma
- Epilepsy (ictal, interictal, postictal)
- Neoplasm (intracranial or extracranial)
- Other brain-space occupying lesions (e.g. abscess)
- Vascular (cerebral or myocardial)
- Haematological (severe anaemia)
- Extracranial insult (hypothermia)

## How would you investigate?

Corroborative history from family/partner (duration of history, drug history, past medical and psychiatric history, alcohol/drug misuse)

An EEG shows excess slow waves in 90% (with the exception of drug withdrawal states), and may show sharp waves and spikes in status epilepticus. It can be a confirmatory test, if there is doubt about the clinical diagnosis.

## Nursing management

- Single room, if disturbed
- Windows that do not allow exits
- Minimal stimulation by noise
- Persistent orientation by nurses and notices (a very disturbed patient may require one-to-one nursing temporarily)
- Minimal visitors – only those the patient knows well
- Some lighting at night
- Reverse dehydration and do not neglect nutrition
- Treat constipation
- Perceptive aids
  Glasses
  Hearing aids

## Investigations

- Look for infections (MSU, CXR, blood and sputum cultures, lumbar puncture if indicated)
- U&Es (hyponatraemia)
- Calcium
- Blood sugar
- Liver and cardiac enzymes
- ECG (silent myocardial infarct)
- CT brain scan ("silent" parietal infarct; predisposing brain disease/damage)

## Second-line investigations

- Therapeutic drug levels (anticonvulsant, lithium)
- Endocrine (TFTs)
- Vitamin deficiency
- Illicit drug screen

## Management

Find the cause and reverse it.

A psychiatric opinion can be useful regarding differential diagnosis and management.

Reduce all drug treatments to a minimum (see section Group 16, Item 2). Avoid antipsychotic drugs unless the patient is a danger to themselves or others, or is distressed. Symptomatic treatments include antipsychotic drugs, initially in small doses, avoiding strong anticholinergics.

## How would you treat delirium symptomatically? (Note, not involving a drug withdrawal or an anticholinergic induced delirium)?

All doses should start low and be titrated depending on age (the doses below are for a non-elderly adult), pre-existing brain damage and response to initial treatment.

- Phenothiazines (with the exception of thioridazine) are best avoided because of their anticholinergic and alpha-blocking actions.
- Haloperidol 1.5 mg stat; 1.5 – 10 mg x3 (liquid or tablet form; beware extrapyramidal side effects)
- Thioridazine 10-25 mg stat; 10 -50 mgm x3 (syrup, suspension or tablet)

## If intramuscular medication is required

- Haloperidol 5–10 mg stat
- Droperidol 5–10 mg stat
- Repeat after one hour if indicated

Almost never give these drugs intravenously. Avoid giving benzodiazepines, unless treating delirium tremens (Group 16, Item 4), or when delirium is due to benzodiazepine withdrawal. If extrapyramidal side effects are likely or present, consider changing to a newer antipsychotic drug, such as risperidone or olanzapine. Once delirium is resolved, tail off antipsychotic medication gradually over one week or so.

## How do you 'section' a patient?

Advice from a psychiatrist should be taken if the patient does not consent to investigation or treatment, to consider 'sectioning' under the Mental Health Act, which might allow treatment to proceed without the patient's consent (see Kumar & Clark, 4th Ed. page. 1146).

## What is the prognosis?

There is often a delay of a few days when the underlying condition has improved, but the brain is still dysfunctioning. Otherwise the prognosis depends on the successful treatment of the main aetiological condition and the state of the pre-existing brain (25% of the elderly with delirium will have an underlying dementia).

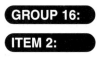

## Psychiatry
## Drugs and poisons as causes of delirium

Delirium can occur in response to excessive or normal doses of many drugs, particularly in the elderly. Some drugs are more likely to cause delirium than others. Drugs with anticholinergic properties are the most likely of all drugs to cause delirium. Anticholinergic delirium is important to diagnose since its treatment is specific to the cause.

### Anticholinergic drugs
- Atropine and Scopolamine (remember eye drops and pre-meds in anaesthesia)
- Other topical cyclopegics and mydriatics
- Antiparkinsonian agents (in both patients with Parkinson's disease and Pseudo-Parkinson's caused by dopamine antagonists.
- Antidepressants (especially tricyclics; amitriptyline most frequently)
- Antipsychotics (commonly the phenothiazines, especially chlorpromazine)
- Antiemetics
- Antihistamines
- Antispasmodics (uncommon)

### What are the physical signs of the anticholinergic state?
- Dilated and poorly reactive pupils (blurred vision)
- Flushed face
- Dry mouth and skin
- Fever
- Tachypnoea
- Tachycardia
- Hypertension
- Urinary retention and diminished bowel sounds

### How would you treat anticholinergic induced delirium?

Oral or intramuscular diazepam (10mg in the adult) can relieve the agitation, and may be all the specific treatment that is required.

Exclude patients with contra-indications of cholinergic therapy (e.g. ischaemic heart disease, asthma, diabetes mellitus, inflammatory bowel disease, bowel or bladder obstruction, glaucoma, pregnancy, hypothyroidism).

• Carefully evaluate and monitor vital signs and mental state
• Intramuscular or sub-cutaneous physostigmine (cholinesterase inhibitor) 1-2 mg (adult dose)
• Observe for cholinergic signs (miosis, sweating, salivation, bradycardia, lachrymation). If noted, review diagnosis
• Repeat physostigmine administration if necessary (two-hourly)

Beware: Cholinergic syndrome and toxicity (heart block, bronchospasm, respiratory failure); have atropine available.

**Remember**
Check doses with a senior and British National Formulary

### Other drugs causing delirium

**Therapeutic drugs affecting the brain**

• Benzodiazepines (although withdrawal is a more common cause; see below)
• Barbiturates (withdrawal again more commonly)
• Other hypnotics (chloral hydrate)
• Lithium (usually a sign of toxicity)
• Anticonvulsants (usually a sign of toxicity)
• Dopamine and its agonists (Levodopa and bromocriptine)

**Cardiac Drugs**

• Digoxin (check level)
• Calcium channel blockers
• Antiarrhythmics (lignocaine)
• Betablockers (especially propranolol; use cardioselective blockers)

**Antibiotics**

• Antimalarials (quinacrine, chloroquine and mefloquine)
• Antibiotics (uncommon)
• Associated diarrhoea (leading to dehydration)

**Gastro-intestinal drugs**

• $H_2$ antagonists (cimetidine most commonly reported)
• Bismuth

**Anti-inflammatory**

• Nonsteroidal anti-inflammatories (NSAIDs)
• Corticosteroids (differential diagnosis of affective and paranoid psychoses)
• Interferons

**Chemotherapeutic agents**

• L-Asparaginase
• Methotrexate
• Vincristine

**Anaesthetic agents**

• Ketamine

**'Recreational' drugs**

• Alcohol (toxic levels)
• Amphetamine
• Ecstasy (Methylene dioxymethamphetamine, MDMA; an amphetamine like drug)
• Lysergic acid (LSD) and other hallucinogens (magic mushrooms)
• Cannabis (toxic doses)
• Cocaine
• Phencyclidine ("Angel dust"; chemically related to ketamine)

**Poisons**

Exposure may be occupational, environmental or by deliberate self-ingestion. The following are some of the most commonly seen in this country:

• Methanol (rough sleepers)
• Solvents (adolescents)
• Carbon monoxide
• Plant alkaloids
• Many industrial chemicals (always find out the occupation)

### How do you treat drug/poison induced delirium?

Stop the delivery of the drug or poison. If in doubt, stop all non-essential medication, and/or reduce the dose.

There are some specific treatments (e.g. Hyperbaric or mask-delivered oxygen for CO poisoning).

General measures are covered in the section on delirium ( Group 16, Item 1)

### Drug Withdrawal

- Alcohol (see Group 16, Item 4)
- Sedatives
  - benzodiazepines
  - barbiturates

### Clinical presentation of sedative withdrawal (beyond delirium)

- Mental – Anxiety, irritability, agitation, insomnia, nightmares
- Arousal – Tremor, sweating, tachycardia, sensitivity to light, noise and touch, muscle tension, uncommonly convulsions (with the exception of barbiturate withdrawal)
- Physical – Nausea, anorexia , 'flu-like' symptoms, metallic taste

### Treatment of sedative withdrawal

- Replace the original class of drug in adequate doses
- Try to use a long-acting drug (e.g. diazepam), but sometimes the original drug itself is required
- Therapeutic drug cessation can be achieved gradually later, but the patient should be closely monitored and supported

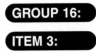

## Psychiatry
## Dementia

*(see also Group 7, Item 4)*

Dementia is the commonest organic brain syndrome seen in elderly inpatients. Seven per cent of people over the age of 65, and 20% over the age of 80 have a dementing illness. Treatable causes can be found in 10% of patients with definite dementia, but that figure is considerably higher if the pseudodementia of depressive illness is included.

Dementia is a global acquired progressive deterioration of intellect, memory, and personality. Altered ('clouded') consciousness is not usually involved, in contrast to delirium, although dementia is often an underlying predisposition for delirium, (see Group 16, Item 1)

### How does dementia present?

- Loss of memory, especially short term
- Episodes of increasing "confusion"
- Falls, with or without head injury
- Wandering and getting lost (getting into the wrong bed), especially at night
- Insomnia
- Weight loss
- Slow recovery and mobilisation after injury (hip fracture) or illness (myocardial infarct, pneumonia)
- Incontinence
- Difficulty dressing (parietal lesion of dressing dyspraxia)
- Behavioural disinhibition (frontal lobe sign)
- Severe extra pyramidal reaction to dopamine antagonists (Lewy body dementia)

### What are the causes?

The commonest causes in the over 65s are Alzheimer's disease, multi-infarct dementia, Lewy body disease, and Parkinson's disease. Below 65 consider AIDS and alcohol. Less common causes include prion diseases (Creutzfeldt-Jakob), Huntington's, frontotemporal dementia (Pick's).

### Examination

Cardiovascular, neurological and endocrine system to exclude secondary causes

Depressed affect

Simple cognitive screening bed-side tests

**Investigations**

- A corroborative history (duration, presentation, mood, alcohol, past history)
- Mini Mental State Examination (a simple bed-side screening test of memory (see Group 7, Item 4)
- Intelligence Quotient (IQ) (performed by a psychologist) to confirm cognitive decline
- Blood tests
  - gamma Glutamyl transpeptidase and mean corpuscular volume (evidence of excess alcohol)
  - urea and creatinine
  - liver enzymes
  - free T4 and TSH
  - VDRL
  - haemoglobin
  - ESR or CRP
  - auto-immune screen to include ANA
  - serum electrophoresis
  - BSL
  - B12 and red cell folate
  - calcium
- HIV testing after counselling in at-risk group
- MSU
- CXR
- CT brain scan (tumour, sub-dural haematoma, normal pressure hydrocephalus and infarcts; confirms generalised cerebral atrophy)
- ECG (arrhythmias)
- EEG (diffuse slow waves are rare before 75 in normal health. A normal EEG would suggest an alternative diagnosis)
- Consider lumbar puncture, if diagnosis is unclear

- Orientation in place and person
- Attention and concentration: Ask the patient to recite the days of the week, or the months of the year, backwards (should be 100% accurate)
- Verbal short-term memory: Teach patient to immediately recite a name and address accurately (a test of registration: they should be able to do this in two attempts). Then ask them to recall the name and address five minutes later (test of memory recall; they should recall 95% of the individual items)
- Premorbid intelligence: (necessary to judge whether there has been a deterioration in intellect). Ask level of education achieved and occupation

## How would you manage a case of dementia?

- Treat any reversible cause
- Stop anticholinergic drugs, if possible
- Involve a psychiatrist early regarding diagnosis and management
- Cholinergic therapy may be indicated in early Alzheimer's disease, e.g. donepezil
- Low dose haloperidol can help agitation and any accompanying delusions
- Short-acting hypnotics, such as temazepam, can help insomnia
- While on the ward, ensure adequate fluids, nutrition and treatment of constipation and any other reversible causes of incontinence
- If possible, discharge home as soon as possible to avoid disorientating experience of admission
- Involve the nearest relatives only.

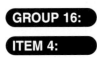

## GROUP 16:
## ITEM 4:

# Psychiatry
# Delirium tremens (DT)

Delirium tremens is the most severe form of alcohol withdrawal syndrome, and is a medical emergency because of the significant complications that can arise. It often occurs on the second or third day after admission, due to suddenly stopping drinking, although it can occur after a significant reduction in drinking.

## CASE HISTORY

A 49-year-old man was admitted via A&E to the orthopaedic ward having had a fall and fractured his pelvis. On the third day after admission he became disorientated and restless with visual hallucinations. The orthopaedic SHO wants your advice.

A full history elicits that he had been a heavy drinker for 10 or more years and obviously had had no alcohol since the fall. You think he has DTs – particularly as he had had a similar episode in the past.

## Remember

Complications of DTs
- Co-morbid illness or trauma (infection, dehydration, head injury)
- Hypoglycaemia
- Electrolyte disturbances (sodium, potassium, magnesium)
- Co-morbid encephalopathy (Wernicke/Korsakoff's)
- Convulsions
- Coma
- Death

### What are the clinical features of DTs?
- Coarse tremor (which may affect the whole body)
- Disorientation in place and time
- Anxiety (often severe)
- Motor restlessness
- Nausea and/or diarrhoea
- Insomnia
- Nightmares
- Excessive sympathetic drive
  – sweating
  – tachycardia
  – hypertension
  – low grade fever
- Reduced attention
- Illusions (visual)
- Hallucinations (classically visual, but may be tactile or auditory; small animals [insects, spiders, rats] advance menacingly towards and over the patient)
- Persecutory delusions

### How would you treat DTs?

• Admit the patient to an acute medical bed
• General measures (see section on delirium, Group 16, Item 1)
• Particularly treat electrolyte and fluid imbalances
• Treat any co-morbid disorder
• Oral thiamine 200 mgm daily even in the absence of Wernicke/Korsakoff encephalopathy.
• Parenteral high dose thiamine is necessary in the presence of a thiamine related encephalopathy

---

**Investigations**

• Serum urea and electrolytes (especially hypokalaemia)
• Calcium and magnesium
• Gamma glutamyl transpeptidase
• Aspartate transferase
• Bilirubin
• Glucose
• Haemoglobin
• Mean corpuscular volume
• Mid stream urine
• If necessary, appropriate x-rays to exclude infection (CXR) and trauma (CT brain scan if indicated: ?sub-dural)

---

### Specific drug therapy

Follow a protocol if your hospital has one.

Oral treatment is preferred unless the patient is severely distressed and disturbed. Doses suggested below may not be adequate to control the initial condition, and more may be required.

Diazepam 20 mgm x4 orally; or
Chlordiazepoxide 20 mgm x4 orally; or
Chlormethiazole 1-2 capsules x4 orally is used in some centres, but this drug can cause significant problems with dependence and adverse effects.

Slow intravenous infusion of 0.8 % solution of chlormethiazole is employed in some centres for the acutely distressed patient. Great care should be taken to avoid oversedation, hypotension and respiratory depression in this situation. The patient must be constantly monitored and resuscitation facilities must be available.

Prophylactic anticonvulsants (phenytoin or carbamazepine) should be given when there is a previous history of withdrawal convulsions.

If the patient has improved after two or three days of this treatment, the dose of the antidelirious medication should be tapered to nothing over the next seven days, depending on clinical response. More gradual tapering should occur with a history of convulsions.

### Long-term care

This primarily involves maintaining abstenance from alchohol. Acamprosate (Group 5, Item 7) has been shown to be helpful.

**GROUP 16:**

**ITEM 5:**

# Psychiatry
# Acute depression

*(see also Group 7, Item 5)*

Depressive illness is common. It is an important condition to recognise since it often goes undetected or inadequately treated. The central symptom is most often low mood. This is accompanied by a number of associated symptoms reflecting the impact of the condition on an individual's behaviour, thinking and perception. These symptoms become more marked as the severity of the condition increases.

Much depressive illness has an insidious onset and may never reach the attention of acute medical or specialist services.

### Acute presentations of depression can be associated with:

- Suicide attempt (see Group 16, Item 6)
- Concurrent physical illness
- Weight loss
- Self neglect
- Behavioural change with functional impairment at work, home or socially
- Uncharacteristic behaviour (e.g. the onset of heavy drinking, shop-lifting in the elderly)
- Development of psychotic symptoms

### CASE HISTORY

A 66-year-old woman is admitted to a medical ward for investigation of anaemia. Her husband died six months previously. The ward nurses have noted that she has been despondent, reluctant to care for herself and her nutritional intake has been poor. You suspect she may have a **depressive illness.**

### How would you assess this case?

- Accurate diagnosis requires a detailed history, with a reliable corroborative account if possible, and mental state examination
- Mode of presentation can give clues to possible depressive illness
- Factors which increase vulnerability to develop depression:
  - Previous history of depression
  - Family history of depression or suicide
  - Stress/life events particularly with separation or loss ⎫
  - Social isolation ⎬ all common in the
  - Physical illness especially chronic painful illness ⎭ elderly
  - Some medications can trigger depression

---

**Information**

Depression can be broadly categorised:

- Mild – low mood often associated with anxiety symptoms
- Moderate – increasingly low mood, depressive thinking (e.g. suicidal) with biological symptoms (sleep disturbance with early morning waking, mood worse in the morning, reduced appetite, weight and libido)
- Severe – more intense low mood, suicidal thoughts with development of psychotic symptoms, including delusions and hallucinations (Most often associated with suicide)

– Alcohol/substance abuse

## How do you identify a severe case?

In moderate to severe depression, mental state examination may reveal:

- Depressed facial appearance, tearfulness, reduced expression, poor eye contact, retardation of movement or agitation
- Speech may be slow and impoverished
- Low mood, anhedonia (loss of interest or pleasure), reduced motivation or energy
- Suicidal thoughts may be present and should always be enquired for and explored carefully
  - have you had any desperate thoughts?
  - do you feel that life is not worth living?

Mood congruent thoughts may include pessimism, feelings of guilt, worthlessness, self-reproach, poverty, hopelessness (often associated with suicidal contemplation). In severe depression thoughts may reach delusional intensity and may be associated with perceptual abnormalities e.g. condemnatory auditory hallucinations. Tests of cognitive function may be poorly performed due to impaired memory and concentration. In the elderly with severe depression this may give the impression of a dementia (pseudodementia)

## How would you manage this case?.

Exclude physical cause. This patient has an anaemia which is being investigated.

Consider possible organic causes of depressive symptoms.

- Endocrine
  - hypothyroidism
  - Cushing's syndrome
  - hyperparathyroidism
  - Addison's disease
  - hypercalcaemia
- Infections
  - viral illness
  - hepatitis
  - HIV
- Metabolic
  - anaemia (particularly $B_{12}$ and iron deficient)
  - renal disease
  - cancer
- Neurological
  - MS
  - brain tumour
  - Parkinson's disease

## Investigations
- Full blood screen, including FBC, U+E, creatinine, thyroid function tests, liver function tests, serum calcium.
- A CXR may also be helpful.

– post stroke
– dementias

- Drugs
(many drugs have the potential to cause depressive symptoms – check data sheet)
– steroids
– L.dopa
– antihypertensives
– regular use of stimulants

### Further management depends on the severity

Mild depression may respond to counselling and attempts to resolve problems leading to depression.

Moderate to severe depressive illness is more likely to present acutely.

- Establish if the patient is at risk (see Group 16, Item 6)
- Referral to psychiatric team. Psychiatric admission considered on the basis of severity and risk, if necessary using Mental Health Act (see Kumar & Clark 4th edition, Table 19.37, p1146).
- Identify support and communicate
- Inform GP

### What medication would you consider and how would you begin treatment?

In prescribing antidepressants the following should be considered (See British National Formulary – doses and side-effects)

- A psychiatric opinion will often be appropriate
- Medication is most effective in moderate and severe depression
- Compliance is essential. Good prescribing practice includes explanation of:
  – the diagnosis
  – the likelihood of response to appropriate treatment (around 2/3 respond well)
  – possible side effects which can often occur before benefits
  – delay of two to three weeks before treatment begins to take effect
- Older tricyclic and related antidepressants have proven efficacy but significant side-effects (e.g. anticholinergic, postural hypotension, cardiotoxic in overdose) and have largely been superceded by new generation drugs. They can still be useful if newer agents aren't tolerated, sedation is desirable or if previous beneficial response. Avoid large prescriptions
- Most commonly prescribed of newer antidepressants are selective serotonin reuptake inhibitors (SSRIs). Associated with nausea but better tolerated and less toxic in overdose

## Remember
- Severe depression can be life endangering (e.g. acutely suicidal, not eating or drinking).
- Refer to the psychiatric team who may consider the use of emergency ECT treatment.

- Difficult to predict which antidepressant will be best tolerated in view of range of side effects and significant individual variations
- Elderly patients often require lower starting dose and more gradual dose increase
- As a general rule, treatment should continue for at least six months after recovery from acute episode

---

**GROUP 16:**

**ITEM 6:**

# Psychiatry
# Suicide and deliberate self harm (DSH)

Patients presenting to hospital having attempted self harm comprise around 10% of acute medical admissions in the UK. The most common method is drug overdose which is associated with recent alcohol consumption in up to 50% of cases.

The majority of deliberate self harm (DSH) does not represent a serious suicide attempt. Motivations include:

- Escape from overwhelming stress
- To effect a change in personal circumstances
- Wish to die (serious suicidal intent evident in up to a fifth of DSH presentation)

Many of the components of the assessment of deliberate self harm can be applied to patients who describe having 'suicidal thoughts'.

### How would you manage a case of deliberate self harm?

- Attend to immediate medical requirements (overdose see Group 13, Item 1). Most patients will be admitted to hospital after overdose for specific treatment or observation. Patients may underestimate or understate the number of tablets taken
- When medical condition stable, interview if possible with collateral history from reliable informants aiming to:

### Identify mental illness

- Most completed suicides are associated with a psychiatric diagnosis most often a depressive illness (see Group 16, Item 5). Many suicide victims visit their GP in the preceding weeks
- Conversely, clear psychiatric illness is evident in less than 1/3rd of DSH presentations. Most occur after a life event with up to half following a relationship problem. Commonest diagnoses

**Remember**

- Dependants who may be at risk (e.g. young children at home). Inform social worker if necessary
- Some hospitals have dedicated staff who assess all patients. In these situations your task is to identify those who are in need of immediate attention or treatment

include depression, alcohol dependence, personality disorders (borderline, antisocial)

### Detect patients at risk of completed suicide:

- Serious suicide attempts form a minority of DSH presentations but individuals who harm themselves have a greatly increased risk of suicide compared to the general population
- A high proportion of suicide victims have a previous history of DSH
- An indication of risk should be documented in the notes with an appropriate plan of action

### Features associated with increased suicide risk

- Demographic – socially isolated (divorced, widowed, never married); male (rates in young men increasing alarmingly); older age, minority groups e.g. young Asian women; unemployed; low socio-economic class, certain professions (doctors, dentists, vets, farmers), individuals with access to means (drug users, gun owners)
- The attempt – Planning: taking care of affairs (cancelled appointments, final acts e.g. suicide note – content of which can be helpful).
- Circumstances: performed in isolation, steps to avoid detection.
- Method: violent, severe OD or believed likely to be lethal.
- The history – present or previous psychiatric diagnosis (particularly depression, schizophrenia), recent hospital discharge, previous DSH, recent life event (e.g. bereavement, retirement, divorce) physical illness (chronic painful illness, CNS disorders (MS, epilepsy), cancer, HIV), family history of psychiatric illness/suicide, alcohol/drug misuse, impulsive personality
- The mental state – agitation, depressed mood, suicidal thoughts, hopelessness, delusion, hallucinations, insight in early schizophrenia

### Exploring suicidal thoughts

Never avoid detailed but tactful questions concerning suicidal ideas and intentions.

Responses need to be assessed in the context of the overall presentation especially if the patient is unforthcoming.

Establish:

- Thoughts about episode of self harm
- Does patient wish to die – ask questions to assess underlying mental state e.g.
  - how do you see the future?
  - do you see things as completely hopeless?
  - do you feel you'd be better off dead?
- Plans for further attempts (method, circumstances)

- Reasons for not wishing to complete suicide (e.g. change in circumstances, family, dependants)
- Alternative methods of dealing with distress

### Identify means of preventing recurrence

(the most significant factor predictive of repetition is the number of previous episodes). Assess:

- current and previous coping resources
- level of support – identify important relationships
- possible precipitants (current problems, recent events) and means of addressing them

### Psychiatric liaison referral

Consider:

- Although hospitals often have dedicated staff to assess all deliberate self harm presentations in liaison with the psychiatric team, it is important to recognise individuals in need of immediate attention or treatment
- Most do not require further psychiatric intervention
- If a significant psychiatric disorder is identified management can be initiated as an inpatient or outpatient in communication with the patient's GP
- High risk cases or those with severe symptoms will require psychiatric admission – if necessary using compulsory admission eg section 5 (2) Mental Health Act (MHA). Level of risk and nursing observation required should be communicated and documented

### Difficult management problems

Repeated presenters (eg self laceration, overdose, actual or threatened)

- Behaviour often related to borderline personality disorder in the absence of other clear psychiatric diagnosis
- Planned consistent multidisciplinary response coordinated through psychiatric team can sometimes help
- Reduction in maladaptive behaviour may occur in response to provision of key support worker, counselling, psychotherapy or enhanced social suport
- Occasional psychiatric crisis admissions may be required but kept to minimum in favour of longer term strategies
- Low dose antipsychotic medication may be helpful to reduce arousal and distress, avoiding large prescriptions

Refusal of medical treatment

- Explain clearly risks of not having treatment
- Assess capacity to make informed decision and record it

• If treatment is considered necessary attempt persuasion/negotiation if possible including a friend or relative

Management decisions and clear reasons should be carefully documented and discussed with senior colleague

The Mental Health Act can be used to detain a patient who is refusing medical treatment in hospital if they are exhibiting symptoms of mental disorder.

Patients unwilling to remain in hospital for further assessment

• If considered at risk, appropriate staff should attempt to hold in hospital under common law to allow urgent mental health assessment by psychiatrist and approved social worker. Reasons should be carefully documented.

• Intoxicated or violent patients
  – Assistance of security or police may be necessary
  – Assessment will be more accurate if the patient is given time for the effects of alcohol intoxication to subside. This can only happen as long as the patient or others are not put at risk. Behaviour may then settle.

• Assess underlying cause

• Consider psychiatric opinion if underlying psychiatric disorder is thought likely

---

**Remember**

• Enforced physical treatment is given under common law and not sanctioned by use of the Mental Health Act. Decision to go ahead depends on consideration of:
  – reasonable professional practice and a doctor's duty of care to the patient
  – necessity of the treatment to save life, prevent a serious incident or a deterioration in health
  – decision to treat being in the patient's best interests.

**GROUP 16:**

**ITEM 7:**

# Psychiatry
# Acute anxiety

## CASE HISTORY 1

You are called to the A&E to see a breathless young woman. She is acutely distressed and breathing rapidly. She feels light-headed and has parasthesiae in her hands and feet.

Differential diagnoses should include a respiratory emergency (asthma, pulmonary embolus, and pneumothorax).

**Panic attack** (see also Group 11, Item 4) is suggested by:

- Extreme fear
- Subjective complaint of difficulty breathing in rather than out
- Respiratory alkalosis (causing tetany and relative hypocalcaemia)
- Arterial blood gases will show hypocapnia and normal oxygen levels.
- Sweating
- Emotional trigger (shock)
- Environmental trigger (crowd phobia)

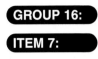

**Information**

The patient can be educated about panic attacks when better and how to prevent them (seek behaviour therapy for phobias) and use of a paper bag during an attack

## Management

Hyperventilation is best treated by rebreathing into a paper bag in order to increase $pCO_2$.

Alternatives include giving a minor tranquilliser

Lorazepam 1-2 mgm, orally or I/M

Diazepam 5-10 mgm orally

This can be repeated one hour later if necessary

## CASE HISTORY 2

Nursing staff inform you that a 55-year-old man is refusing to have any more haemodialysis having just started this treatment. A **phobic reaction to dialysis** is suggested by avoidance, abnormal fear and sympathetic overdrive, during dialysis or talking about it. Depressive illness is a common association of anxiety and should always be excluded (see Group 16, Item 5). These phobias are also common in oncology (vomit phobia with chemotherapy).

### How would you manage this patient?

- Support and sympathy with explanation of the phobia
- Minor tranquilliser (see above) short-term only: two to three weeks of diazepam 5 mg x 3 (long half-life drugs are better)
- Ask a psychologist to consider graded exposure therapy

- Consider a selective serotonin reuptake inhibitor (sertraline, citalopram, paroxetine, fluoxetine) in the presence of comorbid depressive illness

### What are the physical symptoms and signs of anxiety?

- Dilated pupils
- Photosensitivity (may be wearing dark glasses)
- Phonosensitivity (cannot bear any noise)
- Dry mouth
- Flushed face and neck
- Sweating
- Hyperventilation
- Associated hypocapnia and respiratory alkalosis causing relative hypocalcaemia (tingling or numbness in extremities and face, light-headedness tetany (see Group 14, Item 20).
- Tachycardia (pulse may be as high as 140 bpm)
- Nausea
- Diarrhoea
- Frequency of micturition

### What are the psychological symptoms of anxiety?

- Excessive fear
- Derealisation (patient feels that the environment is less real and solid, with a feeling of detachment)
- Fear of collapse
- Catastrophic thinking ('I'm about to die from a heart attack')

### Always look for the following associations

- Phobias (abnormal fear and avoidance of particular situations or things)
- Depressive illness (see Group 16, Item 5)
- Obsessive compulsive disorder (repetitive ruminations which are inconsistent with the personality, along with repeated behaviours; checking excessively or hand-washing because of fears of germs)

**GROUP 16:**

**ITEM 8:**

# Psychiatry
# Opiate dependence

Drugs in this group include: diamorphine (heroin), morphine, pethidine, methadone, dihydrocodeine and buprenorphine.

### Effects of opiate use
• Euphoria
• Analgesia
• Relaxation
• Drowsiness

Heroin addicts are 16 times more likely to die than individuals of equivalent age chiefly as a result of overdose. They frequently present in the acute hospital setting.

## CASE HISTORY 1

You are called to see a 23-year-old man admitted 24 hours previously after a road traffic accident. He is verbally abusing nursing staff and wants to leave against medical advice. He is demanding methadone stating that he is a heroin addict.

### How would you assess this man?
• Attempt to defuse the situation and prevent an escalation of disturbed behaviour
• Take history of drug use including each drug taken, amount and route.
• Obtain information from other sources:
  – previously or currently attended drug support agencies if patient admits to having received help. They may be able to tell you if the patient has a regular prescription for methadone
  – corroborative history from reliable other informant with patient's consent
• Examine for evidence of opiate abuse:
Withdrawal symptoms begin within 12 hours of last use and increase in severity over the first 48 hours. With longer acting opioids such as methadone, onset of withdrawal symptoms can be delayed and their duration increased. Opiate withdrawal is uncomplicated by other drugs, subjectively unpleasant but not life-threatening, and can present with:
  – agitation
  – anxiety
  – low mood
  – restlessness

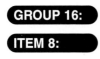

### Information
Information concerning previous notification and treatment of opiate addicts from the Home Office Drugs branch including the doctors' helpline, is NO longer available.

– tachycardia
– sweating
– 'goose flesh'
– dilated pupils
– yawning
– sneezing
– vomiting
– lacrimation
– rhinorrhoea

• Look for evidence of recent drug use e.g. needle marks, phlebitis, skin abscesses.
• (Subjective complaints include craving, poor sleep [which can last months], abdominal cramps, nausea, diarrhoea, musculoskeletal pain.)

### How would you investigate?

• Send urine for drug screen
• Consider infection screen (risk of hepatitis B, C, HIV)

### How would you manage and treat this patient?

**Prescribing methadone.**

• Oral methadone mixture should be considered if you are satisfied a significant habit exists
• If possible, seek advice from local specialist drug unit
• Department of Health has published guidelines on clinical management of drug misuse and dependence (HMSO 1991) – a copy may be available from hospital pharmacy
• Any registered medical practitioner can prescribe methadone. A Home office licence is only required to prescribe certain drugs (heroin, cocaine, dipipanone) in treating addiction.
• Methadone tablets should not generally be prescribed in view of their potential for abuse.
• Dose required to control withdrawal can be carefully titrated in hospital. Start at low dose of methadone e.g. 10 mls (1mg per 1ml mixture). Consider further 10 mls at four hourly intervals until withdrawal symptoms controlled to establish daily requirement
• Doses above 40 mls daily should only be considered with great caution unless there is reliable information that the patient has been receiving higher regular prescription – but even in this case dose should be gradually titrated upwards.

**Symptomatic treatment of withdrawal symptoms may be indicated and includes:**

• Ibuprofen for pain
• Loperamide for diarrhoea
• Patients may demand more methadone than required to control withdrawal symptoms in order to promote sleep. This

**Remember**

• Avoid high doses – methadone overdose causes respiratory arrest – patients can overstate their requirements and physical tolerance to opiates can change quickly

should be avoided. Short-term use of hypnotic medication is an alternative. Diazepam also helps muscle spasm and anxiety.
- Observe for evidence of withdrawal from other drugs e.g.
  - Alcohol – DTs (see Group 16, Item 4)
  - Benzodiazepines – risk of convulsions
- Comorbid psychiatric disorder can be present:
  - Depressive illness (see Group 16, Item 5)
  - Psychotic symptoms (if polydrug abuse includes stimulants or hallucinogenic drugs)

### When condition stable

Consider gradual reduction in methadone by 10% per day if aiming for abstinence. The patient may wish to remain on methadone in the longer term if already receiving regular prescription prior to admission or if requesting referral to local drug support agency. Discuss this with the patient. The reduction regime may need to be flexible to secure co-operation.

If indicated, request assessment from the local drug service. On discharge, if ongoing drug support required, arrange planned transfer of care particularly with regard to taking over prescribing. The patient's GP should be informed and may be willing to prescribe. Avoid giving large prescriptions. Methadone should generally be prescribed as a daily collection.

**Remember**

Patients should be warned of the risks even of relatively low doses particularly if there are children in the home (5 to 10ml could be lethal for a child).

### Should you notify this patient?

Doctors are no longer legally obliged to notify substance misusers encountered in clinical practice to the Home Office. However, the Department of Health through the Regional Health Authority keeps anonymous records of substance misusers. Details on providing information without obligation for these databanks should be available locally.

### CASE HISTORY 2

A young man is rushed to A&E in a comatose state. His girlfriend tells you he used heroin after an abstinence of four weeks.

### How do you proceed?

**Heroin overdose**, causing life threatening respiratory depression, can occur after a period of abstinence as physical tolerance is reduced.

- Urgent cardiorespiratory support
- Assess evidence of opiate toxicity (an acute medical emergency)
  - impairment of conscious level
  - respiratory depression
  - bradycardia

**Remember**

All patients need to be monitored in hospital for at least 24 hours even if they make a brisk recovery.

– miosis

– hypothermia

• Examine for other causes of impaired consciousness (e.g. head injury)

• Administer opiate antagonist naloxone. IV Naloxone has a high affinity for opiate receptors and reverses the signs of toxicity by displacing ingested opiates. Life-threatening symptoms may recur in view of the relatively short half-life of naloxone which may need to be readministered depending on the half life of the opiate taken. (e.g. half life of methadone is over 24 hours).

**GROUP 16:**

**ITEM 9:**

# Psychiatry

# Disturbed patient

## Examples of disturbed behaviour:

• Agitation

• Overactivity

• Communicating distress e.g. self injury or mutilation, threatening self harm.

• Unpredictable behaviour

• Intimidating or violent conduct

The individual or others may be at risk

## Organic mental disorders

• **Dementia**

– Patients can be restless, aggressive and may wander because of disorientation. May be exaggerated by co-existent physical conditions e.g. acute infection, constipation.

• **Delirium** (see Group 16, Item 1).

– Arising from a number of causes and commonly associated with disturbed behaviour due to misinterpretation of surroundings. Conscious level is impaired often with fearfulness, perceptual abnormalities (visual or auditory hallucination) and abnormal thinking (e.g. persecutory delusions)

• **Epilepsy**

– Ictal (e.g. temporal lobe) or post ictal

## Other psychiatric disorders

• **Major psychoses**

– Schizophrenia – delusional thinking or abnormal sensory experience (e.g. auditory hallucination) may be causing behaviour

– Manic psychosis – elevation in mood can be associated with hyperactive and disorganised behaviour

• **Anxiety and depression** (see Group 16, Item 5).

– Can be associated with agitation, restlessness and high arousal. Major depression is associated with suicidality and self harm

## Substance misuse

– Alcohol intoxication or withdrawal (see delirium tremens Group 16, Item 4). Abuse of other drugs e.g. stimulants, hallucinogenics, solvents

## Physical illness

Individuals may have a physical cause to explain their disturbed behaviour e.g. chronic pain, side-effects of medication

## No physical or psychiatric disorder

Some individuals may have a propensity to violence or anger in the absence of any underlying medical explanation. Certain 'personality disorders' are associated with self mutilating or cutting, explosive or antisocial conduct.

## CASE HISTORY 1

A young man walks into A&E. He is unkempt, preoccupied and suspicious. His behaviour is bizarre, disorganised and unpredictable. He has been argumentative and intimidating, causing distress to other patients.

## Management

• Aim to identify cause (see above) and take control of the situation

• Of paramount concern is the safety of the patient, other patients, yourself and colleagues

• Disturbed patients should be assessed in a safe area with adequate staff support (medical, nursing, security) and access to a panic alarm

• Consider the possibility that the patient may be concealing a weapon

• Specific management depends on the severity of the disturbed behaviour and the cause

• Clues to the diagnosis can often be found by carefully observing an uncooperative patient even from a distance while awaiting staff support e.g. Impairment of the conscious level may suggest delirium, drug intoxication. Smell of alcohol may be apparent. A major psychotic mental illness may be suggested from the appearance, behaviour and speech e.g. preoccupation, suspiciousness, overactivity, thought disorder, delusional ideas

- Additional background information from reliable informants is invaluable though not always possible

Following initial assessment of the situation, and with appropriate staff support:

### Use interpersonal skills

- Approach the patient in a non-confrontational manner avoiding invasion of their personal space – disturbed patients may misinterpret their surroundings and the motives of others
- Sensitive questions or statements may be helpful
- Offer advice and reassurance
- Attempt to interview the patient in a safe setting

### If the patient settles and co-operates

- Expand assessment and plan appropriate management depending on the cause of the disturbed behaviour

### If patient remains uncooperative

If presentation suggests mental health problem, request an urgent mental health assessment. An approved social worker and two doctors one of whom is approved under the mental health act (often the duty psychiatrist) are required to consider detention of the patient on mental health grounds. If this is appropriate the patient will be transferred to the psychiatric team. Should the patient's behaviour be considered to present a risk to themselves or others before this can be completed, the use of restraint and possibly medication (see below) under common law should be considered. The reasons for taking this step should be clearly documented and suitable staff should be available.

### Following implementation of mental health act

If the patients behaviour remains disturbed and a risk to themselves or others, safe restraint should be used as a co-ordinated response by suitably trained nursing staff.

### Medication

Reduction in arousal can be achieved by a carefully regime of antipsychotic medication starting at a low dose and administering in accordance with response. Giving medication to a potentially resistive and aroused patient is not without risk which must be outweighed by risks of inaction and clearly documented. The dose of antipsychotic medication can be reduced by combining with a benzodiazepine which promotes sedation and can be used in the immediate short term situation. *It is important to begin with a low dose and increase this gradually.* A suitable regime may be

- Droperidol 5 mg i.m stat
- Lorazepam 1-2 mg im stat
- Oral medication possibly in liquid form should be offered in the first instance. Vital signs (pulse, temperature, blood pressure, conscious level) should be monitored.
- While the behaviour continues to present a risk, the dose may be repeated at intervals of 30 minutes to one hour until the patient is settled, subject to regular monitoring of vital signs.

### When the patient is more settled

Further assessment can be carried out to establish an accurate diagnosis prior to starting regular treatment.

### If no physical or psychiatric cause is identified

The assistance of security or the police may be required.

---

### ⚠ Remember

Particular caution should be used in patients who have never received antipsychotic medication previously because of the possibility of an adverse reaction such as acute dystonia (involuntary muscle contractions involving face, neck, limbs and trunk).

**Fig 16.9.1 Management of a disturbed patient**

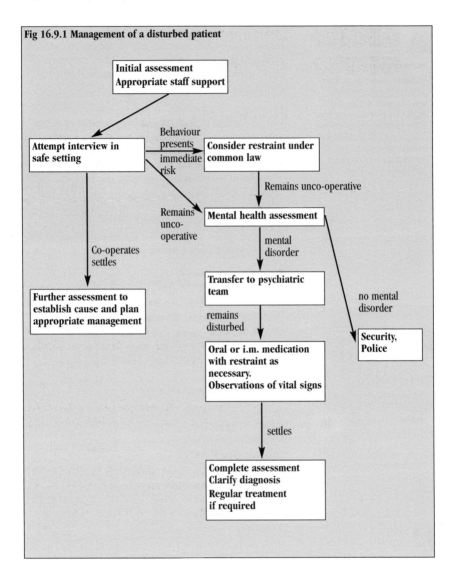

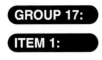

**GROUP 17:**

**ITEM 1:**

# Dermatology
# A swollen red leg

## CASE HISTORY

The A&E officer asks you to come and see a 50-year-old man who is unwell and has a red, swollen leg below his knee. He thinks he needs admitting for anticoagulation for a possible DVT.

On arrival you check if this was of sudden onset or was a chronically swollen leg. You ask if there is a past history of DVTs or whether there are any risk factors such as a long car journey, air travel, or immobility. You also ask about any recent illness e.g. heart failure, blood disorder.

### What should you do next?

You do a full medical examination noting obesity and the presence of any other disorders – heart failure, recent surgery. On examination, – he weighs 102 kg and has a temperature of 38°C. The leg is indeed red, swollen, hot and tender below the knee. You note a small ulcer on the medial side of the leg above the ankle. Dorsalis pedis pulse is palpable.

### What is your diagnosis?

You think that this man's immediate problem is **cellulitis** due probably to streptococci gaining entry via the venous ulcer.

### How do you treat?

You start with penicillin V (or erythromycin) + Flucloxacillin) 500 mg x 4 daily having ascertained that he is not allergic to penicillin. (If the cellulitis is very severe he may require parenteral benzylpenicillin and flucloxacillin, i.e. IV for two to three days + 10 days oral)

### What about the leg ulcer?

See below

The patient's leg improved with antibiotics and he was discharged after two days.

## LEG ULCERATION

Take a full history on associated diseases (diabetes mellitus, rheumatoid arthritis, past history of deep vein thrombosis), family history of venous insufficiency, heart disease, hypertension, sickle cell, scleroderma, varicose veins.

**Investigations**
- Streptococcal titres
- Swab/blood cultures rarely helpful

**Information**

LIPODERMATOSCLEROSIS

Hot and woody hard "atrophic" skin

Long-standing venous disease

Patient well/no pyrexia

## Causes and signs

- Venous insufficiency
  - oedema, venous eczema, skin discolouration (atrophie blanche [scarring], erythema, haemosiderin pigmentation) skin texture, (lipodermatosclerosis), ulcer site: internal malleollus
- Arterial insufficiency
  - ulcer – punched out; site – often lateral or higher up on leg (painful)
  - pulses – absent dorsalis pedis or posterior tibial
  - cool leg
- Vasculitis
- Neuropathic – sensory signs present particularly over pressure sore areas in feet. Common in diabetics.

## Management

**For venous ulcers** – elevation, exercise, compression, dressings. Antibiotics if infected

**For arterial ulcers** – investigate arterial supply, dressings with NO compression

**For vasculitic ulcers** – vasculitic screen, e.g. ANCA, ANA, rheumatoid factor

**For neuropathic ulcers** – keep ulcer clean and remove the pressure point

Note: Operating on varicose veins rarely helps venous insufficiency problems – 'replumbing of the veins cannot be done.'

### Investigations

- General – FBC, U&Es, LFTs, BSL, autoantibodies
- Venous – Doppler ultrasound – always perform before compression
- Arterial – Doppler ultrasound, digital substraction angiography

**GROUP 17:**

**ITEM 2:**

# Dermatology
# Erythema nodosum
(See Group

### Make the diagnosis
- Spontaneous onset and evolution over a few days
- Single or multiple bruise-like patches 1 to 10 cm diameter
- Tender and warm to touch
- Predominantly affecting limbs (shins or lower limbs)
- No age or sex limitation (but young females more common)
- Sometimes associated with arthralgia
- Always do a CXR looking for hilar lymphadenopathy

### Identify the cause
- Drugs
  - oral contraceptives
  - aspirin & NSAIDs
  - sulphonamides

- Infection
  - streptococcal
  - tuberculosis
  - chlamydia

- Sarcoidosis
- Inflammatory bowel disease
- idiopathic
- pregnancy

### Initial treatment
- Tubigrip support bandages
- Aspirin (unless the identified cause)
- Bed rest if severe
- Dapsone/steroids especially if it ulcerates

### Decide when to refer
- Recurrent or unresolving symptoms
- Tuberculosis/leprosy suspected
- Systemically unwell patient

## GROUP 17:

## ITEM 3:

# Dermatology
# Urticaria and angio-oedema

**Urticaria or HIVES** is characterised by short-lived swelling (weals) anywhere on the body which usually itch and except in some subtypes resolve without bruising within 24 hours (often within 10 to 20 minutes). Can form bizarre serpiginous-shaped lesions.

**Angio-oedema** is a deeper form of urticaria affecting the dermis and subcutis usually affecting the mucous membranes e.g. eyes, lips, tongue, genitals and much less commonly the larynx and gastro-intestinal tract. It is commoner in atopics. It is generally not itchy but can be painful and disappears within 72 hours. It may occur in isolation or with urticaria (45% cases).

The incidence of urticaria/angioedema is ≈15% in a person's lifetime.

### Classification of Urticarias

• **Acute**
By definition this lasts < six weeks. Only 2 to 4% cases have an identifiable allergen. IgE mediated. In severest form there is an anaphylactic reaction but may cause urticaria without systemic symptoms.

– Acute idiopathic urticaria and angio-oedema accounts for >90% of urticaria

– Acute allergic – drug reactions, insect bites, foods, can cause this type of reaction, as well as contact urticaria caused by e.g. latex , tomatoes

• **Chronic** – by definition if urticaria persists > six weeks. Only 2 to 4% cases have an identifiable cause and extensive investigation is not indicated. Some cases are autoimmune and functionally significant IgG anti-IgE receptor autoantibody can be demonstrated in patient's serum. In a few patients an acute illness (hepatitis, brucellosis) focal sepsis, dermatophyte or parasitic infections can precipitate a reaction.

• **Physical** – reproducible wealing occurs in response to a specific physical stimulus, e.g. friction, pressure, vibration, delayed pressure, cold, cholinergic, aquagenic, solar. The diagnosis might be suspected from the patient's history or site of urticaria i.e. pressure sites in cases of delayed pressure urticaria.

### Management

• Explanation of condition and likelihood of not identifying specific cause
• Avoidance of non-specific factors e.g. aspirin, NSAIDs
• Antihistamines (non-sedating or combination of daytime non-

sedating $H_1$ blockers and sedating $H_1$ blocker at night)
• Mast cell stabilisers – ketotifen, terbutaline
• Immunotherapy – corticosteroids, IV immunoglobulin. Cyclosporin A for very severe cases – refer to dermatology department.

### Preferred regimes if no contraindications:

• Loratidine 10-20 mg daily Cetarizine 10-20 mg daily. (non-sedative antihystamine)
• Sedative antihistamines e.g. Hydroxyzine 25-50mg at night

### Management of severe angio-oedema

(see Group 13, Item 4)
• Adrenaline 1:1,000 (1mg/ml) subcutaneously. Adult dose 0.5-1.0ml
• IV chlorpheniramine 10-20mg (max 40mg/24 hours)
• IV hydrocortisone succinate (100-300mg)

Adrenaline 1:1000 (1mg/ml) is available on prescription (Epipen) in pre-loaded injections to deliver dose of 0.3 or 0.5mg (adult) or 0.15mg (paediatric) and should be carried out by the patient.

### Hereditary angio oedema (HAE)

Important to recognise as patients may develop laryngeal obstruction. Lesions appear as deep swellings that may have associated enlarging oedematous borders that last up to two to four days. Urticaria does not occur as part of HAE. Patients generally suffer from recurrent attacks of painful angio-oedema. May be precipitated by minor trauma, emotional upset, infections and temperature change. Involvement of the gastro-intestinal tract may simulate a surgical emergency. Inherited in an autosomal dominant fashion with either a functional or absolute deficiency of C1 esterase inhibitor (C1-INH). Acquired forms are seen in SLE or lymphoma.

Patients often have a history of recurrent attacks of abdominal pain since childhood and 80% of cases give a positive family history (for e.g. of sudden death).

### Management

Unresponsive to antihistamines (may exacerbate condition), systemic steroids or adrenaline. Treatment of choice is intravenous (C1 -INH) concentrates. If unavailable fresh frozen plasma can be used. In adults, prophylaxis with attenuated androgens e.g. stanozolol or danazol may be required if episodes are frequent.

# GROUP 17:
# ITEM 4:

# Dermatology
# Sun-induced rash

## Information

**UVA and UVB**

- Medium wavelengths 280-310 nm (UVB) – cause sunburn and long term skin changes e.g. cancer.
- Long wavelengths 310 -400 nm (UVA) – does not cause sunburn (unless high doses through glass) but does cause photodermatoses. It also contributes to long term skin damage.

- Sunscreen preparations protect against UVB. The sun protection factor (SPF) number gives an indication about the amount of time that a person is protected against burning compared to the unprotected skin. Most modern sunscreens protect against both UVA and UVB (utilising reflectants or chemical absorbers).

## CASE HISTORY

A 24-year old-arrived in A&E with blisters on her face and arms. She had fallen asleep on the beach in the sun. She had applied factor 4 sunscreen and was surprised that she had developed an itchy rash. On examination she had papules and a few vesicles over the exposed areas.

### What is the diagnosis?

This is a **polymorphic light eruption** which occurs in 10 to 20% of the population. The rash appears some hours after the exposure and can last several hours or a few days following exposure. She also had evidence of sunburn – remember factor 4 does not protect for very long.

### Differential diagnosis

- Sunscreen allergy leading to photocontact dermatitis (presents as eczema rather than papules/vesicles)
- Solar urticaria (very rare) gives rise to a rash immediately after sun exposure.

### How would you treat this girl?

No treatment was necessary for this young woman as she was virtually asymtomatic. She was given a leaflet on sun exposure and told that her type of rash usually tended to improve over the summer period. If symptomatic, however, application of a topical steroid for one week could be considered.

If the rash becomes worse each year consider desensitising with PUVA each spring or short bursts of oral Prednisolone for one week for an attack.

Always keep SLE and porphyrias in mind for any photosensitivity case where diagnosis is not obvious (+ drug induced photosensitivity)

**GROUP 17:**

**ITEM 5:**

# Dermatology
## Generalised rash or eruption

(**"Erythroderma"** i.e. not an extensive maculopapular rash)

### Clinical

Take a comprehensive history about onset, past history, family history, medication, occupation, other systemic symptoms.

Full skin examination including nails, mouth, genitals, scalp and hair. General examination, temperature, lymph nodes, organomegaly, etc.

### Causes

• Skin diseases which can present as generalised erytheroderma:
• Eeczema
• Psoriasis
• Drug eruption
• Idiopathic
• Cutaneous T-cell lymphoma ( Mycosis Fungoides, Sezary Syndrome)
• Pemphigus foliaceous

### Symptoms

• Chills
• Flu-like symptoms
• Itching
• Burning

### Investigations
• FBC
• U&Es
• LFTs
• CXR
• Skin biopsy (later).

### Are there any complications you should look out for?

Check for:

• High output cardiac failure from increased blood flow
• Hypothermia from heat loss
• Fluid loss
• Hypoalbuminaemia
• Increased BMR
• Capillary leak syndrome in very severe cases of psoriasis can give rise to ARDS (NB. Can be seen in severe drug rash).

### Management

• Bed rest
• Rehydrate, plenty of fluids orally or IV
• Keep warm

### Remember

Erythroderma means red skin. It refers to the clinical state of inflammation or redness of 90% of the skin.

• Moisturise the skin
• Treat as appropriate according to primary skin disease

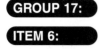

**GROUP 17:**

**ITEM 6:**

# Dermatology
# Pruritus

## Causes

Diseases of the skin associated with pruritus:

• Eczema
• Scabies
• Urticaria
• Psoriasis
• Lichen planus
• Dermatitis herpetiformis
• Pemphigoid

Systemic diseases associated with pruritus:

• Hypothyroidism
• Iron deficiency
• Advanced renal failure
• Liver disease (PBC and Hepatitis C)
• Lymphoma/myeloproliferative disease

## Investigations

• **PRIMARY SKIN DISEASES**
  Do scrapings, direct microscopy (scabies), punch biopsy. (+ IMF)
• **SYSTEMIC DISEASES**
  FBC U&Es, LFTs, Iron, Folate, B12, TFTs, Auto-immune Hepatis screen, Endomysial antibodies

## Management

Treat respective primary skin disease. Ask dermatology department.

• Eczema – moisturisers and topical corticosteroids
• Psoriasis – tar, Vit $D_3$ ointments, mild to moderate topical steroids, Dithranol (causes staining)
• Scabies – Malathion or permethrin
• Lichen planus – topical steroids/oral steroids
• **Systemic diseases** – see individual disease for treatment

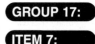

**GROUP 17:**

**ITEM 7:**

# Dermatology

## Cutaneous adverse drug reactions (ADR)

True incidence unknown as many go unreported, but the skin is the most commonly affected organ, involved in 30% of reported ADR.

Pre-existing disease (SLE,CLL,HIV), advancing age (polypharmacy, reduced renal and hepatic clearance), sensitivity to other drugs (e.g. penicillins – 10% cross-reactivity with cephalosporins) can all increase susceptibility to the development of ADRs.

### Classification

**Type A: augmented (~80% of all ADRs)**

• Exaggerated responses to known effects of the drug. Predictable and dose-related. e.g. skin necrosis after extravasation of vincristine, alopecia due to cytotoxic agents, cheilitis due to retinoids, urticaria triggered by opiates causing mast cell degranulation.

**Type B: unpredictable/bizarre**

• Idiosyncratic and therefore more difficult to diagnose (see below)

**Type C: associated with prolonged therapy/cumulative**

• e.g. analgesic nephropathy, chloroquine retinopathy, skin thinning, striae and purpura due to oral/topical/inhaled steroids.

**Type D: delayed reactions**

• arsenical keratoses, squamous cell carcinoma with azathioprine, (tends only to be with 2-3 drug immuno suppression, not single drug) teratogenicity due to retinoids.

**PHYSIOLOGY BOX**
There are a number of mechanisms but the pathogenesis of many cutaneous ADRs remains unknown.

| Type 1<br>Immediate, IgE-mediated hypersensitivity | **Examples**<br>urticaria and anaphylaxis due to penicillins |
|---|---|
| **Type II**<br>cytotoxic | allergic thrombocytopenic purpura |
| **Type III**<br>Immune complex formation | Morbilliform maculo-papular rash. Serum sickness, vasculitis e.g. allopurinol and penicillin |
| **Type IV**<br>Cell mediated | Morbilliform maculo-papular rash, allergic contact dermatitis to topical medicaments, erythema multiforme, toxic epidermal necrolysis, Lichenoid drug eruption |

Cutaneous ADRs can also be categorised morphologically into three groups:

• Skin reactions specific to drugs
• Rashes potentially caused by drugs
• Established skin disease exacerbated by drugs

### Skin reactions specific to drugs

Fixed drug eruptions are very rare. Develop within 24 hours of drug ingestion and are sharply demarcated, round, red, oedematous (and sometimes bullous) plaques which become violaceous or hyperpigmented with time. Lesions recur at the same site on re-exposure to the drug.

### Pigmentation caused by drugs

• Long-term amiodarone or chlorpromazine
  – purple/slate grey pigmentation on sun-exposed sites
• Long-term minocycline
  – blue/black pigmentation of skin, nails, buccal mucosa, scars (may be irreversible)
• Mepacrine
  – reversible yellow skin pigmentation
• Bleomycin
  – flagellate erythema then hyper-pigmentation of trunk

## Rashes potentially caused by drugs

There are many different reaction patterns and only a few common ones will be considered here.

### Maculopapular/exanthematic eruptions (see Table 17.7.1)

Commonest type of cutaneous ADR. Thought to be a cell mediated reaction (may also be Immune complex) involving CD8 T cells. Widespread, symmetrical, itchy eruption. Macules and papules may become confluent and develop into a sheet like erythema +/– fever and eosinophilia. When due to a drug it usually begins on the trunk. Suspect a viral aetiology if it starts on the face and moves down and if there is associated lymphadenopathy and conjunctivitis. After withdrawal of the drug, it usually settles over two weeks.

Note: If this eruption has progressed rapidly over 24 hours it may herald the onset of:

**Erythroderma** (synonym exfoliative dermatitis) in which > 90% of the skin surface is erythematous and inflamed. Ten per cent of cases are drug induced (e.g. sulphonamides, sulphonylureas, penicillins, barbiturates, allopurinol, gold, mercury, arsenicals) (see Group 17, Item 3).

**Toxic epidermal necrolysis.** The development of vesicles and/or bullae and skin tenderness raise this possibility. (May then be followed by "sheeting off" of the epidermis, see below).

### Photosensitivity (see Table 17.7.1)

Reactions range from erythema to blistering and characteristically spare the submental area, finger webs, under-eyebrow area and triangle of skin behind the ear lobe.

### Lichenoid reactions (see Table 17.7.1)

Similar to idiopathic lichen planus, but often more widespread and rarely involves mucous membranes.

**Table 17.7.1 Common drug associations**

| Maculopapular eruption | Photosensitivity | Lichenoid eruption |
| --- | --- | --- |
| antibiotics | thiazides | gold |
| (penicillins, sulphonamides) | sulphonamides | β blockers |
| anticonvulsants | amiodarone | quinine/antimalarials |
| (carbamazepine, phenytoin) | tetracycline | thiazides |
| NSAIDs | nalidixic acid | |
| allopurinol | | |
| gold | | |

**The Spectrum of Erythema Multiforme (EM), Stevens-Johnson Syndrome (SJS) And Toxic Epidermal Necrolysis (TEN)**

The classification of these diseases is confusing in the literature.

### Erythema Multiforme (EM) Minor

Ten per cent of cases are drug related (majority are post-infectious e.g. HSV, mycoplasma). Mild and self-limiting, usually resolves within two to four weeks. Characterised by target lesions of a central dusky erythema (sometimes with blistering), pale oedematous ring, peripheral erythematous ring. These usually occur acrally (extremities) and symmetrically on extensor surfaces. May involve palms and soles. Mucosal involvement may be present but is mild and limited to the oral cavity.

### Stevens-Johnson Syndrome (SJS) (also called EM Major)

More severe and extensive eruption. Widespread atypical target lesions may appear on the trunk and in which epidermal necrosis may result in the formation of blisters and epidermal detachment involving<10% of body surface area. At least two mucosal surfaces are involved (oral, ocular, genital) Mucosal lesions often more prominent than skin lesions. Systemic toxicity may occur. Usually resolves within six weeks.

### Stevens-Johnson syndrome/toxic epidermal necrolysis (sjs/ten) overlap

When the extent of epidermal detachment is between 10 to 30% of the body surface area, in the presence of other features of SJS, this is considered an SJS/TEN overlap.

### Toxic Epidermal necrolysis (TEN)

Sudden onset (usually evolves over 24 to 48 hours) widespread morbilliform or confluent dusky erythema with skin tenderness, followed by widespread blistering (necrolysis) of the skin with histologic evidence of full thickness epidermal necrosis, subepidermal separation and a sparse or absent dermal infiltrate. Nickolsky +ve. Mucous membrane involvement usually severe including ocular, genital, oral, nasopharynx and GIT. Mortality 20 to 30%

Adverse prognostic factors include:

• Age >60 years
• Area of involved skin > 50%
• Plasma urea >17 mmol/l
• Neutropenia <1.0 x 10$^9$/l
• Idiopathic nature of TEN

If extensive predict:
　– ventilation
　– Contact ITU

### Treatment of TEN

• Early high dose Immuno-suppression
• Analgesia (opiate)
• Dressings / Human skin bank

**Remember**

All cases of TEN should be considered drug induced and suspected drug(s) should be stopped immediately. Commonest drugs responsible are sulphonamides, penicillins, anticonvulsants and NSAIDS.

**Investigations**

These are of little help!

- Blood eosinophilia (may be found in toxic erythema but is non-specific)
- Biopsy 'may suggest but not prove a drug aetiology':
  - lots of eosinophils, common
  - 'lichenoid pattern, rare
  - SLE pattern, rare
  - vascuilitis, sometimes
- Blood level of drug (may be useful to check for overdosage)
- If a fixed drug eruption is suspected re-challenge may be helpful (in other situations it is rarely justifiable for fear of precipitating a more severe reaction)
- Patch testing is always helpful in patients with suspected allergic contact dermatitis (type IV hypersensitivity reactions).

- Clinitron bed
- ITU-supportive therapy

**Established skin disease exacerbated by drugs**

- Psoriasis – can be destabilised by lithium and possibly ß blockers and antimalarials
- Acne – can be aggravated by progesterone-containing contraceptives, lithium and corticosteroids
- Rosacea – worse with topical steroids
- Peri-oral dermatitis (POD) – caused and exacerbated by topical steroids

**Diagnosis of Adverse Drug Reaction**

The key elements to diagnosis are a meticulous drug history and a high index of suspicion.

- Exclude other causes from history and examination
- Take a careful drug history. Remember to ask about over-the-counter preparations e.g. laxatives, tonics and cough medicines), vitamins and complementary treatments
- Start and stop dates of medication and relationship to onset of the rash
- When the eruption begins from seven to 21 days after the first administration of a drug or within 48 hours if the drug has caused a similar reaction in the past, this is highly suggestive of an ADR
- The timing is incompatible with an ADR if the drug was started after the onset of cutaneous or mucous membrane signs. If the onset is within 24 hours of the first dose, or more than 21 days after stopping the drug, a drug aetiology is doubtful. If there are several drugs, each should be considered as a potential cause
- Consult drug information /CSM for previous reports

**Treatment**

- Withdraw drug(s). Symptomatic treatment with oral antihistamines, topical steroids and moisturisers
- Severe reactions (SJS and TEN) require supportive therapy and monitoring of infection, fluid balance and temperature. Patients may need ITU. Use of systemic immunosuppression may be considered if patients are seen within the first 24 hours of onset.
- Dressings – leave on
- Clinitron bed
- Opiate analgesia
- Give written information to patient and GP

The following flow diagram may be used as a guide to referral:

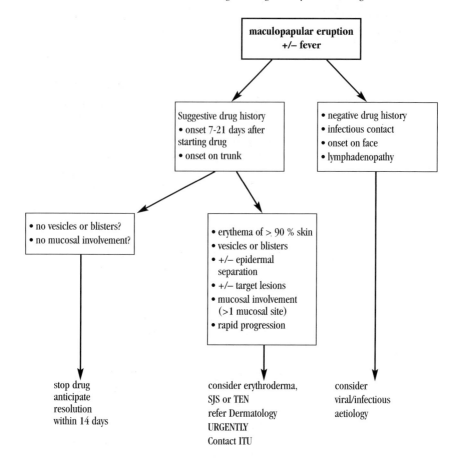

**maculopapular eruption +/− fever**

Suggestive drug history
- onset 7-21 days after starting drug
- onset on trunk

- negative drug history
- infectious contact
- onset on face
- lymphadenopathy

- no vesicles or blisters?
- no mucosal involvement?

- erythema of > 90 % skin
- vesicles or blisters
- +/− epidermal separation
- +/− target lesions
- mucosal involvement (>1 mucosal site)
- rapid progression

stop drug
anticipate resolution within 14 days

consider erythroderma, SJS or TEN refer Dermatology URGENTLY Contact ITU

consider viral/infectious aetiology

SJS=Stevens-Johnson Syndrome, TEN=toxic epidermal necrolysis

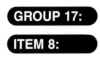

## Dermatology
## HIV and the skin

### Why is the skin relevant in HIV infection?

- Up to 90 per cent of HIV +ve patients will develop a muco-cutaneous disease
- 30-40 per cent of people with AIDS will suffer from three different dermatoses
- A rash may be the presenting sign of HIV infection or AIDS (remember that up to 30 per cent receive their diagnosis of AIDS and HIV at the same time, suggesting a large pool of undiagnosed patients)

### What dermatoses have commonly been the presenting illness of HIV (or indeed other causes of immunosuppression)?

- Extensive molluscum contagiosum in an adult
- Kaposi's sarcoma
- Extensive seborrhoeic dermatitis
- Pruritic Papular Eruption (PPE) of HIV
- Extensive oro-pharyngeal candida
- Hairy leucoplakia

### Why is the skin so frequently affected?

The exact mechanisms are not known but the following are probably important:

- Immune deficiency (increased infection)
- Poor immune surveillance (increased skin tumours)
- Post infective (Reiter's syndrome)
- Auto-antibodies (Sjogren's syndrome, polymyositis, ITP, pemphigoid, vitiligo, alopecia areata)
- Aberrant immune function TH1 to TH2 switch (eczema, pruritis, PPE)
- GVHD (Lichen planus, erythroderma)

### What type of rashes are seen?

A huge number of different rashes may be seen, which can be arbitrarily divided:

- Cutaneous infection
- Opportunistic infection
- Malignancy (BCC, SCC, KS, malignant melanoma)
- Papulosquamous/Inflammatory
- Oral lesions

## How would you diagnose the rashes?

The diagnosis can be difficult as frequently the rash is very extensive or there is an atypical clinical presentation. One should always have a low index for doing:

- Skin biopsies (both for all the relevant stains and for culture for bacteria, fungi, viruses and AFBs)
- Skin swabs
- Serology screens
- Investigation of other 'organs' such as blood, stools, sputum, bone marrow etc. Furthermore treatment is often problematic as HIV rashes (even those that are common in immunocompetent people) tend to be resistant to standard therapies and the use of immunosuppressive drugs is usually contraindicated.

## What cutaneous infections are seen in HIV and immunocompetent people?

See box.

Molluscum normally only occur in children. In HIV they occur in adults, in large numbers, and are often 'giant' in size.

Fungal: Candida (in flexural areas, white, macerated, with satellite lesions). Tinea ('ringworm' – anywhere including nails) – take scrapings and swab for culture.

Other: Scabies (often extensive or 'crusted' can look like crusted eczema and is very infectious as patients are teeming with mites).

## What opportunistic infections occur in the immunocompromised and how would you distinguish between them?

A variety of normally non-pathogenic organisms have been described in AIDS and other immunosuppressed patients. Clinically they are difficult to distinguish.

- Cutaneous CMV may present with blisters, ulcers or necrotic lesion.
- Fungi are common culprits and may present with nodules (often deep subcutaneous) or scaly papules.
- Crytococcus is seen in the UK whereas histoplasma is commoner in the US.
- Non-tuberculous or 'atypical' mycobacteria are a particular problem in advanced AIDS and may present with papules, nodules, ulcers or sporotrichosis-like lesions.

These infections may be localised to the skin but can also represent a systemic infection. Malaise, fever, abdominal pain, headache or diarrhoea may be non-specifically suggestive of the latter. Biopsy and culture is the best way to diagnose these rashes.

---

**Information**

Cutaneous infections in HIV

Bacterial: Impetigo (staph aureus), cellulitis/erysipelas (streptococcus). Clinically, these infections tend to look much the same as in immunocompetent individuals.

Viral: Herpes (may present with blisters, often extensive and ulcerative, especially peri-anally and orally).

Shingles/VZV (often painful, verrucous and extending over more than 1 dermatome).

---

**Information**

Failure to diagnose scabies may lead to a high proportion of medical staff (including medical students!) becoming infected.

---

### What is hairy leucoplakia due to and what does it look like?

It is due to Epstein-Barr virus in an immunosuppressed patient and is almost unique to HIV patients. It is a relatively late sign of HIV disease. Clinically white plaques appear on the sides of the tongue. Vertical ridging or corrugations are seen within the plaques. Unlike candida, there are no small satellite lesions around the edge and the white material cannot be scraped off leaving raw areas underneath

### What types of malignancy occur in immunocompromised patients?

- The two commonest types of skin cancers (BCC and SCC) appear to be increased in HIV +ve patients. They look the same as in immunocompetent patients.
- Malignant melanoma may be increased in prevalence. The clinical appearance is typical.
- Kaposi's sarcoma is commoner and more severe in AIDS patients than in classical KS or African KS. It presents as purplish brown plaques and nodules (see the film Philadelphia). The nose, palate and genitalia seem common sites but remember they can spread internally. KS is predominantly seen in homosexuals with AIDS and for unexplained reasons the incidence has declined somewhat. There is a strong link between Herpes Virus type 8 and the development of all types of KS although there may be other important factors involved, as not all people with HHV type 8 get KS.
- Lymphomas are more common with HIV and may present with lymphadenopathy.

### What are the commoner 'papulo-squamous' dermatoses encountered in HIV patients?

The commonest 'papulo-squamous' dermatoses encountered are:

- Seborrhoeic dermatitis        80%
- Unexplained pruritis          40%
- Xerosis, ichthyosis           30%
- Pruritic papular eruption (PPE) 20%
- Eczema                        10%
- Psoriasis                     5%
- Drug rashes                   20%

These rashes become more common (and severe) with progression of the disease.

### Seborrhoeic dermatitis

Itchy, red and scaly eczematous rash in the seborrhoeic areas (sides of nose, around eyes, forehead, scalp, over sternum, glans penis). This looks similar to seborrheic dermatitis in immunocompetent patients but is often more extensive. It may appear in early 'asymptomatic' HIV disease.

Therapy: topical miconazole/hydrocortisone cream, emollients, ketoconazole shampoo. If resistant consider topical lithium and oral itraconazole.

### Pruritus and xerosis (dry skin)

These often go together and the aetiology is unclear. Again they may be early manifestations of HIV disease.

Therapy: emollients, bath oils, aqueous cream as soap substitute.

Sedating antihistamines (e.g. hydroxyzine or chlorpheniramine). Consider 0.5% menthol in aqueous cream or crotamiton.

### PPE (Pruritic Papular Eruption)

A unique papular and (at times) pustular eruption centred on hair follicles. This is intensely itchy and usually involves the upper trunk and back and the proximal arms. Papules tend to arise, grow in size, frequently have the top scratched off and then recede as other new lesions arise. Skin biopsy reveals a lymphohistiocytic infiltrate around blood vessels and hair follicles often accompanied by eosinophils.

The so-called unique HIV rash 'eosinophilic folliculitis' is probably a variant of PPE.

PPE tends to appear in more advanced HIV disease and becomes worse as CD4 counts fall.

Therapy: medium strength topical steroids, oral antihistamines and low dose long-term antibiotics (as used in acne) may help. UVB therapy is very effective for resistant cases.

### Eczema

The prevalence of eczema is probably increased in HIV patients reflecting the eosinophilia and high IgE levels that are commonly seen. It looks similar to eczema in immunocompetent patients.

Therapy: is as for normal eczema but avoiding systemic immunosuppressants such as prednisolone and cyclosporin.

### Psoriasis

The prevalence of psoriasis is increased in HIV (5% v 2% in the normal population). Thirty per cent may get psoriatic arthropathy (v 5% of normal psoriatics). The disease can be typical with red, scaly plaques on elbows and knees, and scaling in the scalp. However psoriasis frequently becomes severe and widespread in HIV patients. They may become erythrodermic or develop pustular psoriasis, especially on the soles of the feet. When the latter happens there is clearly an overlap with Reiter's syndrome.

Therapy: topical steroids, calcipotriol (a synthetic Vit $D_3$ analogue) and tar compounds will help mild cases. UVB or PUVA are useful for more advanced disease. While there is some in vitro evidence that phototherapy may promote HIV replication, this has not been shown to be a problem in clinical practice.

Oral drugs to consider for severe disease are acitretin or anti-retroviral drugs.

The other drugs used in 'normal' psoriasis (methotrexate, cyclosporin, hydroxyurea) are best avoided as they probably accelerate disease progression.

# Notes

# Notes

# Notes

# Notes

# Notes

# Notes

# Notes